Food and Nutrition in the Middle East, 1970-1986

Bibliographies and Indexes in Science and Technology

Publishing Opportunities for Energy Research: A Descriptive Guide to Selective Serials in the Social and Technical Sciences
Roberta A. Scull, compiler

Toxic and Hazardous Materials: A Sourcebook and Guide to Information Sources
James K. Webster, editor

Three Mile Island: A Selectively Annotated Bibliography
M. Sandra Wood and Suzanne M. Shultz, compilers

Food and Nutrition in the Middle East, 1970-1986

An Annotated Bibliography

Compiled by

Gail G. Harrison,
Osman M. Galal,
and
Mary E. Mohs

Bibliographies and Indexes in Science and Technology, Number 4

Greenwood Press
New York • Westport, Connecticut • London

Library of Congress Cataloging-in-Publication Data

Harrison, Gail.
Food and nutrition in the Middle East, 1970-1986 : an annotated bibliography / compiled by Gail G. Harrison, Osman M. Galal, and Mary E. Mohs.
p. cm. — (Bibliographies and indexes in science and technology, ISSN 0888-7551 ; no. 4)
Includes index.
ISBN 0-313-26188-1 (lib. bdg. : alk. paper)
1. Nutrition—Middle East—Bibliography. 2. Diet—Middle East—Bibliography. I. Galal, Osman. II. Mohs, Mary E. III. Title. IV. Series.
Z5776.N8H37 1988
[TX360.M628]
016.3638'0956—dc19 87-34023

British Library Cataloguing in Publication Data is available.

Library of Congress Catalog Card Number: 87-34023
ISBN: 0-313-26188-1
ISSN: 0888-7551

First published in 1988

Greenwood Press, Inc.
88 Post Road West, Westport, Connecticut 06881

Printed in the United States of America

The paper used in this book complies with the Permanent Paper Standard issued by the National Information Standards Organization (Z39.48-1984).

10 9 8 7 6 5 4 3 2 1

Copyright Acknowledgments

The author and publisher are grateful to the following for granting the use of their material:

Excerpt from M. K. Abdelkhalek et al., "Iron metabolism in Egyptian infants with protein-calorie deficiency" in the *British Journal of Nutrition* 28.Copyright 1972 by The Nutrition Society. Reprinted with the permission of Cambridge University Press.

Excerpt from Galal et al., "Feeding the Child with Diarrhea: A Strategy for Testing a Health Education Message within the Primary Health Care System in Egypt." Reprinted with permission from *Socio-Economic Planning Sciences*, 21(2), Galal, O. M.; Shaheen, F. M.; Harrison, G. G.; Shehab, D.; Ritenbaugh, C. K.; and Burkhalter, B. R., "Feeding the Child with Diarrhea: A Strategy for Testing a Health Education Message within the Primary Health Care System in Egypt," Copyright 1987, Pergamon Journals Ltd.

Contents

Preface

This annotated bibliography is intended as a summary of the recent literature on human nutrition and food in the Middle East. To our knowledge, no one has attempted to bring together under one cover a guide to the literature in this area since the American University of Beirut's 1960-1970 compilation of abstracts, A Decade of Nutrition Research in the Arab World 1960-1970.

This bibliography contains abstracts of works published on nutrition in the Middle East from 1970 through 1986. The geographic scope of this work includes Algeria, Bahrain, Egypt, Ethiopia, Iran, Iraq, Israel, Jordan, Kuwait, Lebanon, Libya, Morocco, Qatar, Saudi Arabia, Somalia, Sudan, Syria, Tunisia, Turkey, United Arab Emirates, North Yemen, and South Yemen. In addition, a few studies are included from some other countries that have substantial Arab and/or Islamic populations (for example, Afghanistan). Some studies focus on the nutrition of Middle Eastern guest workers and their families or of Islamic migrants to Europe. In addition, the larger categories of "developing countries" and "Middle East including Arab world/Islamic world" contain abstracts on relevant inter-country studies, projects, and conferences.

The population focus is on people consuming primarily traditional Middle Eastern diets. Therefore, the studies from Israel that are included focus predominantly on Bedouin and other Arab populations. Studies from Gaza and the West Bank are included under the heading of Israel.

We included only articles related directly to human nutrition or related food science. Plant and animal nutrition studies were included only where findings were directly relevant to human nutrition. Similarly, studies focusing on commercial food products, commercial production of nutrients, and soil characteristics that contain information directly relevant to improving human nutrition were also included.

Materials for this work were obtained from standard library and computer searches and from individual authors' contributions. If abstracts were previously published, we have reproduced the author's abstract verbatim. Where there was no published abstract or where we could not locate the author, we have abstracted the article ourselves. Any errors in interpretation are ours. We have included material predominantly from the English-language literature. For articles in which the original language of publication was not English, we have provided either an English abstract or an English translation of the author's abstract.

Several people worked to bring this bibliography about. The original idea and ongoing responsibility for maintenance of the resource rest with Drs. Harrison and Galal. Ms. Mohs did the bulk of the work involved in abstracting and organizing the bibliography. Dr. Rita Leavell edited many of the abstracts. Jill Durall and Laura Kettel saw to the many details involved in readying the final draft for publication. We thank Sue Theiss, Gayle Croft, Jane Vuturo, and Jennifer Vuturo for assistance in index preparation.

We hope that individuals who are aware of literature that we may have missed will bring it to our attention, so that future editions may be more complete.

Gail G. Harrison
Osman M. Galal
Mary E. Mohs

Egypt

1. Galal, O. M., Shaheen, F. M., Harrison, G. G., Shehab, D., Ritenbaugh, C. K., Burkhalter, B. R. "Feeding the Child With Diarrhea: A Strategy for Testing a Health Education Message Within the Primary Health Care System in Egypt." Socio-Econ. Plann. Sci. 21(2), 1987, pp 139-147.

   Egypt has successfully implemented a nationwide program of oral rehydration therapy (ORT) for acute diarrheal disease which should make a substantial impact on diarrhea-specific mortality. However, ORT alone cannot alleviate or prevent the malnutrition which commonly accompanies diarrhea. Traditional practices in Egypt result in food being withheld from children who have diarrhea, thus contributing to the vicious circle of diarrhea and malnutrition. Early and continued feeding of children with diarrhea has been shown to be effective when practiced; however, it requires specific efforts to educate mothers appropriately. This study was designed to address the operational problem of promoting the nutritional repletion of children with diarrhea. Specifically, the tasks were to design an appropriate and practical message for the education of mothers, to test its delivery through the existing primary health care (PHC) system, and to incorporate it into the nationwide program of diarrheal disease control. A baseline survey of knowledge, attitudes, and practice (KAP) of mothers and health center professionals was carried out in July 1985 in three areas of Egypt. A simple educational message was developed based on knowledge of existing practices, consistency with existing mass media messages, and the addition of a component specific to this project. The message was delivered through the PHC system for three months. No special infrastructure or training was developed; the directors of several programs in three governorates simply incorporated the message into their existing systems of information flow and training. A second KAP survey was conducted in the same centers in December 1985. The follow-up survey indicated several significant findings. Of mothers who had attended any PHC center in the previous three months, 78% reported that a staff member had talked to them about feeding their child during and after diarrhea. Behavioral differences were also reported. There was a statistically significant increase in the proportion who continued to give breast milk during diarrhea and a significant increase in ORT use. Health care providers in the follow-up survey reported giving more, and more appropriate, dietary advice. In conclusion, the PHC system, with no additional infrastructure, was able to successfully incorporate this educational component. The message has now been adopted by the mass media and other health education channels. (Authors' abstract)

2. Borschel, M. W., Elkin, R. G., Kirksey, A., Story, J. A., Galal, O., Harrison, G. G., and Jerome, N. W. "Fatty acid composition of mature human milk of Egyptian and American women." Am. J. Clin. Nutr. 14(3), September 1986, pp 330-5.

   Fatty acid composition of mature human milk of rural Egyptian and American women was determined by gas-liquid chromatography. Milk of Egyptian women contained significantly higher percentages of capric, lauric, myristic, linoleic and arachidonic acids, saturated fatty acids (SFA), and polyunsaturated fatty acids (PUFA). Conversely, milk of American women contained higher percentages of stearic and oleic acids, total unsaturated fatty acids, and monounsaturated fatty acids. The PUFA:SFA ratio in Egyptian samples was 0.54 +/- 0.18 compared to 0.47 +/- 0.22 in American samples. Increased percentages of medium-chain SFA in Egyptian milk suggested increased mammary gland lipid synthesis. Analysis of Egyptian diets indicated high-carbohydrate and low-fat intakes may have resulted in limited availability and incorporation of dietary fatty acids into milk triglycerides. Thus, increased percentages of medium-chain SFA observed in Egyptian milk may reflect mammary gland synthesis in an attempt to maintain lipid concentrations in milk.

3. Serdula, M. K., Seward, J., Marks, J. S., Staehling, N., Galal, O., and Trowbridge, F.L. "Seasonal differences in breast-feeding in rural Egypt." Am. J. Clin. Nutr. 44(3), September 1986, pp 405-9.

   Two surveys in Upper and Lower rural Egypt allowed an analysis of the seasonality of infant feeding. The first, with 937 children, was conducted during the relatively cool season of low diarrhea incidence in January-April 1978; the second, with 976 children, during a hot season which has a high diarrhea incidence in August-September 1980. Of the infants 6-11 months old, the exclusively breast-fed proportion was greater in the hot-season survey (40% vs 16% in Lower Egypt, p less than 0.01; 36% vs 22% in Upper Egypt, p less than 0.01). Of the children 12-17 months old, a higher proportion were completely weaned during the hot season in Lower Egypt only (28% vs 14%, p less than 0.01). This difference being explained by an increase in pregnancy rates during the hot season which results in less breast-feeding. These seasonal variations must be considered in the interpretation of any infant-feeding surveys.

4. Zaki, A. M., DuPont, H. L., el Alamy, M. A., Arafat, R. R., Amin, K., Awad, M. M., Bassiouni, L., Imam, I. Z., el Malih, G. S., and el Marsafie, A., et al. "The detection of enteropathogens in acute diarrhea in a family cohort population in rural Egypt. Am. J. Trop. Med. Hyg. 35(3), September 1986, pp 1013-22.

   In 8 villages of rural northeastern Egypt, a 2-year study of the etiologic agents associated with episodes of diarrhea was carried out. Stool specimens (3,243) from 3,513 episodes of diarrhea were processed for enteropathogens. The most commonly identified agents in the group with diarrhea were Giardia lamblia (44%), heat stable enterotoxin (ST)-producing enterotoxigenic Escherichia coli (ETEC) (15%), heat labile toxin (LT)-producing ETEC (12%), enteropathogenic E. coli (EPEC) (4%), rotavirus (3%), Shigella (2%) and Salmonella (1%). Isolation rates were increased in cases compared to controls for all agents except G. lamblia and EPEC strains. Rotavirus, Salmonella and ST-producing ETEC were more frequently isolated during cooler months and Shigella and LT-ETEC occurred more commonly in warmer months. Campylobacter, EPEC, Giardia and E. histolytica did not show a discernable seasonal pattern.

5. Anonymous "Workshop on identification and prioritization of nutritional problems in Egypt." A joint project by the Nutrition Institute of the Ministry of Health and the United Nations Children's Fund, Cairo, Egypt, October 1984.

   This workshop was the first in the series and concentrated on identifying Egypt's nutritional problems and the sectors involved; setting priorities; recommending broad courses of action; and formulating nutrition policy recommendations for future development plans. The workshop involved a broad cross-section of representatives from relevant government sectors and international agencies which assured recommendations that could be implemented at a variety of levels.

6. Arafa, A. M., and Hussein, L. "The assessment of the vitamin B6 status among Egyptian school children by measuring the urinary cystathionine excretion." Int. J. Vitam. Nutr. Res. 54(4), 1984, pp 321-7.

Assessing their vitamin B6 status a metabolic study was carried out on 19 school boys and girls (age 7-13 years). The study was divided in five different periods, basal (A), post-methionine loading (B), one (C) and two (D) week after oral vitamin B6 therapy (50 mg/day) and post-methionine. Mean cystathionine excretion (beta mol/24 h) increased significantly (p less than 0.01) at stage B compared to mean values obtained at stage A. The deficit in the vitamin B6 nutriture was corrected by Vitamin B6 therapy and utilization of administered methionine.

7. Brink, E. W., El-Sayed Aly, H., Dakroury, A. M., Said, A. K., Ghoneme, F. M., Hussein, M. A., and Shaheen, F. M., et al. "The Egyptian National Nutrition Survey, 1978" Bull WHO 61(5), 1983, pp 853-860.

The Egyptian National Nutrition Survey, conducted during January-April 1978, quantified the protein-energy and anaemia status of young children from urban and rural areas. The close correspondence between the distribution of weight-for-height measurements of children in the survey and reference children showed that the protein-energy intake of Egyptian children was adequate. The prevalence of chronic undernutrition (less than 90% of the height-for-age reference median) and of anaemia decreased with urbanization, and was highest among children in the 12-47 months age range. Anaemia was more common among chronically undernourished children than among children of normal stature. (Authors' abstract)

8. El-Kirdassy, Z. H., Dakroury, A. M., Salama, F. M., Hegazy, M. I., and Abdel-Failil, A. A. "Fat composition of some Egyptian foods-cholesterol and fatty acids content of beef meat organs and adipose tissue." Bull. Egypt. Soc. Physiol. Sci. 3(2), 1983, pp 153-165.

A total of 25 samples of beef muscle, heart, liver, kidney and adipose tissue, with 5 samples from each type, were collected from Cairo Slaughterhouse from healthy animals available for human consumption. The samples were immediately transferred to the laboratory and the lipids were extracted for the determination of total cholesterol, phospholipids and fatty acids composition.

Results obtained showed that the kidney had the highest cholesterol value, while the muscle and adipose tissue had the lowest values. On the other hand, phospholipid contents of liver, heart and kidney were higher than the values of muscle and adipose tissue. The kidney contained the highest percent of total saturated fatty acids, while the heart contained the lowest value. Moderate values were observed in muscle meat, liver and adipose tissue. The highest U/S ratio was found in heart (1.98) and in muscle (1.79), while the adipose tissue, liver and kidney showed values of 1.63, 1.59 and 1.06, respectively. (Authors' abstract)

9. El-Nahry, F. I., Bassily, N. S., and Tharrwat, S. A. "Detoxificaion and nutritional evaluation of solvent-extracted

Egyptian cottonseed meal." Die Nahrung 27(6), 1983, pp 537-544.

Attempts at degossypolization of the solvent-extracted Egyptian cottonseed meal (CSM) and evaluation of its nutritional value as a possible protein supplement for human feeding were undertaken. Three methods were applied for degossypolization: steaming, addition of iron(II)-sulphate dihydrate, and steaming after addition of iron(II)-sulphate dihydrate. Steaming was done for varying periods of time. Nutritional evaluation was undertaken by chemical analysis and by feeding experiments. Chemically, the third method for degossypolization was the most effective. Feed efficiency and protein efficiency for diets containing 15% and 10% levels of CSM protein indicated that all treatments used for detoxification caused a decrease in diet and protein quality. Diets containing iron-supplemented CSM at the same level were the best of all. Mixing CSM with casein to form a diet containing 10% protein increases the protein quality of both casein and CSM. (Authors' abstract)

10. El-Shafei, M. M., Kamal, M. A. M., Abbassi, M. H., Said, A. K. "The effect of baking on availability of essential amino acids in wheat." Die Nahrung 27(1), 1983, pp 45-53.

Lysine availability in wheat flour and bread was determined by the growth response method on rats, using regression analysis relating gain in body weight and/or in body water to lysine consumed at two extractions, 87% and 72%. The availability of nitrogen and of essential amino acids were also determined by the balance trials method (fecal analysis method) with rats.

The results of the growth method show that baking increases lysine availability on the basis of body water gain. Extraction levels also affect lysine availability on the basis of change in body water. Wheat flour and bread of 72% extraction had more lysine availability values than the 87% extraction on the basis of moisture gain. Results of balance trials show that neither the extraction level nor the baking has a significant effect on essential amino acids availability.

A fairly good correlation is obtained for wheat flour and bread for the two extractions. Values of change in weight, food efficiency, PER, NPR and true digestibility showed that baking and level of extraction of wheat has no significant effect on the nutritive value of wheat investigated in the present study. (Authors' abstract)

11. Fahmy, K. A., Abdel Aziz, M. T., El-Raziky, E. S., El-Nahry, F., Zakria, S., and Tharwat, S. "Effect of protein of diet on murine schistosomiasis." Nutr. Rep. Int. 27(1), January 1983, pp 59-65.

Sixty albino mice infected with Schistosoma mansoni, in the stage of hepatosplenomegaly without fibrosis, were the subject of this study. Sixty uninfected mice constituted the controls. Test and control animals were divided into three dietary groups and given casein standard diets containing 5%, 10% and 20% protein, respectively. Growth rate and food intake were lower in infected animals than in uninfected animals. At a low dietary protein (5% and 10%), total serum proteins, albumin, A/G ratio, tryptophan and phenylalanine of infected animals were depressed, while the ratio of non-essential/essential amino acid was elevated. At the high dietary protein (20%), serum proteins were high while the non-essential/essential amino acid ratio was somewhat lower. (Authors' abstract)

12. Hegazi, M. I., and Marquardt, R. R. "Development of a simple procedure for the complete extraction of vicine and convicine from fababeans (Vicia faba L.)" J. Sci. Food Agric. 34, 1983, pp 100-188.

Egyptian foods prepared from fababeans contain variable and relatively high concentrations of vicine. Vicine and convicine can be readily extracted from whole or dehulled fababeans. The rate and completeness of extraction depends upon size of beans, the presence or absence of testa, the pH, temperature and volume of the aqueous extracting solution, the duration of the extraction procedure and the frequency with which the extracting solution is changed. In a typical experiment, vicine and convicine were almost completely removed from whole or dehulled fababeans when they were extracted at 20 or 40°C with 1% glacial acetic acid (0.17m) or water over a 72h period with changes in the extraction. The low pH of the acid solution prevents the bacterial fermentation that occurs when water is used. Water at temperatures greater than 70°C is a highly effective extracting agent. Extraction of fababeans with acetic acid does not markedly affect the concentration of protein (Nx5.7), fat or fibre. Ash content, however, was reduced by a factor of 2 and the total dry matter content of the extracted beans was reduced by 16-17% in whole beans and 20-21% in dehulled beans. (Authors' abstract)

13. Morcos, S. R., Gabrial, G. N., and Hady, N. A. E. "Supplementary and weaning foods for the Egyptian child." Die Nahrung 27(4), 1983, pp 21-27.

Attempts were made to prepare 5 protein-rich food mixtures to be used as supplementary and weaning foods for children from 6 months of age onwards. They contained vegetable and animal protein sources and were prepared in a way to simplify their use. Potatoes, carrots and peas were the basic ingredients in each mixture. The protein content of the mixtures ranged from 16-20% with a chemical core not less than 50%. The mixtures contained most of the essential amino acids in optimal concentrations, except methionine and cystine which were slightly lower than the amounts recommended by FAO. The nutritive value of each mixture estimated by the slope ratio bioassay procedure was high. They were nutritionally superior to casein, used as a reference protein. They differed slightly when compared with each other. (Authors' abstract)

14. Morcos, S. R., Said, A. K., Gabrial, G. N., and Hady, N. A. "Supplementary and weaning foods for the Egyptian child." Die Nahrung 27(4), 1983, pp 295-304.

Attempts were made to prepare 5 protein rich food mixtures to be used as supplementary and weaning foods for children from 6 months of age onwards. Prepared in a way to simplify their use, potatoes, carrots and peas were the basic ingredients in each mixture. The protein content of the mixtures ranged from 16-20% with a chemical score of no less than 50%. The mixtures contained most of the essential amino acids of optimal concentrations, except methionine and cystine which are slightly lower than the amounts recommended by FAO estimated by the slope ratio bioassay procedure. The nutritive value of each mixture was high. They all were nutritionally superior to casein which was used as a reference protein.

15. Moussa, W. A. "The role of infection in causation of malnutrition in urban areas of Egypt with special reference to diarrheal disease". Urban Health August 1983, pp 44-47.

As part of a comprehensive study on feeding and weaning practices among infants less than two years of age, 274 Cairo and 220 Alexandria infants and young children from low-income sectors were measured for height and weight. 61.7% of the Cairo sample and 67.1% of the Alexandria sample were normal weight for age.

Questionnaires for mothers focussed on the role of infection in a child's food intake reduction or dietary modification with illness. 75% of Cairo and 68.9% of Alexandria children suffered from illness, mainly gastrointestinal and respiratory, in the one month preceeding the study. In Cairo, gastrointestinal illness was greater than respiratory illness, while the opposite was true in Alexandria. In Cairo in a 3 month period, about 60% of those with diarrhea had 2 to 4 attacks, 31.1% more than 5 attacks, and 11.1% only 1 attack. In Alexandria, 78.9% of those with diarrhea had only 1 or 2 attacks. Modified diets during illness were mainly fluids such as tea, caraway and anise concoctions, with no milk intake. Breast feeding continued only if diarrhea was not present. Gradual resumption of ordinary diet occurred after illness ceased. 81.2% of children with illness in Cairo were given a modified diet for less than one week. In Alexandria a smaller percentage used a modified diet, but the duration of use was longer than in Cairo.

16. Thomson, A. M. "Egypt: food security and food aid". Food Policy 8(3), August 1983, pp 178-186.

This article examines the multi-faceted notions of food security and food aid through a case-study of a rather exceptional country in political terms - Egypt. Egypt has achieved a high degree of food security with lessened reliance on domestic production and has become one of the largest recipients of cereal food aid. The analysis considers significant questions about the interdependence of food security and food aid, the maintainability of an externally dependent food system, its implicit resource costs and its internal distribution and equity impact. (Author's abstract)

17. Toma, R. B. "Nutritional status in Egypt (A.R.E.)" Nutr. Rep. Int. 28(2), August 1983, pp 309-316.

Egypt imported 5% of its total food supply in the late 1950s. But in 1980 food imports reached 50%, including over 75% of its total consumption of wheat, 50% of sugar, 70% of cooking oil and 33% of meat products. Some other factors besides increase in population (doubled in less than 30 years) that lead to increase in imported foods are increase in GNP, land erosion and slower rate of productivity. Recommendations are presented to help achieve self-sufficiency both in quantity and quality of food commodities produced. (Adapted from authors' abstract.)

18. Toppozada, H. K., and Ghoneim, S. M. "A hematologic study of pregnant women in free and insurance hospital populations." Int. J. Gynaecol. Obstet. 21(6), December 1983, pp 439-42.

The prevalence of anemia among 631 women in late pregnancy was studied. There were two groups: those in the Medical Insurance Pregnancy Centre of the Alexandria clinic (320) and those in the free government hospitals (311). Related social and demographic observations were also done. Complete medical and obstetric examinations and several laboratory tests were performed. Women in the insurance hospital had lower parity, smaller families, lower crowding index, better income and a healthier hematological picture than women in the free hospitals.

19. Abdel-Fattah, H. M., Kamel, Y. Y., Megalla, S. E., and Hafez, A. H. "Aflatoxin and aflatoxicosis. I. Fungal flora of some food and animal feeds with special references to aflatoxin-producing abilities." Mycopathologia 77(3), March 1982, pp 129-135.

A wide range of fungi, amounting to fifty-six species belonging to twenty-two genera, have been recovered from animal feeds and foodstuffs. The most frequent fungi were Aspergillus niger, and A. flavus, followed by Mucor racemosus, Alternaria alternata, Rhizopus stolonifer, Penicillium corylophilum and P. notatum. Three genera were found to be of moderate occurrence, namely, Mucor, Rhizopus and Alternaria. The three following genera were of low occurrence: Cladosporium, Fusarium, and Neurospora. The fluorescence method of detecting aflatoxin-producing strains demonstrated that only one isolate of A. flavus possesses this property. Certain species of Penicillium and Aspergillus produced fluorescent substances (metabolites) similar in color to B and G aflatoxin. These substances were subsequently proved not to be aflatoxin by (TLC) chromatography. The animal and public health significance of such toxins was also discussed. (Authors' abstract)

20. Anonymous "Egypt: Mothers cut diarrheal deaths in half with homemade treatment". Salubritas 6(1), January 1982. Published by the American Public Health Association and the World Federation of Public Health Associations.

This study was carried out in 1980, and involved more than 29,000 children between one month and five years of age. The Egyptian Ministry of Health, aided by the World Health Organization and U.S. Agency for International Development, mounted an educational program to combat diarrhea-induced dehydration in infants by teaching mothers four ways of using oral rehydration solution (ORS). The four treatment groups were educated in different ways, and two control groups were also maintained. Group 1 received prepackaged Oralyte as a part of regular home visits every 4 to 6 weeks with instructions. Group 2 was instructed to obtain the Oralyte at local shops at a nominal price with instructions. Group 3 was instructed how to prepare ORS at home with granulated sugar, salt and water. Group 4 received a prepackaged sugar and salt mixture at home with usage instructions.

Results showed a 50% reduction in infant mortality with ORS made from household salt and sugar packets. The Oralyte home distribution group also reduced the death rate by 40%. Control groups and the group commercially purchasing Oralyte reduced infant deaths by 12% and 15%, respectively.

21. Bassily, N. S., Michael, K. G., and Said, A. K. "Blood urea content for evaluating dietary protein quality." Die Nahrung 26(9), 1982, pp 759-764.

The protein quality of broad beans was evaluated by using three different methods: the net protein ratio (NPR), the net protein utilization (NPU) and the relative protein value (RPV). Casein was used as a reference protein. The relationship between the values obtained on rats by each method and serum urea concentrations were examined.

Serum urea concentration increased with higher dietary protein content. It showed a positive correlation of 0.70 and 0.60 for broad beans and casein, respectively. NPR values increased by decreasing the level of dietary protein. There was no relationship between the NPR and the serum urea contents in animals fed the casein and broad bean diets. The NPU values indicated that protein utilization was greatest at low dietary protein levels and was decreased with increasing protein content of diet. Serum urea concentration showed an inverse proportion with the NPU values. This was demonstrated by correlations of -0.67 and -0.75 for broad beans and casein, respectively. The highest RPV for broad beans was obtained by using the change in body water and the lowest by using the change in body nitrogen as a response parameter. An inverse relationship existed between serum urea concentration and the RPV for broad beans. (Authors' abstract)

22. Bothina, M. A., El Naggar and Hussein, L. A. "Measurements of arm muscle circumference and skinfold thickness as indicators of the nutritional status of rural Egyptian school students" <u>Nutr. Rep. Int.</u> 25(1), January 1982, pp 57.

The stature, upper arm circumference, and triceps skinfold measurements were taken in 302 boys and 183 girls between 6 and 13 years of age. This study group as school children in a rural primary school. Arm muscle size was computed according to special formula. The results were compared with Jelliffe's standard, and statistical analysis of the data was done. The results of arm circumference, skinfold, and arm muscle diameter showed lower values than published data on age-matched children fed competely balanced diets. The staple foods of this study group were relatively low in calories.

The correlation between the arm muscle diameter and stature was highly significant among both boys and girls studied, which compared with the results reported by other investigators. (Authors' abstract)

23. El-Aaser, A. A., and El-Merzabani, M. M. "Vitamin A, bilharziasis and cancer." <u>Egypt J. Oncology</u> 2, 1982, pp 81-94.

The possible role of vitamin A deficiency, which may be due to parasitic infection such as bilharziasis and/or malnutrition, was reviewed in relation to metaplasia and cancer induction. Studies have shown the induction of keratinization and squamous metaplasia with vitamin A deficiency, and its reversal by vitamin A treatment. Low vitamin A and B-carotene levels have been found in Egyptian cancer patients compared to healthy Egyptian adults. The authors reviewed various animal and human cancer studies utilizing vitamin A treatment and hypothesized possible modes of action of vitamin A.

24. El-Kady, I. A., Abdel-Hafez, S. I., and El-Maraghy, S. S. "Contribution to the fungal flora of cereal grains in Egypt." <u>Mycopathologia</u> 77(2), February 1982, pp 103-109.

Thirty genera, 77 species and 4 varieties were isolated from 25 samples each of barley, wheat, maize and sorghum grains collected from different places in Egypt. The broadest spectrum of genera and species was recorded in wheat (25 genera and 59 species + 4 varieties) followed by barley (21 genera and 52 species + 2 varieties), sorghum (14 genera and 33 species + 2 varieties) and maize grains (11 genera and 29 species + 2 varieties). Aspergillus, Fusarium, Penicillium, and Rhizopus were the most common genera in the four grains, except maize where Penicillum emerged in low frequency. Aspergillus was the main component of the fungal flora of the four grains and contributed 79-94.4% of the gross total count of fungi. From the preceeding genera, A. niger, A. flavus, A. fumigatus, F. oxysporum, P. chyrsogenum, P. corylophilum, P. notatum and R. stolonifer were the most frequent. (Authors' abstract)

25. Elsokkary, I. H. "Contamination of soils and plants by mercury as influenced by the proximity to industries in Alexandria, Egypt." Sci. Total Environ. 23, April 1982, pp 55-60.

The amounts of total Hg in the soils and the edible parts of seven vegetable plant crops grown in unpolluted and polluted soils were studied. The highly polluted soils contained higher levels of Hg (495 ppb) than those in the unpolluted (35 ppb). The topsoil was more highly enriched with Hg than the subsoil as the result of the deposition of Hg particulates produced from the industries. Plants grown in soils near industries contained high levels of Hg up to 262 ppb. The amounts of Hg in the plant species which were grown in winter were higher than those grown in summer. (Author's abstract)

26. Hamdy, B. H., Elnokaly, F., Gaafar, S., Hinaggar, B., and Husein, L. "Effectiveness of periodic oral vitamin A dosage on hypovitaminosis in Egypt." Int. J. Vitam. Nutr. Res. 52(3), 1982, pp 235-240.

Seventy boys, aged 6-13 years, were subjected to a periodic oral vitamin A program. Non-parasitized boys (n = 63) responded to oral treatment with significant increase in plasma retinol level even five weeks after the end of oral treatment. On the other hand, boys infested with parasites, none of whom had originally acceptable plasma-retinol level, did not respond significantly to oral treatment. Vitamin A was found also to have an affect on growth, and there was highly significant correlation between retinol level and percentile weight for age. (Authors' abstract)

27. Hoogstraten, B., Gad-El-Mawla, N., Hamsa, M. R., Abdelaziz, I., and Omar, Y. "Breast cancer in Arabic women." Oncology 39(3), 1982, pp 134-139. S. Karger, AG, Basel.

A case-control study of breast cancer was conducted in Cairo, Egypt and in Kuwait. This is the first such report from Arabic countries and the most significant finding is the small incidence rate of 7.67 per 100,000 in Kuwaiti women, which ranks amongst the lowest thus far reported in the world. Factors which contribute to this low rate are a short period of active menstruation, low family history, first childbirth at very early age and most likely significant dietary factors. More than half of Egyptian women give birth to a child before the age of 20, with 56.5% of controls and 42.3% of patients (p   0.01). Many patients already have extensive disease at time of diagnosis as a result of considerable delay. However, this delay did not result in a high incidence of inflammatory breast carcinoma, such as has been reported in Tunisia. (Authors' abstract)

28. Hussein, L., Flaqz, S. D., Kuhnau, W., and Flatz, G. "Distribution of human adult lactose phenotypes in Egypt." Hum. Hered, 32(2), 1982, pp 94-99. S. Karger, AG, Basel.

Lactose absorption was studied in 570 healthy adolescent and adult males in Egypt. Employing a field version of the mininvasive hydrogen breath test, 156 (27.4%) lactose absorbers and 414 (72.6%) lactose malabsorbers were identified. The age-specific prevalence of the lactose phenotype indicated that lactose repression is complete at the age of 14 years in Egyptians. The regional distribution showed significant differences between the Nile Delta and the northern and southern part of Upper Egypt. The existence of a north-south gradient of decreasing frequencies of the hypolactasia gene from the Nile Delta to the Sudan is suggested. (Authors' abstract)

29. Kasperek "Multi-element analysis of fingernail, scalp hair and water samples from Egypt". Sci. Tot. Environ. 22(2), January 1982, pp 149-168.

Scalp hair, fingernail and water samples collected from different parts of Egypt were analysed by atomic absorption spectrophotometry and neutron activation analysis.

The results for hair showed minimum variation of Zn among different regions; a relatively well-controlled dispersion of values (maximum to minimum 2) for Co, Fe, Mn and Se; an overall inter-regional variation of factors of 7, 10, 6, 4 and 6 for the elements Ag, Cd, Cs, Sc and W, respectively; a steady decline in the concentration of Sc from south (Aswan) to north (Alexandria).

The findings for nail showed a steady decline in the concentration of Fe and Sc from south (Aswan) to north (Alexandria); elevated levels of Cd in samples from Aswan area; and regional variations extending up to factors of 6.5, 3.6, 4.7, 5.9, 4.4, 4.5 and 1.9 for Co, Cr, Cs, Mn, Mo, W, and Zn, respectively.

No unified relationship was observed between the elemental compositions of hair and nail. For Cr, Cs, Fe, Sb and Sc, mean values for hair were lower than in nails. Among the remaining elements the ratio nail/hair was 1 for Ag in Assiut, El Kharga and Alexandria, for Cd in all of the areas with the exception of Aswan, for Co, Mn and Mo in Cairo, for Zn in Cairo and Alexandria, and for W in Alexandria.

The data for water samples reflected highest concentrations of all the measured elements in the Mediterranean sea; a steady increase of the concentration of Cu in drinking water from south to north and for Nile water a similar trend for Ca and Mg; and elevated concentrations of Sb and Mn in river water. No distinct trend for the interrelationship between water and tissue elemental concentrations could be established for the regions around Cairo, Aswan and Alexandria. (Author's abstract)

30. Manieh, M. A., El Sherbini, M., Abd-El-Wahab, M., Ramzy, A. F., and Ali, Sh. A. "Implications of protein-calorie malnutrition in 50 surgically treatable patients." Egypt. J. Oncology 2, 1982,

pp 33-42.

Fifty patients with malignant diseases were randomly selected for a study of their nutritional status. The patients came from the surgical populations of Kasr El Aini and Cairo University Hospitals and from the National Cancer Institute. Nine nutritional parameters were measured, and clinical examinations were done. Forty-four patients were malnourished, representing 88% of the sample studied. Of these, 22% showed mild, 52% showed moderate, and 14% showed severe malnutrition. 87% of these patients showed 3 or more abnormal nutritional values. A prognostic nutritional index was performed. Results showed that 22% had low, 24% had intermediate, and 45% had high risk of complications.

31. Omran, L. A. "Ascaridia galli (Shrank, 1788): An erratic parasite in a fowl's egg albumin." J. Egypt Soc. Parasitol. 12(1), June 1982, pp 167-168.

Ascaridia galli is one of the commonest nematodes of fowls. The infection rate reaches 27.5% in Egyptian fowls. An adult male Ascaridia galli was recovered in the albumin portion of a fowl's egg. 1500 eggs were examined, and no others were found from Assiut. The author concluded that the presence of the parasite in fowl's eggs cannot be considered hazardous to man even if it is taken in with raw infected egg, for it will be destroyed in the stomach during digestion.

32. Said, A. K., El-Shafei, M. M., and Bassily, N. S. "Health and nutritional status of adolescent girls in a Cairo native neighborhood". J. Egypt. Pub. Health Assocation. 57(1,2), 1982, pp 1-12.

A nutrition survey of 57 adolescent girls and young women of low socio-economic class living in Boulac, a native neighborhood of Cairo, was done to investigate their nutritional and health status. Anthropometric, physical and biochemical measurements, and parasite detection were performed, as well as food intake analysis via diet history and 24 hour recall.

Mean heights were lower than standard by 1.8%, and for girls between 15 and 22 years, were 1 to 8% lower than standard. 33% and 9% of adolescent girls were overweight and underweight, respectively. Dry hair and cheilosis were found in 40% of the sample, and one third of the girls showed marked thyroid enlargement. In a sub-sample of 29 girls, the average blood hemoglobin concentration was 12.4 gm%, while 28 urine samples had no urinary bilharziasis and 11 stool samples produced only 2 samples of parasitic ova or cysts. Food intake data showed the daily diet intake to be about 60% of the caloric needs. Bread, rice, macaroni, and potatoes constituted the main sources of calories. The average intake of animal protein was low, as was the average intake of B-complex vitamins, iron, and iodine.

33. Anonymous "Arab Republic of Egypt nutrition status survey II, 1980"-Abstract found in Nutrition Research, 2(633), 1982 under "Country report-Egypt and Middle East". Original report by Nutrition Institute, Ministry of Health, Egypt, March 1981.

A follow-up nutritional status survey of preschool children was performed in the summer of 1980 in two areas, one in Lower Egypt and one in Upper Egypt, which was originally surveyed during the winter of 1978. Both surveys were conducted by the Nutrition Institute, with the technical assistance of the Center for Disease Control, U.S.A. The report presents information regarding prevalence and distribution of acute and chronic protein energy undernutrition and anemia in children 6 through 71 months of age during two periods 18 months apart as well as interaction with diarrheal disease.

Anthropometric data were analysed for 1783 children for the 1980 survey versus 1772 for the 1978 survey. Results indicated an increase in the median height for age of preschool children during the 18 month period, reflecting a small improvement in long term nutrition status. Figures for severe chronic undernutrition (less than 85% of the NCHS/CDC reference median for height) which varied between 3% in Lower Egypt and 5% in Upper Egypt during the 1978 survey, decreased to 2% and 6%, respectively in the 1980 survey. However, there was an increased prevalence of acute wasting. While 6% in Lower Egypt and 15% in Upper Egypt had a weight for age below 75% of standard in 1978, the figures were 11% and 19% respectively in the 1980 survey. Various factors might be involved: economic, social, and disease prevalence, particularly diarrheal disease. The prevalence of recent diarrheal disease was higher in the 1980 survey and children with such a history were thinner and more likely to be wasted than children without diarrhea. Anemia both in mothers and children remained substantial in the 1980 survey and at a comparable level to 1978 survey findings.

34. Anonymous "Economics of the Egyptian rice" M.E.N. Economic Weekly 20(33), August 14, 1981, pp 15.

This is a 1981 report on the economics of rice production in Egypt. Rice is a principal export as well as a nutritive crop whose residue is also used. When an analysis of net yield per feddan is calculated, rice is preferable to cotton, yet secondary to wheat as a profitable Egyptian crop. Egypt exports rice to European, Asian, Arab and African countries, making this an important source of foreign exchange. However, Egypt may have to import rice, reaching 400,000 tons by 1985. Tables are added. (Author's abstract)

35. Aref, K., Soliman, S., Hamam, M., Shaban, M., Koraitim, Y., Kato, A., Hodeib, A., and Sherif, A. No Title-Abstract found in Nutrition Research, 2(632), 1982 under "Country report-Egypt and Middle East". Original article in Gaz. Egypt. Ped. Ass. 29, 1981, pp 103.

Twenty children suffering from pellagra were given hepatic histological and histochemical examinations prior to and during 6 to 7 weeks of treatment. Initial pathological changes included necrotic foci, irregular cords of hepatocyte, and dilated blood sinusoids in all the patients. Fatty infiltration and decreased glycogen stores were also seen in the hepatocytes. Enzyme changes seen included increased activity of acid phosphatase and alphaesterase and decreased activity of succinic dehydrogenase and alkaline phosphatase. All these pathological conditions improved greatly after the 6 to 7 weeks' treatment.

36. Assad, M., and El Katsha, S. "Villagers' participation in formal and informal health services in an Egyptian Delta village". Paper by Senior Research Assistants of Social Research Center, American University in Cairo. Published by The Population Council, West

Asia and North Africa Region, 2, Sharia El Nil, Giza, Arab Republic of Egypt.

A structured interview was conducted of 100 women, 100 men, 50 male youth and 50 female youth randomly selected in one Egyptian village, Babel wa Kafr Hamam. The study examined the various types of formal and informal health care provided and the response of villagers to these services. The study provides an ethnographic account of health-seeking and health-providing behavior, and explores the extent of complementarity and interchangeability among the services via the utilization behavior of individual villagers.

Formal health care was defined as all government-regulated health services, and informal health care took in the services of all other health care providers. Predominant mode, relative costs, varying demands in population segments, detectable change in the relationships of the formal and informal systems, and ways of making formal services more responsive to villagers' needs were evaluated.

37. Awadalla, M. Z., Mekhael, K. G., and Hegazy, M. I. "Evaluation of local varieties of Egyptian rice." Z. Ernaehrungswiss 20(2), June 1981, pp 152-155. Dr. Dietrich Steinkopff Verlag.

The different nutritional ingredients of the Egyptian varieties of rice (Giza 171, Giza 172, and Giza 180) were determined. 1. The nutritive values decreased in polished varieties more than in the hulled ones. 2. A wide variation in the protein content in the different varieties was recognized. 3. Giza 180 could be considered the best Egyptian variety from the nutritional aspect. (Authors' summary)

38. El-Aaser, A. A., and El-Merzabani, M. M. "Biochemical detection of etiologic factors." in Detection of Bladder Cancer Associated with Schistosomiasis. El-Bolkainy and Chu, editors, Al-Ahram Press Cairo, Egypt, pp 157-173.

The biochemical detection of dietary and non-dietary factors involved in the etiology of bilharzial-related bladder cancer in Egypt are presented. Nitrosamine contamination of white cheese as consumed in towns was found to be common. Cottage cheese and salted cheese, consumed by farmers on a daily basis, were found to be commonly contaminated with nitrosamines also, and the contamination increased with length of storage of salted cottage cheese. Vitamin A deficiency was common in Egyptian farmers, as bilharzial infection would disrupt liver function. In addition, Egypt cancer patients have been also found to have low vitamin A parameters compared to healthy adults.

39. El-Hawary, M. F., Soliman, A. A., Nosseir, S. A., and Kholief, T. S. "Biochemical studies on the effect of breast and artifical feeding in newborn Egyptian infants. I. Serum proteins and immunoglobulins in 1 to 4-day-old newborns." Z. Ernaehrungswiss 20(4), December 1981, pp 83-290. Dr. Dietrich Steinkopff Verlag.

Investigations on the effect of colostrum feeding in 1 to 4-day-old newborn infants on serum proteins and their immunoglobulins were carried out. The values for serum total proteins, albumin and gamma globulins were higher in colostrum-fed infants than the artificially-fed group. Immunoglobulin G and immunoglobulin A levels were significantly higher, while immunoglobulin M level was only slightly elevated in the former group. On the other hand, serum total proteins as well as albumin and gamma globulins levels were decreased in lactating compared with non-lactating females, while the alpha and beta globulins levels were higher for lactating than controls. For individual immunoglobulins, IgG level was lower and IgA and IgM levels were higher for lactating than non-lactating females. (Authors' abstract)

40. El-Hawey, A. M., Rozeik, M. S., Sherif, M. H., El-Kholy, A., and Abo-Taleb, S. "Morbidity studies of Schistosomiasis hematobia in Egyptian adults". J. Egypt Soc. Parasitol. II(2), 1981, pp 507-515.

Thirty-six adult male Egyptian patients with active urinary hematobiasis were selected for this study. The aim was to assess the morbidity of such a disease and to find out its relationship to urine egg counts. In addition to clinical examination, the patients underwent urine and stool analyses, hemoglobin and serum creatinine estimations, urine egg counts, urinary system plain X-ray and intravenous pyelogram. The severity of the clinical manifestations was closely related to the parasitic loads. Patients with positive radiological findings had significantly higher mean urine egg counts than those without findings. Renal dysfunctions in this study were minimal and uncommon.

41. El Mougi, M., Mostafa, S., Osman, N. H., and Ahmed, K. A. "Social and medical factors affecting the duration of breast feeding in Egypt." J. Trop. Pediatr. 27(1), February 1981, pp 5-11.

The role of medical and social factors affecting breast feeding duration in different socioeconomic classes was studied. 504 mother-child pairs in which the child was weaned not more than two years previously, were divided into 3 socio-economic groups: 330 urban poor pairs, 104 traditional rural pairs, and 100 urban elite pairs. Interviews with mothers gathered pertinent information on economic, educational, and health factors for them, the child and their husbands.

TR mothers experienced longest breast feeding duration. Duration decreased with higher income per capita, with higher education, and with those working outside the home. These factors in turn were associated with higher socio-economic status. Reasons for cessation of breast feeding differed among groups: Urban poor and traditional rural mothers stopped more due to new pregnancy, while upper elite mothers stopped more due to the adverse effect of contraceptive pills.

42. El-Mougi, M., Mostafa, S., Osman, N. H., and Ahmed, K. A. "Social and medical factors affecting the duration of breast feeding in Egypt". J. Trop. Ped. 27, February 1981, pp 5-11.

504 mother-child pairs were studied: 300 urban poor, from Cairo slum areas; 104 traditional rural, from the villages of Kafr-Tohormous, Al-Kanater, and Kalioub; and 100 urban elite in Cairo. Traditional rural mothers were found to experience the longest duration of breast feeding.

Reasons for stopping breast feeding differed. New pregnancy was the most common major cause in the rural (30.8%) and urban poor (31.7%) groups, while contraceptive pills were the major reason in the urban elite (19%) group. The duration of breast feeding was shorter among those with higher per capita income, with higher education and with work outside the home. Hospital deliveries and deliveries conducted by forceps and/or episiotomy were negatively related to duration of breast feeding. On the other hand, antenatal care of the breasts and use of spoon versus bottle as a method of prelacteal feeding were found to promote breast feeding. Also, night feeding was associated with longer breast feeding. (Adapted from author's summary)

43. El-Saied, H. M., Abdel-Moneim, M. A. "Amino acid distribution of cereals in commercial mill products." Z. Ernaehrungswiss 20(2), June 1981, pp 139-144. Dr. Dietrich Steinkopff Verlag.

The amino acid contents of wheat and rice, as well as their final products produced by commercial milling, were determined quantitatively by the amino acid analyzer. Low quantities of lysine, glycine, arginine, alanine, and aspartic acid were found in flour, whereas more of these amino acids were found in wheat grain. Conversely, more proline, phenylalanine and glutamic acid were found in flour, and less of these amino acids were found in the wheat grain. The proportion of the other amino acids were slightly affected by milling. Low amounts of aspartic acid, serine, glutamic acid, and proline were found in rice bran and germ, whereas more of these amino acids were found in brown and milled rice. Rice bran and germ contained more threonine and cysteine than brown and milled rice. The proportions of other amino acids were only slightly affected by milling, but high content of lysine in germ was noted. (Adapted from authors' abstract.)

44. El-Saied, H. M., Morsi, M. K., and Amer, M. M. "Composition of cocoa shell fat as related to cocoa butter." Z. Ernaehrungswiss 20(2), June 1981, pp 145-151. Dr. Dietrich Steinkopff Verlag.

The physical and chemical constituents of cocoa shell fat (a by-product of the production of cocoa butter at chocolate factories) were almost identical with those of cocoa butter obtained from the same cocoa beans, except for a high acid value. Shell fat contained more phospholipid (as cephalin) than cocoa butter. The lipid classes were almost the same in cocoa butter and shell fat, except the latter contained an additional unidentified constituent. The fatty acids were determined quantitatively by GLC, with the predominant acids in cocoa butter found to be were palmitic and oleic. Small amounts of capric, myristic, palmitoleic and linoleic were found in cocoa butter, with more of these acids except myristic found in shell fat.

Seventeen compounds were detected by GLC in the unsaponifiable matter of both cocoa butter and shell fat, from which eight were identified as C30 hydrocarbon, C32 hydrocarbon, squalene, alpha-tocopherol, cholesterol, campsterol, stigmasterol and beta-gitosterol. The sterols were determined quantitatively, with B-sitosterol, the predominant sterol in both cocoa butter and shell fat. Cocoa butter contained higher values of stigmasterol than shell fat, which contained increased values of campsterol. Low values of cholesterol were found in both samples. Stability of cocoa butter and shell fat towards oxidative rancidity at 100° C was the same (10.5 hrs). (Adapted from authors' abstract.)

45. El-Warraki, A. G., Hussein, M. F., El-Samkary, M. A.,

El-Mahdy, R. M., and El-Nahry, F. I. "Development of high protein biscuits suitable for feeding babies. I-Organoleptic, chemical and bacteriologic tests." Paper presented at the International Conference of New Trends and Techniques Towards Food Supply and Its Preservation, 1981, 30 pages. For copies write to Ain Shams University or Nutrition Institute, Cairo, Egypt.

In an effort to develop suitable protein-rich food mixture for feeding infants and young children, eight formulas and recipes were designed from wheat flour supplemented with some local legume seeds flour and high protein seeds flour. The formulas were processed and packed in biscuits. The resulting biscuits were subjected to organoleptic, chemical and bacteriological tests. Moisture, crude protein, fat, carbohydrate, ash, fiber, thiamine, riboflavin, minerals, total sugars and starch were determined in the different biscuit formulas.

Bacteriological evaluation was conducted by determination of total bacterial, spore forming bacteria, staphylococci, and anaerobic spore formers contents.

Results obtained for organoleptic evaluation showed that, with the exception of formula No. 2, all the other formulas were statistically similar and had reasonable scores. Chemical tests revealed the superiority of these mixtures, as they contained considerable amounts of proteins and fats. Biscuit formulas were found to contain very high amounts of thiamine, riboflavin and minerals. Bacteriological tests showed good sanitary aspects of all formulas which were free from pathogenic organisms. (Authors' abstract)

46. El-Warraki, G., El-Mahdy, R. M., Tharwat, S. A., and El-Nahry, F. I. "Development of high protein biscuits suitable for feeding babies. II-Amino pattern." Paper presented at the International Conference of New Trends and Techniques Towards Food Supply and Its Preservation, 1981, 13 pages. For copies write to Ain Shams University or Nutrition Institute, Cairo, Egypt.

The resulting high protein biscuits formed from the eight formulae previously designed were subjected to amino acid determination. Paper chromatography was used for the separation and identification of the different amino acids in both acidic and alkaline protein hydrolyzates. From the amino acid analysis data, chemical score (C.S.) and dietary protein calories percent (NDP CAL%) were calculated.

The results proved the presence of all amino acids in good pattern in all the biscuits studied. Chemical scores ranged from 64 to 84. They showed lysine to be the first limiting amino acid in most biscuit formulae, while the sulphur-containing amino acids were the first limiting ones in biscuits containing beans.

For the biscuit formulae presented, NDP CAL% were 7.50 to 10.70. (Authors' abstract)

47. El-Warraki, A. G., El-Mahdy, R. M., Therwat, S. A., and El-Nahry, F. I. "Development of high protein biscuits suitable for feeding babies. III-Biological evaluation of their proteins and determination of possible toxic effects." Paper presented at the International Conference of New Trends and Techniques Toward Food Supply and Its Preservation, 1981, 13 pages. For copies write to

Ain Shams University or Nutrition Institute, Cairo, Egypt.

Protein quality of the high protein biscuits was evaluated by determination of protein efficiency, net protein ratio, net protein utilization, biological value and true digestibility coefficient. The biological experiment also covered the determination of toxic effects possibly present.

All biscuit formulae were of high quality protein and can support moderate and good growth for children. They were also free from toxic effects.

The results of those studies proved that one more of these formulae can be chosen for commercial manufacturing at the national level. (Authors' abstract)

48. Farmer, R. G., Gulya, A. J., and Whelan, G. "Traveler's diarrhea: clinical observations." J. Clin. Gastroenterol. 3(1), March 1981, pp 27-29.

An observational study was made of traveler's diarrhea in all members of a 48-person medical seminar group during a trip to Egypt and the Nile in September 1979. In addition to comparing symptoms in those who took antibiotic prophylaxis with doxycycline with those who did not, the study also took into account water and dietary restrictions. Although the study supports the use of prophylactic doxycycline, the response appears to be considerably influenced by dietary or water restrictions. This report emphasizes the need to assess diet and water intake of travelers when conducting trials of medication aimed at preventing traveler's diarrhea. (Adapted from authors' abstract)

49. Gabrial, G. N. "The utilization of faba beans and their role in diet in Egypt". Paper prepared for International Conference on Faba Beans held in Cairo, March 7-11, 1981. Preparation by G.N. Gabrial, Food Science and Nutrition Research Department, National Research Centre, Dokki, Cairo, Egypt.

The broad bean Vicia faba plays an important role in the Egyptian diet. It constitutes the major indispensable meal for the majority of the people, and is served throughout the day in different forms. It is a rich source of protein and amino acids. The national production and consumption of broad bean compared to meats and other nuts, legumes and pulses are discussed. The nutrient composition and factors affecting nutritive values, including amino acid composition, biological value, antinutritive factors and effect of different food preparation methods, are discussed.

50. Gabrial, G. N., El-Nahry, F. I., Awadalla, M. Z., and Girgis, S. M. "Unconventional protein sources: Apricot seed kernels." Z. Ernaehrungswiss 20, 1981, pp 208-215. Dr. Dietrich Steinkopff Venlag.

Hamawy apricot seed kernels (sweet), Amar apricot seed kernels (bitter) and treated Amar apricot kernels (bitterness removed) were evaluated biochemically.

All kernels were found to be high in fat (42.2-50.91%), protein (23.74-25.70%) and fiber (15.08-18.02%). Phosphorus, calcium and iron were determined in all experimental samples.

The three different apricot seed kernels were used for extensive study including the qualitative determination of the amino acid constituents by acid hydrolysis, quantitative determination of some amino acids, and biological evaluation of the kernel proteins for use as new protein sources.

Weanling albino rats failed to grow on diets containing the Amar apricot seed kernels due to low food consumption because of its bitterness. There was however no loss in weight. The Protein Efficiency Ratio data and blood analysis results showed the Hamawy apricot seed kernels to be higher in biological value than treated apricot seed kernels.

The Net Protein Ratio data which accounts for weight, maintenance and growth showed the treated apricot seed kernels to be higher in biological value than both Hamawy and Amar kernels. The Net Protein Ratio for the first two kernels were nearly equal. (Authors' summary)

51. Ghali, Y., El-Nahry, F., El Rahim, E. A. A., and Wasif, M. M. "Effect of carbohydrates on cholesterol level in liver and serum, Part I: Soluble carbohydrates and starch." Paper presented at the First National Congress of Biochemistry, Egypt, 1981, 15 pages. For copies write to Nutrition Institute, Cairo, Egypt.

Glucose, maltose, sucrose and starch were added separately as a sole source of carbohydrate to a diet for rats. Their effects on the average body gain, food efficiency, liver weight, liver/body weight, serum and liver cholesterol with and without addition of cholesterol and bile salts, were investigated.

Starch diet showed the highest food efficiency value, followed by sucrose. The lowest value was given by glucose. Addition of cholesterol and bile salts affected the food efficiency value. Maltose showed the highest value. Starch with the hypercholesterolemic diet showed a decrease in the food efficiency from 0.334 to 0.238. Sucrose without addition of cholesterol or bile salts led to increase in the serum and liver cholesterol. Maltose diet gave the lowest value for serum cholesterol.

Addition of bile salts and cholesterol to the different diets led to a net increase in serum and liver cholesterol. Such increase differs according to the presence of different carbohydrates. In the presence of sucrose and hypercholesterolemic agents, the highest increase in cholesterol was recorded. (Authors' abstract)

52. Ghali, Y., El-Nahry, F. I., Abd El Rahim, E. A., and Wasif, M. M. "Effect of carbohydrates on cholesterol level in liver and serum, Part II: Polysaccharides." Paper presented at the First National Congress of Biochemistry, Egypt, 1981. 15 pages. For copies write to Nutrition Institute, Cairo, Egypt.

In order to study the hypocholesterolemic effect of some polysaccharides in rats, carboxymethyl-cellulose, pectin, fenugreek mucilage and sodium alginate were added separately in 2% and 5% concentrations to the hypercholesterolemic diet containing sucrose. It was found that all the polysaccharides led to a decrease in the cholesterol level in serum and liver.

Pectin showed the most reducing effect (in 2% and 5% level), where the cholesterol decreased in serum and liver to a level equal to that observed in the sucrose diet without addition of cholesterol. This means that the pectin completely inhibited the absorption of the cholesterol and bile salts.

Fenugreek mucilage, separated from fenugreek seeds also had a reducing effect on the serum cholesterol. However, this polysaccharide does not affect the food efficiency as in the case of pectin.

Incorporation of such polysaccharides in the human diet may cause a decrease of cholesterol absorption in a diet rich in cholesterol. (Adapted from authors' abstract)

53. Janowitz, B., Lewis, J. H., Parnell, A., Hefnawi, F., Younis, M. N., and Serour, G. A. "Breast-feeding and child survival in Egypt" J. Biosoc. Sci. 13, 1981, pp 287-297.

The effects of breast-feeding on survival probabilities of children born in 1977 and 1978 were studied. A sample of 2907 women in three Cairo hospitals were interviewed soon after delivering a subsequent infant. The data consisted of breast-feeding and survival information on the previous child, in all cases a full-term liveborn infant. Almost three-quarters of the women reported breast-feeding their last child for 6 months or more, and almost half continued breast-feeding beyond a year.

Regression analysis showed that in the first 12 months, breast feeding was positively correlated with survival. Mother's education was positively correlated with child survival and the effect of breast-feeding. When women were grouped according to level of education, the effect of breast-feeding on child survival was more pronounced the lower the mother's education.

54. Khalil, M., Aref, M., Mahmoud, S., El-Sawy, M., Abdel Hay, M., and Sidrak, M. No Title-Abstract found in Nutrition Research, 2, 1982, pp 631-632, under "Country report-Egypt and Middle East". Original article in Gaz. Egypt. Ped. Ass. 29, 1981, pp 35.

Kwashiorkor patients were compared with normal controls for total phospholipid concentration, phospholipid fractions in serum and platelets, and platelet functions. Results showed significant decreases in total phospholipids, phosphatidylcholine, and sphingomyelin. Platelet total phospholipids were 11.2% of those in serum. Platelet, but not serum concentrations of sphingomyelin, ethanolamine, and phosphatidylcholine were significantly decreased in kwashiorkor patients. Percent of phosphatidyl ethanolamine increased significantly in platelet of kwashiorkor patients. Platelet aggregation and adhesiveness correlated significantly with platelet phosphatidyl ethanolamine in patients who showed purpura. Serum phosphatidylcholine percent was higher than that in platelets.

55. Mansour, N. S., Higashi, G. I., Schinski, V. D., and Murrell, K. D. "A longitudinal study of Schistosoma haematobium infection in Qena Governorate, Upper Egypt 1. Initial epidemiological findings." Am. J. Trop. Med. Hyg. 31(4), 1981, pp 795-805.

This paper describes an epidemiological study conducted as an initial phase of a longitudinal study on the immunology of Schistosoma haematobium in Upper Egypt. Three villages in Qena governorate, a region endemic for S. haematobium only, constituted the study area.

A cross-sectional survey in two of the villages, via urine examination of the family members in every third household, showed an overall prevalence of infection to be 28.7% (29.9% at Khozam and 26.9% at El Ayaisha). All age groups, including infants below 1 year of age, were found to be infected with S. haematobium. The percent infected showed an increase with age in children, reaching a peak of 57-63% in the 11- to 15-year age group. This was followed by a rapid decline and stable prevalence below 28% in adult years. Males and farmers had a higher prevalence rate than females and non-farmers, respectively.

56. Morcos, S. R., Elhawary, Z., and Gabrial, G. N. "Protein-rich food mixtures for feeding the young in Egypt. 1. Formulation." Z. Ernaehrungswiss 20(4), December 1981, pp 275-282. Dr. Dietrich Steinkopff Verlag.

Ten protein-rich food mixtures were assembled, based on popular dishes which could be prepared simply at home. Such mixtures were prepared from seeds or legumes available in the local markets at reasonable prices, including polished rice, decorticated lentils, defatted sesame flour, white or roasted chick peas (dehulled), maize bread, sun flour kernels, fenugreek seeds, wheat (whole grains or parboiled grains), white wheat flour, defatted peanut flour, defatted sesame flour and dry yeast. The protein content of such food mixtures ranged from 17.7% to 23.2%, which is in agreement with recommended values. Defatted sesame flour was incorporated in most of the mixtures in order to correct for their low content of sulphur-containing amino-acids, as it is already known that sesame is a rich source in comparison to other vegetable sources. Further investigations are continuing to determine the nutritive value of the formulated mixtures before feeding them to the children. (Adapted from authors' abstract)

57. Sukkary, Soheir "She is no stranger: The traditional midwife in Egypt." Medical Anthropology Winter 1981, pp 27-34.

The traditional midwives, or dayas, of Egypt play an important role in delivering practical and beneficial health services to women and infants, including nutritional advice. The desirability of utilizing their services in conjuction with the formal MCH (Maternal and Child Health) centers' services is stressed. The progressive attitudes of two Cairo dayas who service poor and middle class Cairo urbanites are discussed. Their desires to acquire modern information and techniques, as well as their attempts to project modernism via trips to the hairdresser and seamstress, are also described. The author advocates licensing of dayas and linking them to MCH centers. Dayas may also be usefule in spreading the concept of family planning under the notion of 'spacing' babies for the mother's health and other benefits of life style.

58. Abdel Kader, M. M., Abdou, I. A., Said, A. K., and Bassily, N. S. "An estimate of endogenous nitrogen excretion in subjects on varying protein intakes." Med. J. Cairo Univ. 48(1), 1980, pp 57-61.

Data of total urinary and urea nitrogen in previous studies were used to estimate non-urea nitrogen, which was found to be almost constant over protein intakes above and below maintenance requirements. Moreover, it was used to calculate the total urinary nitrogen output at theoretically zero nitrogen intake. It was found to be a satisfactory approximation to the value obtained from subjects maintained on a practically protein-free diet. (Authors' abstract)

59. Abdel-Wahab, M. F., Strickland, G. T., El-Sahly, A., Ahmed, L., Zaharia, S., El-Kady, N., and Mahmoud, S. "Schistosomiasis mansoni in an Egyptian village in the Nile delta." Am. J. Trop. Med. Hyg. 29(5), 1980, pp 868-874.

This was an epidemiologic, clinical, and laboratory study of 537 subjects from Kafr Tarana, a Nile delta village of 900 people. The long-term morbidity produced by schistosomiasis was determined at the village level. None of the subjects had Schistosoma hematobium. There was a high prevalence of S. mansoni infection: 74% total, males 78%, females 68%. Age groups between 10 and 40 years showed peak prevalence and intensity of infection. Most villagers over 40 were still excreting large numbers of eggs. Field-working women had prevalence and intensity rates similar to those of men, which were 37% greater than those of women staying exclusively at home. Clinical parameters were studied, and follow-up studies to evaluate methods of reducing prevalence and intensity of infection were mentioned.

60. Aly, H. E., Hussein, M. A., Ghoneme, F., Salib, F., and El-Ghorab, M. "Nutrition status of preschool children in Matrouh Governorate." Publication of the Nutrition Institute, 16 Kasr el-Ainy, Cairo, Egypt. July 1980, 7 pages.

The National Nutrition Survey conducted for Egypt in 1978 did not include the frontier governorates: Red Sea, New Valley, Matrouh and Sinai. These were surveyed by the National Institute at a later stage (1979), except Sinai. The goal was to provide information concerning the nutrition status of young children in the frontier region that could be used for determining local policies and priorities. This report presents the nutritional state of preschool children in Matrouh, which is one of the four frontier governorates and is located in the northwest part of Egypt along the Mediterranean sea, west of Alexandria.

The nutrition status of preschool children in Matrouh is characterized by a high prevalence of stunting. Wasting and concurrent wasting and stunting are observed in infancy and the 2nd year of life. The prevalence of anemia is greater during infancy than the following years. Anaemia is also prevalent among mothers, especially during pregnancy. (Adapted from authors' summary)

61. Aly, H. E., Moussa, W. A., Demian, H. G., Hasanyn, S. A., and Said, A. K. "Anthropometric measurements of Cairo school children. A follow-up study." J. Egypt. Pub. Health Assoc. 55(3,4), 1980, pp 143-165.

A comprehensive nutritional survey of Cairo school children, 6-20 years of age, was carried out 13 years after a previous similar one to detect changes in growth and nutritional states during that period.

Heights and weights of Cairo school children followed the same pattern as the Americans. However, they were retarded by less than one standard deviation than the Iowa standard. Means weights and heights of Cairo school children in 1975 were more than those reported in 1962 survey. School boys and girls with normal weight for height for age (90-110% of Std.) constituted about 50-58% of the total sample. Overweight and obesity (110% of Std.) were more in girls than in boys, and more in 1975 than in 1962 survey.

The mean values for left mid-arm circumference and triceps skinfold thickness followed the same pattern as reference standards. However, they were lower for boys and girls except at the 12-15 years of age period. On the other hand, the triceps skinfold thickness values were higher till the age of 15 years for boys and 17 years for girls, and became lower thereafter. This may denote depletion of fat stores after puberty. (Authors' summary)

62. Anderson, J. E., Aly, H. E., Dakroury, A. H., Said, A. K., Hussein, M. A., El-Ghorab, M. I., Miller, D. C., and Brink, E. W. "Family planning use and child health in the Arab Republic of Egypt." Report for U.S. Department of HEW, Public Health Service, CDC. 1980

The 1978 Nutrition Survey of the Arab Republic of Egypt (ARE) provides a chance to look at the prevalence of contraceptive use in that country. Moreover, the survey provides an unusual opportunity to link anthropometric and medical measurements of the nutritional status of children with the contraceptive practice of their mothers. In the ARE Nutrition Survey about 1 in 5 mothers interviewed were current contraceptive users; there was wide variation in use by area of residence and socioeconomic status. A positive association was found between current contraceptive use and measures of child health, an association that was maintained when residence, social status, and other background variables were controlled statistically. Although a fully developed causal model cannot be evaluated from these data, the data suggest that contraceptive use and child health are related, and that the connection could be evaluated further in future studies. (Authors' abstract)

63. Awadalla, M. Z., El-Gedaily, A. M., El-Shamy, A. E., and El-Aziz, K. A. "Studies on some Egyptian foods. Part 1: Biochemical and biological evaluation." Z. Ernaehrungswiss 19(4), December 1980, pp 244-247. Dr. Dietrich Steinkopff Verlag.

General chemical analysis of some Egyptian legumes (Lupinus termis and fenugreek seeds) and biological evaluation for their proteins were investigated. Results showed that Lupinus termis and fenugreek seeds have high protein contents, with the exception of germinated fenugreek. They are good sources of calcium and phosphorus. Raw seeds gave low PER and NPR values. However, these values increased after roasting or germination. (Authors' abstract)

64. Awadalla, M. Z., El-Gedaily, A. M., El-Shamy, A. E., and El-Aziz, K. A. "Studies on some Egyptian foods. Part 2: The effect of protein on blood constitutents of rats." Z. Ernaehrungswiss 19(4), December 1980, pp 248-250. Dr. Dietrich Steinkopff Verlag.

This study was undertaken to evaluate the changes of the blood constitutents of rats fed different proteins (Lupinus termis, Guiza 1 and 2, balady, and fenugreek seeds raw, roasted, and germinated). The total serum protein for animals fed casein was slightly higher than those fed other proteins. Total serum protein of animals fed roasted and germinated fenugreek and Lupinus termis was higher than those fed raw seeds. The albumin/globulin ratios showed a similar trend. The ratio of nonessential to essential free serum amino acids of rats fed a non-protein diet was higher than those fed a protein. Lupinus termis and fenugreek seeds are good sources of protein. Treatment of seeds either by heat or germination improves the nutritive value of the proteins. (Adapted from authors' abstract).

65. Behairy, F., Elissa, A., Eldiwani, K., Abdin, F., Abdel Hafiz, A., and Malky, F. No Title-Abstract found in Nutrition Resarch, 2, 1982, p 631, under "Country report-Egypt and Middle East". Original article in Gaz. Egypt. Ped. Ass. 28, 1980, p 191.

Renal function tests together with renal biopsy were performed on 45 infants and children suffering from PCM (kwashiorkor, marasmus and marasmic kwashiorkor). Glomerular filtration rate was impaired in PCM, especially the kwashiorkor group. Renal tubular concentration was also impaired as evidenced by the constant low specific gravity of urine in all types of malnutrition. Blood serium uric acid concentration was reduced. Proteinuria and hypoalbuminemia were pronounced in PCM with edema. Renal biopsies revealed dilation and rigidity of glomerular capillaries, variability of glomerular size and thickening of the basement membrane. The tubules were dilated and their walls were thin and showed cloudy swelling with frequent vascular degeneration. Interstitial fibrosis was seen in a few caes from the kwashiorkor group only. This study revealed that significant morphologic changes occur in the kidney in severe PCM. Impaired renal function is most pronounced in kwashiorkor, confirming the relation between histopathologic changes and deranged renal function. (Authors' abstract)

66. Behairy, F. E., El-Garhy, M., El-Mougy, M., El-Diwany, K., Khalifa, E., and Soliman, A. No Title-Abstract found in Nutrition Research, 2, 1982, p 631, under "Country report-Egypt and Middle East". Original article in Gaz. Egypt. Ped. Ass. 28, 1980, p 233.

A study of the effects of birth interval on the child's physical growth using various anthropometric measurements, was carried out on 838 infants and children, aged 0-24 months. Cases were divided at 3 months' intervals into 8 groups. Anthropometric measurements included body weight, length, head circumference, chest circumference, subscapular and triceps skin fold thickness and mid-upper arm circumference. As one moved from one age group to an older one, the gain in each body measurement was greater for infants following long birth interval in relation to their age matched cases following short birth interval. A statistically significant difference was present throughout nearly all of the second year of life indicating that children delivered following a long birth interval had better growth. Children with malnutrition, delayed teething, or rickets had significantly shorter mean birth interval than others.

67. Domyatic, H., Heneidy, F., Khalafallah, Bahgat, N. and Shenawy, R. No Title-Abstract found in Nutrition Research 2, 1982, p 631, under "Country report-Egypt and Middle East". Original article in Gaz. Egypt. Ped. Ass. 28, 1980, p 11.

Two groups of children, 58 normal controls and 38 protein-calorie malnutrition patients, were compared for serum glycoproteins.

Protein-calories malnournished patients showed elevated alpha acid glycoprotein and decreases in the serum globulin fractions of transferrin, alpha macroglobulin, and alpha antitrypsin ceruloplasmin, while hepatoglobin was not changed. Serum IgG and A decreased significantly, but serum IgM did not in malnournished children. The relationship of serum glycoproteins to increased susceptibility of protein-calorie malnourished children to infections and their role in modulating lymphocyte responsiveness were discussed.

68. El-Ashwah, L. T., Eid, N. M., and Said, A. K. "Utilization of yeast in nutrition I-Nucleic acid removal and flavor improvement." Egypt. J. Microbiol. 15(1,2), 1980, pp 81-90.

Heat shock treatment of compressed Baker's yeast was done to reduce its nucleic acids content from 10.5% to 2.22%, considered a safe level. 17.6% of crude protein was also lost by this treatment, but since the nonprotein nitrogen was lost in even higher amounts, the true protein content actually increased from 32% to 42% after heat treatment. Various organic solvents were used to extract crude yeast fat from medicinal yeast in order to improve its acceptability. Ethyl ether was found to be the most suitable solvent, as it produced the highest yield of extracted fats and waxes and gave the most preferred yeast flavor. Different solvents gave different values for total fatty acids in yeast fats. The major fatty acid present was oleic acid, at 41.4%. Linoleic acid represented 20.9%, and palmitoleic acid represented 23% of fatty acids present.

69. El-Ashwah, L. T., Eid, N. M., and Said, A. K. "Utilization of yeast in nutrition II-evaluation of yeast protein and its potential use as a food supplement." Egypt J. Microbiol. 15(1,2) 1980, pp 91-98.

Since a 1970 pilot study had demonstrated that protein and purine intakes of various socio-economic classes were deficient compared to PAG recommendations, a study was conducted to determine how efficacious heat-shock treated crude Baker's yeast could be as a protein supplement. Biological evaluation (NPR, NPU, and BV) was done on albino rats. Results showed that yeast proteins were lower than that of casein but improved after heat treatment to almost the same value as casein. Essential amino acid composition was not significantly changed by heat treatment. Total sulphur amino acids were the most limiting, but lysine was well represented. Authors suggested that heat-treated Baker's yeast could be used to supplement lysine deficient diets. Heat-shock treatment reduced the nucleic acid content from 10.5% to 2.22%, a safe level.

70. El-Nahry, F. I., Mourad, F. E., Abdel Khalik, S. M., and Bassily, N. S. "Chemical composition and protein quality of lentils (Lens) consumed in Egypt." Qual. Plant-Pl. Fds. Hum Nutr. 30, 1980, pp 87-95.

Three local cultivars of lentil (Lens) seeds (Giza 9, Family 91, and Family 195), as well as one imported Pakistani variety, were studied. Moisture, protein, fat, carbohydrate, ash, fiber, thiamine, riboflavin, amino acids and some protein fractions were determined on the unpeeled and peeled seeds. The protein quality was evaluated by determining the protein efficiency ratio, net protein utilization, biological value, and true digestibility coefficient. All components were increased by peeling, except the ash, fiber content, and residual nitrogen content of the insoluble protein fraction. The latter was markedly decreased by peeling. Giza 9 lentil seeds were found to contain the highest protein and thiamine contents. They showed the highest protein quality and proved to be nutritionally superior to other varieties. Generally, the three local cultivars were found to be chemically and biologically superior to the imported Pakistani cultivar. (Authors' abstract)

71. El-Nahry, F. I., Saddik, M. F., and El-Sherbeeny, M. R. "Biological evaluation of basterami proteins" Egypt. J. Food Sci. 8(1,2), 1980 pp 55-60.

Protein biological value of basterami (Egyptian pastrami) samples with and without casing was studied by determination of protein efficiency ratio (PER), net protein ratio (NPR) and serum analysis at 5 and 10% levels of protein intake.

Biological evaluation of basterami proteins showed them to be nearly the same as those of casein. PER of basterami did not differ greatly by increased level of protein intake from 5 to 10%, while NPR was reduced. PER and NPR values for basterami without casing were much higher than those of basterami with casing. This may be due to the presence of large amounts of fenugreek in the casing. Serum analysis did not differ greatly in rats fed whole basterami or basterami without casing. (Authors' abstract)

72. El-Sayed, W. A., Shehab, A. H., Mourad, F. E., El-Nahry, F. I., and Said, A. K. "Biochemical and biological evaluation of pigeon meats: Effect of type, age and sex." Die Nahrung, 24(9), 1980, pp 821-828.

The nutritional quality of edible portions from certain kinds of pigeons that exist in Egypt was studied by determining their biochemical composition and by biological evaluation. Pigeon meats are in general fatty. They have a high energy value and contain all essential amino acids in amounts and proportions required by the human body. They are excellent sources for vitamins and minerals, particularly B_1, B_2, calcium, phosphorus and iron. The nutritive value of pigeon proteins is rather good. No significant differences were encountered due to variations of type or sex. (Authors' abstract)

73. Hefnawi, F., El-Zayat, A. F., and Yacout, M. M. "Physiologic studies of menstrual blood loss. I. Range and consistency of menstrual blood loss in and iron requirements of menstruating Egyptian women." Int. J. Gynaecol. Obstet. 17(4), January-February 1980, pp 343-348.

Two physiologic studies of menstrual blood loss in Egyptian women are presented. In the first, an attempt was made to establish the normal range of menstrual blood loss of Egyptian women, to test their individual consistency in the amount of menstrual blood loss, and to determine the iron requirements needed to compensate for iron loss and to prevent iron deficiency anemia in menstruating Egyptian women. In the second, physiologic and other variables affecting the magnitude of menstrual blood loss in Egyptian women were investigated. (Authors' abstract)

74. Liorstad, M. H. "Computerizing nutrition surveys in the field." Food Nutr. (Roma, 6(2), 1980, pp 24-26. (Food and Agriculture

organization of the United Nations.)

Use of microcomputers in the field in household surveys to increase the efficiency of data checking and to speed up data transfer and analysis has been successful in Egypt. Where speed of execution and reliability of results are important survey characteristics, the technique offers a possibility to improve considerably on conventional methods. (Author's abstract)

75. Morsy, Soheir A. "Body concepts and health care: Illustration from an Egyptian village". Human Organization, 39(1), Spring 1980, pp 92-96.

This anthropoligical paper focuses on the beliefs about body and illness held by the villagers of Fatiha, Egypt. The use of informal, traditional healers is compared with the formal, urban-oriented health care system, especially in the approach to psycho social illnesses. The author explores the effect of local concepts on the villagers' use of formal and informal health services and possible improvements in responsiveness of the formal health care system.

76. Nofal, M. A., El-Nahry, F. I., and Shaker, A. M. "Carob seeds oil" Annals Agr. Sci (Moshtohor) 14, 1980, pp 149-160.

Carob seeds oil (2.07%) was extracted with diethyl ether. Some of its physical and chemical characteristics were determined. The keeping quality of the crude oil was studied by Swift stability test. Refractive index and infrared spectroscopy were applied to study the effect of the autoxidation reactions on the oil. The oil under study had no antimicrobial activity against some tested bacteria. Furthermore, food efficiency ratio for rats fed carob seeds oil was compared with that of control animals (cotton seed oil). The nutritional studies prove the absence of any toxic factor and suggest the use of the oil for edible purposes. (Authors' abstract)

77. Nofal, M. A., El Nahry, F. I., and Shaker, A. M. H. "Studies on carob and tamarind pulps and their extracts." Annals Agr. Sci (Moshtohor) 14, 1980, pp 161-169.

The chemical composition of carob and tarnarind pulps was determined. Total carbohydrates were found to be the main constituent in both pulps. Carob pulps can be considered an iron-rich food, as their iron content was much higher than those of tamarind pulps. Carob and tamarind pulps were extracted by some solvents using cold and hot extraction. The solvents used were: water, ethanol and water/ethanol mixture (1:0. The antimicrobial activities of the obtained extracts were studied.

Carob and tamarind extracts produced by hot water extraction were found to contain considerable amounts of protein and high amounts of minerals which reflect their importance as refreshing drinks. The concentration of both extracts that preferred by the consumers was estimated by sensory evaluation. (Authors' abstract)

78. Saddik, M. F., El-Nahry, F. I., El-Ghorab, M. I., Nourad, F. E., and El-Banna, N. "Biochemical and microbiological studies on some locally manufactured meat products." Egypt. J. Food Sci. 8(1), 1980, pp 4-54.

Samples of sausages, luncheon meat and basterami (Egyptian pastrami) obtained from different meat factories and grocery stores in Cairo were analyzed to determine their nutritive values. Samples of basterami were examined bacteriologically. Results showed that the examined meat products are rich in protein, fat and phosphorus, but poor in calcium. Iron was found in fair amounts. Bacteriological examination of basterami showed that the coating contained 41.75×10^4 counts/g while the meat had 60.75×10^5/g. The results also indicated that coliforms were present in five coating samples at different titres ranging from 10^3 to 10^6. Meat products, such as sausages, luncheon meat and basterami are excellent food items that contain a wide variety of easily digested nutrients. (Adapted from authors' abstract)

79. Said, A. K., Hamdy, A. A., Hanna, M. L., Tadros, I., and Abdou, I. A. "Aswan nutriture survey. IV--Diet intake and food habits." J. Egypt Public Health Assoc. 55(1-2), 1980, pp 1-8.

Food consumption studies were undertaken for a total of 112 families and 256 subjects from different population groups in various Aswan regions. The findings showed:

1. Low consumption of animal protein and animal fat, lowest in New Nuba region.
2. High consumption of plant proteins and plant oils, particularly in rural and New Nuba regions.
3. More carbohydrate consumption, mainly bread, especially in rural and New Nuba areas.
4. Average daily intakes of calories, proteins, calcium, iron, vitamin A, riboflavin, niacin, and ascorbic acid below the daily requirements of school children of various age and sex groups.

Accordingly, suitable applied nutrition programs were strongly recommended. (Authors' abstract)

80. Said, A. K., Moussa, W. A., Demian, H. G., Aref, N. M., and Aly, H. E. "Follow-up study of nutritional deficiencies among Cairo school children." J. Egypt. Pub. Health Assoc. 55(5,6) 1980, pp 255-263.

A sample of 3460 Cairo school boys and girls were studied for deficiency signs, haemoglobin concentration and parasitic infection. The aim was to compare the health and nutritional status of Cairo school children with similar data reported 13 years earlier. Prevalences of most deficiency signs and parasitic infections were lower in the present survey. This could be due to better health awareness and medical care. However, the blood haemoglobin levels were slightly lower. (Authors' summary)

81. Samy, M. S. "Some mineral content of Egyptian feedstuffs." Z. Ernaehrungswiss 19(4), December 1980, pp 272-275. Dr. Dietrich Steinkopff Verlag.

Determination of five minerals for the more common Egyptian feedstuffs was conducted. Bone and fish meals contained the highest amounts of calcium, 33.43 and 0.25%, while wheat and corn grains contained the lowest amounts, 0.04 and 0.02%, respectively. Bone and meat meals contained the highest amounts of phosphorus, 12.31% and 5.06%, while corn grains and wheat straw contained the lowest amounts, 0.26 and 0.23%, respectively. Meat and fish meals contained the highest amounts of sulfur, 0.89 and 0.68%, while wheat straw and bone meal contained the lowest amounts, 0.20% and 0.18%, respectively. Rice and wheat brans contained the highest amounts of manganese, 395.3 and 99.8 mg/kg, while corn grains and dried skim milk contained the highest amounts of iron, 0.127 and 0.084%. Barley and dried skim milk contained the lowest amounts, 0.004 for each feed material, respectively. (Author's abstract)

82. Abdel Kader, M. M., Said, A. K., Bassily, N. S., and Abdou, I. A. "Protein requirements for Egyptians II. Nitrogen balance and utilization in healthy adult young men." Egypt. J. Physiol. Sci. 6(1,2), pp 23-30.

The purpose of this study was to estimate the protein requirements for healthy adult male Egyptians and, moreover, to evaluate the assumption made in estimating minimum protein requirements by the factorial method suggested by the FAO/WHO Expert group in 1965.

A series of nitrogen balance studies were carried out. Twenty subjects were maintained for two weeks on a protein-free diet to which varying levels of egg protein were added. Caloric intakes were adjusted to maintain constant body weight.

The minimum requirement to keep healthy adult Egyptian young men in nitrogen equilibrium was estimated to be 3.56 g N/day from whole egg. Net protein utilization was 79% and the biological value of whole egg protein at maintenance requirement was 78%. (Authors' abstract)

83. Abdel-Nasser, M., Mahmoud, S. A., Makawi, A., and Ali, F. S. "Studies on nodulation of soyabean in Egypt. I. Selection of an efficient strain of Rhizobium japonicum." Zentralbl. Bakteriol. (Naturwiss) 134(8), 1979.

Studies on nodulation of soyabean were conducted with "Okadin", a commercial soyabean inoculum, and 23 strains of R. japonicum. Both field and pot experiments were done. The pot runs were done using sterilized sand cultures. Results showed that the non-inoculated plants failed to form nodules possibly because they did not have adequate densities of effective soyabean-rhizobia strains. Egyptian soil conditions were cited as being a factor in the low densities of the strains. Results also showed that the strains of R. japonicum varied in nodulation effectiveness, so that use of an efficient strain was important.

84. Abdel-Nasser, M., Mahmoud, S. A., Makawi, A., and Ali, F. S. "Studies on nodulation of soyabeans in Egypt. II. Effect of seed-diffusates on Rhizobium japonicum." Zentralbl. Bakteriol. (Naturwiss) 134(7), 1979, pp 600-603.

Antibacterial substances were studied in the growth inhibition zones of Rhizobium japonicum (E 45). Seeds were surface-sterilized or autoclaved, and seed coats, dicotyledones, and cotyledona were also studied, in the Harosoy soyabean. The antibacterial substances were water-soluble or partially insoluble, and were thermostable at 121 degrees C. they were in the whole seed. Physical and chemical seed treatments done to ameliorate the inhibitive effects of the seed-diffusates showed that they could be inactivated by germination for 12 hours or more before inoculation, and by some chemical treatments. This was done to produce successful nodulation.

85. Aly, H. E., Dakroury, A. H., Said, A. K., Hussein, M. A., and El-Ghorab, M. I., et al. "Use of nutrition surveys for family planning program evaluation. The case of the Arab Republic of Egypt nutrition status." J. Egypt Public Health Assoc. 54(5-6), 1979, pp 290-312.

A nutrition survey containing data on contraceptive use by mothers has the potential for studying the links between family planning use and child health. In the 1978 Arab Republic of Egypt Nutrition Status Survey, about one in five mothers interviewed were found to be contraceptive users; there was wide variation in use by area of residence and socioeconomic status. A positive association was found between current contraceptive use and measures of child health, an association that was maintained when residence, social status, and other background variables were controlled statistically. With the addition of a small number of questions relating to fertility in future surveys, it will be possible to study further the relationship between family planning use and one important program goal - improved child health. (Authors' abstract)

86. Aly, H. E., Moussa, W. A., and Hammam, A. "Effect of supramine on rehabilitation of children suffering from different forms of protein energy malnutrition." Ain Shams Med. J. 30(5,6), September, November 1979, pp 301-313.

Supramine, a grain- and legume-based mixture was tested as the main source of dietary protein rehabilitation of children with protein energy malnutrition (PEM). The study sample consisted of 50 children aged 3 to 24 months, including 15 cases of severe PEM and 35 cases of moderate PEM. The indicators of nutritional status included various anthropometric measurements, clinical findings and hemoglobin levels.

The children were followed for a minimum period of 6 months. All cases showed a marked improvement in nutritional status while of supramine as the main source of dietary protein. Severe cases of PEM change to a classification of mild to moderate PEM within 4-6 week period. Moderate cases improved to the normal state or a mild degree of PEM within the period of rehabilitation.

The deletrious effect of infection, in particular gastro-enteritis, on the nutritional status of the sample was emphasized. (Adapted from authors' abstract)

87. El-Aaser, A. A., El-Merzabani, M. M., and Zakhary, N. I. "A study on the aetiological factors of bilharzial bladder cancer in Egypt--2. Nitrosamines and their precursors in Egyptian dairy products." Eur. J. Cancer 15(3), March 1979, pp 293-298.

Nitrosamine concentrations in samples of Egyptian milk, yoghurt, and four types of cheese were measured. Deliberate chemical nitrosation of these foods was done, and nitrosamine concentrations again measured. Nitrosamine contamination at g x 10^{-9} level was found in 2, 3, and 7 out of 10 samples of milk, cottage cheese, and white cheese, and in 6 out of 9 samples of salted chesse respectively. After nitrosation, increasing amounts of volatile and nonvolatile nitrosamines were found, particularly in salted cottage cheese and in blue cheese. Authors suggested that the high daily consumption of salted cheese in rural areas together with high bilharzial infestation in urinary bladders of Egyptian farmers possibly combined to produce the high incidence of bladder cancer seen among them.

88. Hegazi, N. A., and Vlassak, K. "Cell morphology and flagellation of nitrogen-fixing spirilla." Folia Microbiol. (Praha) 23(5), 1979, pp 376-378.

Maize and sugar-cane rhizosphere of plants grown in Egyptian and Belgian soils were used to isolate 20 strains of nitrogen-fixing spirilla. Two morphological groups were detected by electron microscopic studies. One group showed long spiral rods which probably possessed a bipolar tuft of flagella. The other group showed short and thick curved rods with a unipolar flagellum.

89. Hoogstraal, H., Meegan, J. M., Khalil, G. M., and Adham, F. K. "The Rift Valley fever epizootic in Egypt 1977-78. 2. Ecological and entomological studies." Trans. R. Soc. Trop. Med. Hyg. 73(6), 1979, pp 624-629.

Epidemiological factors related to the introduction, spread and maintenance of Rift Valley fever (RVF) virus were studied during the 1977-1978 epizootic in Egypt. Culex pipiens is the most ubiquitous and prevalent mosquito species in the Nile Valley and Delta. Isolation of RVF virus from unengorged C. pipiens, and demonstration of laboratory transmission of the virus by this species, strongly implicate it as the chief vector in Egypt. Virus transmission to man also occurs by contamination when handling infected meat and by inhaling natural virus aerosols. Wild rodents apparently do not serve as RVF virus reservoirs. Domestic sheep, cattle, buffaloes, camels, goats, donkeys and dogs act as amplifying hosts. Over 30% of the camels sampled at the southern border of Egypt were serologically positive for antibodies to RVF virus, and it appears likely that the virus was introduced into Egypt, either by these animals or by other vehicles from the south. (Authors' abstract)

90. Mahgoub, A., Idle, J. R., and Smith, R. L. "A population and familial study of the defective alicyclic hydroxylation of debrisoquine among Egyptians". Xenobiotica 9(1), January 1979, pp 51-56.

1. Debrisoquine hydroxylation exhibited profound variation in 72 Egyptian volunteers. 2. The frequency distribution histogram of the metabolic ratio (ratio unchanged drug: 4-hydroxy metabolite in 0-8 hr urine) was polymodal. 3. From family data it was possible to define more clearly than before the heterozygous characteristics. 4. Egyptians appear in general to be more extensive oxidizers of debrisoquine than do English subjects. 5. Ramadan fasting was found to lower the absorption of debrisoquine. (Authors' abstract)

91. Mansour, M. M., Mikhail, M. D., Farid, M. S. Z., and Bassily, S. "Chronic salmonella septicemia and malabsorption of vitamin A." Am. J. Clin. Nutr. 32(2) February 1979, pp 319-324.

Vitamin A absorption was studied in 15 patients with chronic salmonella bacteremia, in 11 patients with active S. mansoni infection, and in 10 healthy Egyptians with no evidence of any infection using a vitamin A tolerance test. Clinical examination showed no signs of vitamin A deficiency in any subject. Mean fasting vitamin A and carotene levels in the patient groups were significantly lower than in the controls; Salmonella bacteremia patients showed lower levels than S. mansoni patients. After the test dose was given, the mean peak vitamin A rise was significantly lower in the salmonella infected group. After therapy, both patient groups showed significant increase in the mean fasting vitamin A and carotene levels. Vitamin A absorption of the salmonella infected group and the S. mansoni infected group increased significantly and slightly, respectively. Gross impairment of vitamin A absorption by chronic salmonellosis was indicated and might be signficant in the prevalence of vitamin A deficiency among populations with borderline vitamin A intakes.

92. Moselhi, M., El-Gazzar, R., Abdel-Kader, H. M., El-Sadik, Y., and El-Dakhakhny, A. A. "Clinical and biological investigations among grain handlers." J. Egypt Public Health Assoc. 54(5-6), 1979, pp 396-414.

A study conducted in grain silos located in Alexandria included dust survey, clinical examination and some biological investigations. Clinical examination of 80 grain handlers showed that the predominant symptoms were chronic cough (58.8%), dyspnea associated with exposure to grain dust (50.0%) wheezing (17.5%) and grain fever (6.25%); diminished vital capacity (7.5%) and decreased forced expiratory volume in the first second (24%) were also shown. The prevalence of dermatitis (6.25%), peptic ulcer (3.75%) and pulmonary fibrosis (5.0%) did not differ from that in the general population. Dust survey indicated that the airborne dust concentration and its histamine content may play a role in the development of respiratory symptoms.

Results of the biological investigations revealed significant decrease of serum beta-globulins and increased gamma fraction, significant increase of immunoglobulins IgG and IgE, neutrophilia and lymphopenia among the workers exposed to grain dust.

Of the predisposing factors, smoking was the most important one accounting for the increased prevalence of abnormal respiratory findings. Duration of exposure and concentration of grain dust seem to potentiate the effect of smoking among grain handlers. (Authors' abstract)

93. Moubasher, A. H., Abdel-Kader, M. I., and El-Kady, I. A. "Toxigenic fungi isolated from Roquefort cheese." Mycopathologia 66(3), February 28, 1979, pp 187-190.

To evalute the potential for mycotoxin production by fungi contaminating blue-veined cheese, as well as by the ripening fungus Penicillium roqueforti, the fungal flora of six of local and imported brands were determined. A total of 19 fungi were isolated from the six brands tested. Fourteen of the isolates were toxic to chicken embryos. The toxigenic fungi produced the following mycotoxins: Aspergillus fumigatus, kolic acid; A. versicolor, sterigmatocystin; Penicillium roqueforti, panicillic acid and unidentified toxic metabolites. (Authors' abstract)

94. Ragheb, S., and Smith, E. W. "Beliefs and customs regarding breast feeding among Egyptian women in Alexandria." Int. J. Nurs. Stud. 16(1), 1979, pp 73-83.

A random sample of 88 lactating Egyptian women was interviewed to elucidate their beliefs and superstitions regarding breast feeding, use of supplementary infant foods, and influences on lactation. The study's purpose was to identify these beliefs so nurses could use the information to help mothers provide good infant nutrition and to promote beneficial changes in areas needing it. Problem customs identified included lack of antenatal breast care for breast feeding preparation, several days' delay in the start of lactation after giving childbirth, late start of supplemental feeding as well as lack of knowledge about appropriate supplemental foods and their preparation, and the habit of abrupt weaning. Most beliefs, however, were seen to be harmless, and many promoted good nutrition and mother-child interaction.

95. Said, A. K., Morsy, M. H., and Abdou, I. A. "Aswan Nutriture Survey Part III-Dental caries among population groups of Aswan Governorate." J. Egypt. Pub. Health Assoc. 65(1,2), 1979, pp 15-22.

Dental examination of 3862 individuals from various Aswan regions showed that general condition of the teeth is poor, as has been reported from other areas of Egypt. Dental caries were generally more prevalent in rural areas, and increased with age, with no clear sex predominance.

Due to the poor condition of the teeth, the prevalence of gingivitis is expected to be high. No filled teeth were encountered, indicating a need for immediate attention for dental care and oral hygiene. (Adapted from authors' summary)

96. Abdel Kader, M. M., Said, A. K., Hussein, M. A., Bassily, N. S., and Abdou, I. A. "Protein requirements for Egyptians - I - Obligatory nitrogen losses in urine and feces of healthy adult young men." Egypt. J. Physiol. Sci. 6(1,2), 1979, pp 13-21.

Forty subjects were maintained on an essentially protein-free diet for 14 days to estimate their obligatory nitrogen losses in urine and feces as a step for assessing their protein requirements. Caloric intakes were adjusted to maintain constant body weight. Urinary nitrogen excretion for the subjects dropped sharply during the first three days, then declined gradually to reach a study level after the tenth day.

The average daily loss in the period between the eleventh and fourteenth days was considered to represent the endogenous nitrogen loss. It amounted to 2.13 g nitrogen/day or 1.14 mg N/basal Kcal. The endogenous nitrogen excretion per basal K. calorie followed a normal distribution. The mean obligatory fecal nitrogen loss during the last 8 days of the experimental period was 0.66 g/day. (Authors' abstract)

97. Samy, M. S. "Chemical analysis of linseed meal produced in Egypt." Z. Ernaehrungswiss 18(1), March 1979, pp 23-25. Dr. Dietrich Steinkopff Verlag.

Representative samples of linseed meal were collected from nineteen oil mills in Egypt. The averages of nutrients in the samples were moisture 6.55 ± 0.22, dry matter 93.45 ± 0.22, ether extract 11.19 ± 0.60, crude protein 26.97 ± 0.59, crude fiber 11.13 ± 0.43, nitrogen-free extract 36.10 ± 0.60, ash 8.0 ± 0.38, calcium 0.39 ± 0.03, and phosphorus 0.89 ± 0.04. The average of the calculated calorific value was 435.81 +/- 3.16 kcal per 100 gram of the meal. (Adapted from author's abstract)

98. Siam, M. A., Michael, S. A., and Ghoneim, N. H. "Studies on the isolation of the infective stages of Trichinella spiralis and Toxoplasma gondii from fresh and processed pork in Egypt." J. Egypt Public Health Assoc. 54(3), 1979, pp 163-170.

Trials were undertaken to isolate the infective stages of Trichinella spiralis (the larvae) and Toxoplasma gondii (the cystic form) from fresh and processed pork.

The examination of 100 fresh pork samples and 100 processed pork samples, revealed that:

1) 3% of the fresh pork contained the infective Trichinella spiralis larvae.
2) 2% of the fresh pork samples contained the infective Toxoplasma gondii cysts.
3) From the processed pork samples, no Trichinella larvae or Toxoplasma cysts were isolated. (Authors' abstract)

99. Abd-el-Dahab, M. K., el-Goorani, M. A., and Wagih, E. E. "Race identification of Pseudomonas solanacearum E.F. Smith in Egypt." Zentralbl. Bakteriol. Parasitenkd. Infektionskr. Hyg. 133(3), 1978, pp 211-216.

Twenty one isolates of Pseudomonas solanacearum E.F. Smith, which does not occur on hosts other than potato in Egypt, were obtained from diseased potato tubers collected from different localities in Egypt and used in this study. These 21 isolates were found to be pathogenic to potato plants, but were not pathogenic to tobacco and banana plants. All the 21 isolates caused only a yellowish discoloration of the infiltrated area of tobacco leaves by 48 hours after inoculation and produced low melanin pigments on a tyrosine agar medium. These results indicate that the obtained isolates belong to Race 3. Biochemical studies, performed on five representative isolates, indicated that they all belong to the biochemical biotype II. The results obtained in the present investigation appear to be the first record of P. solanacearum races in Egypt. (Adapted from authors' abstract)

100. Abd-el-Fattah, M., Gabrial, G. N., Shalaby, S. M., and Morcos, S. R. "An epidemiological and biochemical study on osteomalacia among pregnant women in Egypt." Z. Ernaehrungswiss 17(3), September 1978, pp 140-144. Dr. Dietrich Steinkopff Verlag.

Two hundred thirty pregnant women of low socio-economic standard were evaluated for nutritional status and state of calcium and bone mineralization. Social, environmental, dietary and biological factors of the women were also investigated to determine their possible role in osteomalacia. Results revealed a low nutritional status was associated with biochemical abnormality denoting an impaired calcium state and defective bone mineralization. The low intake of available calcium and lack of supplements or inadequate supplements are suggested to be the main factors in causing the low state of calcium. (Adapted from authors' abstract)

101. Abdel-Rahman, A. H., and Youssef, S. A. "Fortification of some Egyptian foods with soybean". J. Am. Oil Chem. Soc. 55(4), April 1978, pp 338A-340A.

Flours from full fat and defatted soybeans were made in the laboratory and used as supplements to Egyptian bread and two popular legume foods (lentil soup and falafil). The effect of fortification level on water absorption, dough rheology, loaf quality and major chemical constituents of fino (pulp) and Arabic (flat) breads was investigated.

Water absorption was slightly affected and dough mixing time, stability and calorimetric values increased, but the mixing tolerance index was decreased by adding defatted soy flour to wheat flour. Loaves were slightly smaller in volume than the control at high levels of defatted soy flour. Bread score and panel evaluation showed deterioration of fino bread characteristics above 6% and Arabic bread above 8% defatted soy flour, but above only 3% full fat soy. Organoleptic properties of the enriched lentil soup and falafil were similar to those of control at a level of 25% and 50% respectively for full fat soy and of 40% and 60% for defatted soy flour.

The most favorable change of the chemical composition of lentil soup and falafil was the increased protein content. Also, increasing the level of defatted soy flour increased ash content and decreased the level of fat absorption by fried falafil. On the other hand, increasing the level of full fat soy may replace the addition of shortening to lentil soup to make it more palatable. (Adapted from authors' abstract).

102. Abdel-Salam, F. E., Aboul-Seoud, A. A., and Radwan, M. A. H. "Effect of liver meal as animal protein source on the feeding of growing chicks." Egypt. J. Nutr. 2(1), January 1978, pp 31-42

Ninety one-week-old male Dokki 4 chicks were fed 6 different treatment diets containing: (1) plant protein (20 percent crude protein) as a control, (2) 0.2 percent L-lycine supplement, (3) 6 percent imported fish meal, and (4), (5) and (6) containing 2, 4 and 6 percent local liver meal, respectively. The feeding experiment continued to age 8 weeks.

The results indicated that 0.2 percent L-lysine supplement to a plant protein diet (21 percent crude protein and 2670 Kcal metabolizable energy per Kg. diet) did not show significant increase in final live weight of chicks over unsupplemented plant protein diet (20 percent crude protein). Both animal protein sources showed significant increase over the supplemented and the unsupplemented diets. Six percent fish meal would give on calculated basis the same live weight as 3.4 percent dietary liver meal while 0.2 L-lysine would give the same weight as 0.9 percent liver meal.

Although higher feeding cost was reported for 6 percent local liver meal diet, the acceleration of growth rate and better feed efficiency would compensate for this. The superiority of local liver meal used in the present study is probably due to other factors than total amino acids content. (Adapted from authors' summary)

103. Basmy, K., Deib, H. A. F., and Kamel, A. M. "Protein content in the diet therapy of viral hepatitis." Egypt. J. Nutr. 2(1), January 1978, pp 95-106.

A study was conducted on 476 viral hepatitis patients to determine the effect of supplementary proteins in the diet on the course of the disease in moderate, mild, and severe cases. Initial protein restriction was beneficial in severe cases. Mild and moderate cases improved more quickly with high protein supplementation. Thus dietary therapy was shown to be of benefit in treatment of viral hepatitis.

104. Darwish, N. M., Eid, E. E., Fahmy, S. I., and Kamel, N. "Standard anthropometric measurements for children attending day care centers in Alexandria". Bulletin of the High Institute of Public Health of Alexandria, 8(2), 1978.

This study was done to develop local anthropometric norms for preschool children in Alexandria, and to evaluate them compared to previously published local and international measurements for the same age. Three hundred ninety boys and three hundred sixty girls under six years of age who attended seven nurseries were randomly selected. They represented varying income levels and residential districts.

Seven standardized anthropometric measurements were used, including weight, height, triceps and subscapular skinfolds, midarm circumference, head circumference, and chest circumference. The mean and % values by age and sex were presented. Most of the measurements obtained were very close to those previously reported for American children of the same age, and were greater than those previously obtained locally in a study which had assessed children of lower socioeconomic levels only.

105. El Fattah, M. A., Nasser, S. S., and Afifi, Z. E. "Breast feeding and its impact on the infants health and development." Egypt. J. Nutr. 2(1), January 1978, pp 57-64.

Two hundred infants under 6 months of age, attending the M.C.H. Centre and health office, were surveyed for type of feeding, influencing factors in type of feeding, and impact of type of feeding on the infant's health, growth and development. All infants were of a low socio-economic background. Breastfeeding, either complete or partial, was the main infant feeding practice in 82.5% of the group.

The completely breast-fed infants showed the best growth and development, with weight comparable to standard weight for age for up to the 5th month. The mixed and artificially-fed infants showed lower body weight forage and more development of protein-energy malnutrition during the early months of life, including the severest degrees. The best-fed infants showed the lowest incidence of diarrhea and respiratory and skin infections. None of them was suffering from gastroenteritis during the survey, although it was frequently encountered among the artifically-fed ones. (Adapted from authors' abstract).

106. El-Halaly, A. F., Abo-El-Dhab, M. K., El-Goorani, M. A., and Gabr, M. R. "Identification of Erwinia sp., causing stalk rot of maize in Egypt". Zentralbl. Bakteriol. (Naturwiss) 133(7-8), 1978, pp 680-685.

The physiologic characteristics, pathogenic propensities, and sensitivity towards certain antibiotics of the causal bacterium of stalk rot of maize in Egypt were studied. Different isolates of Erwinia carotovora and E. atroseptica were included for comparative studies. The antibiotic sensitivity tests (including erythromycin) were of no value in differentiating between E. cardotovora and E.

atroseptica. The cultures of the causal bacterium of stalk rot of maize showed physiological characteristics similar to those known for E. chrysanthami. The pathogenic propensities of E. chrysanthami isolates suggest the presence of a number of pathotypes of E. chrysanthami. The proposal of Hartman and Kelman to identify maize stalk rot pathogen as E. chrysanthami (corn pathotype) seems, therefore, to be the most appropriate for this bacterium. (Adapted from authors' abstract)

107. El-Mahdy, A. R. A., Moustfa, E. K., and Mohamed, M. S. "Nitrogen solubility of Vicia faba bean proteins as affected by various Egyptian cooking methods." Egypt. J. Nutr. 2(1), January 1978, pp 15-29.

Factors affecting the extractability of Vicia faba bean nitrogen were studied. The optimum particle size, meal to solvent ratio and extraction duration were found to be 60 mesh, 1:50 and one hour respectively. The nitrogen solubility increased outside the pH range of 4 to 6, and the iso-electric points were in the pH ranges 5.65 to 6.30 and 3.40 to 4.30.

Heat processing of germinated, dry decorticated, and dry whole beans to prepare nabet, bean porridge (Bisara) and canned stewed and home-style stewed beans (Medamis) respectively, lowered the nitrogen extracted by the different solvents used--0.1 M hydrochloric acid, 0.01 M sodium hydroxide, 0.5 M sodium chloride, distilled water, 70% ethyl alcohol, 0.8 M trichloroacetic acid, "TCA" and 0.2 M phosphate buffer pH 8.0. Both TCA and ethyl-alcohol soluble nitrogen increased as a function of heat treatment. The presence of testa enhanced this effect in lowering the nitrogen solubility in the different solvents. (Adapted from authors' abstract.)

108. El-Nahry, F. I., El-Ghorab, M. I., Younes, R. "Nutritive value of local varieties of fresh and sundried okra (Hibiscus Esculentus) pods and seeds." Qual. Plant.-Pl. Fds. Hum. Nutr. 28(3), 1978, pp 227-231.

The nutritive value of Egyptian varieties of fresh and sun-dried okra pods as well as okra seeds were studied. These varieties were: Baladi, Eskandarani, and Gold Coast. Pods of the three varieties were shown to contain approximately the same amount of water. Fiber and ash were quite high while carbohydrate and fat contents were low. Fresh and sun-dried okra pods were found to contain high amounts of calcium and iron.

Sun-drying decreased water content, while other components increased considerably. Seeds were found to contain high concentration of protein, fat, ash, fiber, phosphorous, and iron. (Authors' abstract)

109. Fattah, M. A., and Ismail, A. M. "The interrelationship between the nutritional status, parasitic infection and anemia among children in a rural community." Egypt. J. Nutr. 2(1), January 1978, pp 43-56.

A nutritional study was carried out on 470 rural school children aged 6 through 11 years attending Manial Sheiha primary mixed school (Giza Governorate). Each child was investigated for socio-economic condition, nutritional status by weight and height, signs of nutritional deficiency, haemoglobin level and urine and stool examination for parasites. Most children came from families of low socio-economic standard. Their weights and heights were below the standards of both Egyptian and American children. Signs of nutritional deficiencies were found in 18.5% of the children examined. Anaemia was found among 62.6% of children. Urinary schistosomiasis was found to affect 31.9%, ascaris 26%, hymenolepis nana 6.9%, ancylostoma 4.8%, and amoebic cysts 7.5%. It was also found that 95.5% of the anaemic children were infected with one or more parasites.

Recommendations for promotion of the nutritional status of school children are suggested to be based on a package of 3 services or programs, i.e., a school feeding program, an effective school health program and a health and nutrition education program. (Adapted from authors' summary)

110. Hamid, G. A., El-Mougi, M., El-Badrawy, F., and El-Mossallami, M. A. "An epidemiological study of energy protein malnutrition in a rural community in Egypt." J. Egypt Med. Assoc. 61(9-10), 1978, pp 613-620.

The birth to 6-year-old child population of Sendion village in Qualyubeya Governorate, 1527 children, was studied for prevalence and degree of protein-energy malnutrition (PEM). 211 males and 193 females, or 25.11% and 28.09% respectively, had various degrees of PEM. Total prevalence rate was 26.45%. Severe malnutrition occurred in 6.35%, underweight or mild PEM in 20.1% of children. Of the malnourished children, 75.99% were underweight, 14.35% marasmic, 8.66% kwashiorkoric, and 1% suffered from marasmic kwashiorkor. The prevalance of PEM in first 6 months of life was 13.6%, in the second 6 months 23.2%, and 32.6 to 35.2% from 12 to 47 months. From 48 to 72 months, a marked drop in PEM occurred. Birth order was not related to prevalence. Artificial or mixed feeding, large family size, and female sex were related to increased prevalence of PEM.

111. Helali, E. A., and El-Erian, A. F. M. "Some aspects of using milk-replacers, containing hydrogenated marine fat, as applied to feeding of buffalo calves." Egypt. J. Nutr. 2(1), January 1978, pp 77-84.

Twenty-eight, recently-born buffalo calves were fed milk replacers with four different fat compositions until calves were weaned at a weight from 90-95 kgs (100-120 days). Safarol (crude hydrogenated marine fat) and Sandarit (edible marine fat), either with or without linseed oil, were used in the milk replacers. The calves were weighed each week and daily gain was calculated. After weaning, calves were slaughtered to determine carcass percentages. Digestibility coefficient % of each fat was calculated. Results concluded that differences in daily gain were found to be significant; the best results for daily gain, consumption of milk-replacers and digestibility of fat were obtained with milk-replacer containing 2.5% SANDARIT and 2.5% linseed oil which has higher unsaturated fatty acid (C : 18 : 1, C : 20 : 1 and C : 22 : 1). (Calves from this group showed higher vitality); and tests indicate that SANDARIT edible marine fat is better suited than SAFAROL crude hydrogenated marine fat as fat ingredient in milk-replacers for buffalo calves, either as the single fat component or mixed with an equal percentage of linseed oil. (Adapted from authors' abstract)

112. Hussein, F. H., Helmy, O., Khattab, A., El-Sokari, S., and Moawad, Z. "Some anthropometric studies of normal and marasmic Egyptian children." J. Egypt Med. Assoc. 61(7-8), 1978, pp 471-484.

To provide standards and to test validity of anthropometry as a diagnostic tool for early marasmus, 300 normal and 80 marasmic children were measured for height, weight, head circumference, upper arm circumference, and triceps, biceps, subscapular, and supracristal skinfolds. Normal females showed slightly lower curves for body length, head circumference, body weight, upper arm circumference and biceps skinfolds, and slightly higher values for subscapular and supracristal skinfolds than normal males. Measurements were generally less than those of American children. Except for height, the above measurements were slightly (head circumference) to markedly (all others) lower in marasmic children than in normal cases in both sexes. The single best indicative measurement for marasmus was the upper arm circumference.

113. Hussein, M. A., Ghazi, C., Bassiuny, N. M., Fayad, I., and Nelson, C. "Influence of cultural and traditional beliefs of mothers in an Egyptian village upon their nutrition habits and child feeding." Egypt. J. Nutr. 2(1), January 1978, pp 85-93.

A sample of 100 women villagers attending Shoubrament health center were studied to show the influence of cultural and traditional beliefs of mothers upon their nutrition habits during pregnancy and lactation, and their behaviour towards feeding their children in health and disease.

The data was obtained using a questionnaire. The results showed that some of the deeply impregnated traditions could be nutritionally valuable and others could be disastrous. (Authors' summary)

114. Ibrahim, A. M., el-Hawary, M. F., and Sakr, R. "Protein-calorie malnutrition (PCM) in Egypt immunological changes in salivary protein in PCM." Z. Ernaehrungswiss 17(3), September 1978, pp 145-152. Dr. Dietrich Steinkopff Verlag.

Whole saliva protein as well as the separated protein components were estimated in normal and malnourished Egyptian infants and young children. In normal children, eight protein components (albumin, alpha-1-antitrypsin, haptoglobin, beta-lipoprotein, transferrin, IgA, IgM and IgG) were detected, while in PCM cases two more components (prealbumin and alpha-2-macroglobulin) were found. The results also showed that the level of salivary protein components was markedly increased in edematous cases. In non-edematous cases, the level of these constituents was slightly increased in 3rd grade marasmus, but diminished in 2nd grade. It was concluded that the elevation of protein components in saliva of edematous cases could be a result of severe glandular tissue involvement as compared to controls and non-edematous cases. The value of IgA immunoglobulin as specific antibody originating from blood plasma and/or salivary glands may be used to reflect the extent of tissue affection in salivary glands of malnourished cases. (Adapted from authors' abstract)

115. Mekhael, K. G. "Comparative study of some trace elements in fresh and salt water in Egypt and their effect on the rate of growth and blood constitution of experimental animals." (Ph.D. Thesis) Write High Institute of Public Health, Alexandria University, Alexandria

Egypt for copies. 1978. 175 pages.

Natural fresh waters at different localities of River Nile satisfied the WHO standard limits except for high iron content, especially Oases well waters. Brackish waters are not suitable for human consumption from the chemical point of view. Treated waters satisfied the standard limits, and thus are suitable for human consumption. Biological studies showed a bad effect of the high amounts of dietary iron and zinc on the rate of growth and blood constitution, contrary to high dietary copper content. (Author's abstract)

116. Mohamed, A. M., el-Sharkawi, F. M., and el-Fiki, S. A. "Prevalence of schistosomiasis among fishermen of Lake Maryut." Egypt J. Bilharz. 5(1-2), 1978, pp 85-90.

A survey of schistosomiasis among the fishermen of Lake Maryut showed Schistosoma mansoni to be more prevalent than S. haematobium. The snail Biomphalaria alexandrina was frequently found around the lake, especially in areas of low salinity, with an inverse relation between the number of snails and the salinity of the water. The salinity of Lake Maryut seems to be decreasing over time as a result of the increased discharge of agricultural and domestic waste into the lake, and the authors suspect schistosomasis may increase among the fishermen. Bulinus truncatus snails were not found during this survey.

117. Nasser, S., El Fattah, M. A., and Emam, Z. "Maternal factors influencing feeding". Egypt. J. Nutr. 2(1), January 1978, pp 65-76.

Two-hundred mothers 17 - 40 years of age, with infants below 6 months of age, attending 2 MCH Centers of El Darb El Ahmar Health Center during July and August 1977 were examined. Clinical and anthropometric examinations, a sociodemographic questionnaire,and a survey of infant feeding rationale and method were conducted. Exclusive breast-feeding was practiced among 58.5% of studied infants; 17.5% were partially breastfed and 17.5% were artifically fed. Insufficient milk secretion at 6 months accounted for 80% of mixed feeding cases, twins and maternal employment resulted in 6.52% each, contraceptive pill usage 4.35%, and caesarian section 2.17%. Maternal causes for bottle feeding at 6 months were spontaneous secretion cessation 31.4%, maternal diseases 22.9%, contraceptive pill 20%, maternal employment 8.6%, caesarian section 5.7%. Infant causes were refusal of breast 8.6%, and infant's disease 2.9%. 93.5% of mothers were unemployed, most were illiterate; per capita monthly income was 0.5 to 13.6 L.E. Illiteracy rate was highest among breastfeeding mothers, less for mixed feeding mothers, and least for bottle feeding mothers. Mean age of mothers partially or completely breastfeeding their infants was higher than those artificially feeding. 50% of mothers artificially feeding were primiparas and 20% were second paras. Multiparas and grand-multiparas comprised 82.9% and 80.4% respectively, of those who completely or partially breastfed. Previous lactation influenced present feeding habits. In 8.45% of breastfed cases, maternal body weight was below 90% of standard weight for height, and infant PEM of these women was 36.4%, as compared to 24.4% in cases where the mother's weight was standard.

118. Nawar, Isis A. "The structure of human diet in different income levels in an Egyptian new village in Abis zone. I-Sources of energy" In: Paper by Dr. Isis A. Nawar, Associate Professor,

Division of Home Economics Department of Agricultural Extension, Faculty of Agriculture, Alexandria University, Alexandria, Egypt. (Unpublished)

A pilot study was conducted to identify the general trends of caloric consumption in different income levels in families in the eighth village in Abis Zone, a newly reclaimed area in the northwest of Egypt. Four income categories were based on monthly income per person in the family, and for each income level caloric amounts were calculated for fats, carbohydrates, and proteins.

Consumption increased as income increased, with total caloric intake still fairly low, especially in lower income groups, compared to FAO/WHO 1974 recommendations. The share of carbohydrate as starch and sugar, fat, and protein in the total energy supply varied with income. A gradual increase in proportion derived from lipid, total protein, animal protein, and sugar occurred as income increased. A decline in proportion of starch-derived calories, overall carbohydrate calories, and plant-derived protein calories occurred with increasing income.

119. Nawar, Isis A. "The structure of human diet in different income levels in an Egyptian new village in Abis zone. II-Protein and amino acids-Dietary concern" In: Paper by Dr. Isis A. Nawar, Associate Professor, Division of Home Economics Department of Agricultural Extension, Faculty of Agriculture, Alexandria University, Alexandria, Egypt. (Unpublished)

All families of the eighth village of Abis zone in northwest Egypt were interviewed for socioeconomic and dietary information to determine the protein and amino acid intakes and evaluate the quality of protein as affected by income.

Data showed a gradual increase in dietary protein with increase in income, and total protein intake was fairly adequate in all income levels. Mean intakes of essential amino acids lysine, threonine, tryptophan, and total sulfur amino acids were lower than those consumed in the USA. Isoleucine and valine levels were acceptable, and leucine and total aromatic amino acids were high. The ratio of essential amino acids to non-essential amino acids was increased with increasing income level, as was the ratio of essential amino acids to total nitrogen.

120. Nawar, Isis A. "The structure of human diet in different income levels in an Egyptian new village in Abis zone. III-Iron intake" In: Paper by Dr. Isis A. Nawar, Associate Professor, Division of Home Economics Department of Agricultural Extension, Faculty of Agriculture, Alexandria University, Alexandria, Egypt. (Unpublished)

A study on all the families of the eighth village of Abis zone in northwest Egypt was done to investigate iron intake and its sources as affected by income. Interviews established monthly income levels and food intakes. Hemoglobin levels were also determined.

Total iron intake varied with income level, being 15.5 mg/day in the lowest income level and 17.5 mg/day in the highest income level. Plant sources furnished 94.6% in the lowest and 92.3% in the highest income level. Proportion of iron furnished by plant:animal sources was 14:1 compared to .9:1 in the USA. Hemoglobin levels showed a majority of women and almost half of girls having anemia. Men, boys and infants followed in decreasing order of prevalence of anemia.

121. Nawar, Isis A. "The structure of human diet in different income levels in an Egyptian new village in Abis zone. IV-Calcium and phosphorus intakes" In: Paper by Dr. Isis A. Nawar, Associate Professor, Division of Home Economics Department of Agricultural Extension, Faculty of Agriculture, Alexandria University, Alexandria, Egypt. (Unpublished)

This study was done to determine intakes of, sources of, and ratio between calcium and phosphorus in the eighth village in Abis zone in Egypt. Interviews of all village families established socioeconomic and dietary information.

Data indicated that calcium intakes were low, especially in the low income groups, with values below FAO 1974 requirements by 30% in high income and 50% in low income groups. Milk furnished only 16.7% of total calcium intake, while grains were the major source of calcium. Intakes of phosphorus exceeded recommended dietary allowances in all income levels. The average Ca:P ratio was 1:7. This was due to the low Ca:P ratio of the legumes and grain staples eaten, and is conducive to suboptimal calcium utilization.

122. Said, A. K., and Abdou, I. A. "Aswan nutriture survey. Part I--Heights and weights of population groups of Aswan governorate." J. Egypt Public Health Assoc. 53(1-2), 1978, pp 17-42.

A representative sample of about 1% of the Aswan governorate population was surveyed in urban and rural regions. The objective was to evaluate the health and nutritional status of population groups 10 years after a previous survey. This survey included 4405 individuals from 112 families, including workers, nursery children, school children, and pregnant and nursing mothers. The growth retardation observed in the previous survey was still in existence and not improved after 10 years. It was more marked among school boys of rural and New Nuba areas and could be attributed to environmental conditions, particularly nutritional and dietary factors, rather than to heredity. It was sometimes intensified by secondary factors such as parasitic and bacterial infections. (Adapted from a authors' abstract)

123. Said, A. K., and Abdou, I. A. "Aswan nutriture survey. Part 2-Nutritional status of various population groups of Aswan Governorate." J. Egypt Public Health Assoc. 53(5-6), 1978, pp 303-326.

A nutritional survey was carried out on a random sample of 4405 people in Aswan Governorate during 1971 via anthropometric measurements and clinical examinations. In 1415 of the people, hemoglobin determinations, urine and stool examinations for parasites, a dietary survey, and socieconomic investigations were also included. Nutrient deficiency was prevalant among all groups, particularly lip and tongue manifestations, indicating multiple-vitamin-B deficiency with a strong riboflavin component and iron deficiency. Skin signs indicating vitamin A deficiency were few. Thyroid enlargement was common among female adolescents and among pregnant and lactating mothers, but was considered not to constitute endemic goiter. Average hemoglobin (Hb) concentration was lowest among nursery children at 11.8 g/100 ml blood. Of the subsample, 18.3% were anemic with blood Hb below 11.2 g/100 ml.

Primary school children had lower Hb than children over 13 years of age, with an overall average of 12.2 g/100 ml for boys and 12.6 g/100 ml for girls. Urinary bilharziasis incidence was highest among rural males, and was 19% overall. It was thus higher than in 1962, and averaged 23.5% among males and 10.4% among females.

124. Salib, A. G., El-Nahry, F., and Osman, M. A. "Preliminary studies on the biological value of some marine algae. Annals Agr. Science (Moshtohor) 9, 1978, pp 73-84.

Amino acids of five common Egyptian algae species were determined by gas liquid chromatography: Pterodadia capillaceae, Jania Sp (Red algae), Sargassum lenifolium, Hofperis scoparia (Brown algae), and Ulva lactuca (Green algae). Average contents of dicarboxylic acids (glutamic and aspartic acids) present in Red algae exceeded two times the average content of those in Green and Brown algae. However, Green algae were characterized by a high content of S-containing amino acids. Arginine was found in lower quantities in Brown algae as compared to Red and Green species. These algae species contained considerable amounts of crude proteins, ranging from 14.22% to 21.60% (on dry basis).

These algae species are deficient in lysine and tryptophan when compared with the whole hen's egg (WHO, 1965). Tryptophan is the limiting amino acid in Jania Sp. (Red algae) with a protein score of 38; lysine is the limiting amino acid in the other algae. There is no remarkable difference between the algae species in their protein score, 45-47 (FAO, 1957). Biological assay was carried out by feeding albino rats on diets containing algae protein (5% level). An algae toxin was eliminated by extraction with ether, followed by boiling with water. After toxin removal, the biological value of proteins ranged from 48.91 to 57.63. These algae can be used for animal feed after elimination of toxicity. Further treatments are needed in order to use these algae species in human nutrition. (Adapted from authors' abstract)

125. Abdin, Z. H., Waly, G., Salem, A., and Abul-Fadl, M. A. "Serum electrolytes in protein malnutrition and their reflection on the clinical electrocardiographic findings." J. Egypt Med. Assoc. 60(1-2), 1977, pp 101-108.

Forty Egyptian children with Kwashiorkor between 1 and 3 years of age were assessed via urine, stools, Hb%, serum proteins and electrolytes, ECG, and skiagrams of the heart and chest with C/T ratio. Tetany was seen rarely, but somatic vibrations occured in some ECGs. Hb% ranged from 45 to 70% and serum proteins ranged from 3.6 to 5.0 gm/dl. P, R, and T wave changes showed a characteristic Embryonic or Foetal pattern, possibly associated with small cardiac muscle size. Right ventricular preponderance was seen, with no ST changes. There was little congestive heart failure, but moderate hypocalcemia was present. Authors suggested that electrolyte supplementation including magnesium be included in therapy for kwashiorkor.

126. Aly, H. E. "Nutritional problems in Egypt" Practical Approaches to Combat Malnutrition with Special Reference to Mothers and Children Cairo, Egypt. Publication of Proceedings of IUNS Conference held May 25-29, 1977. pp 22-40

Past and current nutritional problems in Egypt were compared and national nutrition trends were determined. Results from nutritional surveys were presented, particularly concerning maternal and young child nutrition and health. The percentage of monthly income devoted to food expenditure rose from 55% to more than 70%, while a downward trend in breastfeeding from 100% to 89.5% was noted.

Survey data indicated severe malnutrition in rural Upper Egypt, particularly among two-year-old children. Repeated diarrheal episodes and their inadequate nutritional treatment contributed to a high, early childhood protein-energy malnutrition incidence. Improvement was noted in growth of school-age children in the decade preceding 1975. Anemia, rickets, goiter, and ariboflavinosis were cited as containing national nutrition problems in children.

127. Darwish, N. M., Shehab, S. K., El-Nahry, F. I., and Agamy, N. "Protein biological value and amino acid content of brain of local meat productive animals." <u>Die Nahrung</u> 21(8), 1977, pp 739-747.

This work compared the amino acid content and biological value of brain of camel, sheep, cow and buffalo and the effect of age on the concentration of different amino acids. Both cow and sheep brain contained higher concentrations of amino acids as compared with either buffalo or camel, with similar concentrations of phenylalanine, tyrosine, arginine, and ornithine. The effect of aging on the concentrations of phenylalanine, valine + methionine, and tyrosine, was also similar. Both ornithine and arginine concentations in brain decreased with aging. Camel brain was found to contain the lowest concentrations of all investigated amino acids. Camel and buffalo brains were found to contain similar concentrations of phenylalanine, arginine, and tyrosine, and the changes in cystine + cysteine, ornithine, tyrosine, and phenylalanine concentrations in brain with aging was also similar. In evaluating the biological value of brain, the NPU method gave more precise information than the PER method. The NPU results showed that for the investigated species, cow brain had the highest NPU value, followed in order by buffalo, sheep, and camel. (Authors' abstract).

128. El-Hinnawy, S., Khaled, G. M., Hamed, A. S., El-Nahry, F. I., and Saad, S. A. M. "Biochemical and biological studies on some local leaf proteins." <u>Annals Agric.Sci.</u> (Ain Shams Univ.) <u>Research Bulletin</u> #782, 1977, pp 1-16.

The local leaves of turnip greens and sweet potatoes grown in Egypt were biochemically investigated to determine their possible use in leaf protein concentrates.

Total nitrogen and crude protein content of turnip leaves were twice that found in sweet potato leaves. The percentage of proteins isolated from both turnip and sweet potato leaves was lower with Guha's method than with Byer's method. However, Guha's method produced a higher percentage yield for both leaves. The following amino acids were isolated from both turnip and sweet potato leaf protein: glutamic, alanine, aspartic, proline, histidine, arginine, threonine, leucine, isoleucine, valine, serine, glycine, tyrosine, cystine, methionine and lysine.

The net protein utilization by body nitrogen determination was 53.07 ± 4.49 and 26.02 ± 6.44 for the isolated leaf proteins and turnip leaves respectively. The protein efficency ratio and the net protein ratio for the isolated turnip green leaf protein were 2.82 and 3.48, respectively. Values for turnip leaves and turnip leaves supplied with methionine and lysine were 0.78, 1.50 and 2.03, 2.73 for protein efficiency ratio and net protein ratio, respectively. Protein efficiency ratio for casein was 3.19 and its net protein ratio was 3.81. (Adapted from authors' abstract)

129. El-Kirdassy, Z. H., El-Safouri, S. A., and Abdel-Galil, A. M. "Biochemical studies on Egyptian buffalo meat Part I. Determination of phosphorus, calcium and magnesium". Die Nahrung 21(4), 1977, pp 281-287.

The effect of age, sex, season and cut on the phosphorus, calcium and magnesium contents of buffalo meat was studied in 128 samples. Statistical analysis for the data showed significant difference to 0.01 level for phosphorus in relation to sex and in dry season in relation to sex. There was also a significant difference for both calcium and magnesium in relation to season and also for both male and female in relation to season. At 0.05 level, phosphorus showed a significant difference in green season in relation to sex and at 0.1 level in relation to season. (Authors' abstract, Akademie Verlag.)

130. El-Kirdassy, Z. H., El-Safouri, S. A., and Abdel-Galil, A. M. "Biochemical studies on Egyptian buffalo meat. Part 2. Determination of iron, zinc and copper". Die Nahrung 21(4), 1977, pp 289-295.

A total of 128 samples of Egyptian buffalo meat were collected from animals differing in age, sex, season and cuts. The samples were analyzed for iron, zinc and copper contents. Statistical analysis of the data obtained showed that zinc and copper differed significantly at 0.01 level in relation to cut variation. For females, they differed also at the same level in relation to season. Zinc differed significantly at 0.01 level seasonally and in male in relation to season. On the other hand, copper differed significantly at 0.05 level for green season in relation to sex. Iron and copper showed significant differences at 0.1 level due to sex and in dry season in relation to sex, respectively. (Authors' abstract)

131. El-Kirdassy, Z. H., El-Safouri, S. A., and Abdel-Galil, A. M. "Biochemical studies on Egyptian buffalo meat. Part 3. Determination of sodium, potassium and chloride". Die Nahrung 21(4), 1977, pp 297-302.

Sodium, potassium and chloride contents of buffalo meat were studied in 128 samples. Statistical analysis of the data obtained showed significant difference at 0.01 level for sodium, potassium and chloride in relation to season and for female in relation to season. Sodium and potassium differed significantly at 0.01 level in male animals in relation to season and chloride differed at this level for green season in relation to sex. At 0.05 level sodium showed a significant difference in cut, while chloride showed a variation of this level due to dry season in relation to sex. (Authors' abstract)

132. El-Kirdassy, Z. H., and Abdel-Galil, A. M. "Determination of pH, moisture, carbohydrates and ash of Egyptian buffalo meat." Die Nahrung 21(7), 1977, pp 567-573.

A total of 128 samples of Egyptian buffalo meat was analyzed for its pH value, moisture, carbohydrates and ash content. Statistical analysis of the data obtained showed significant difference of 0.01 level for moisture in relation to sex and cut (abdomen and thigh). There was also significant difference at 0.05 level for moisture in dry season in relation to sex and for ash in relation to cut. At 0.1 level moisture showed a significant difference at 0.1 level in female in relation to season. (Authors' abstract)

133. El-Kirdassy, Z. H., and Abdel-Galil, A. M. "Protein, amino acid contents and protein efficiency ratio of Egyptian buffalo meat under different biological conditions." Die Nahrung 21(7), 1977, pp 575-581.

The effect of age, sex, season and cut variations on protein, amino acids content and protein efficiency ratio (P.E.R.) of Egyptian buffalo meat was studied in 128 samples under different biological conditions. Statistical analysis for the data obtained showed significant difference at 0.01 level for protein in relation to cut (abdomen and thigh), male in relation to season, and dry season in relation to sex. There was also significant difference at 0.05 level for green season in relation to sex. Protein showed a significant difference at 0.1 level due to sex variation. There was a difference in the amino acids content of young and old animals during dry season in both cuts. Young animals had higher values than old ones in most of the amino acids investigated. There was also an obvious difference in the amino acids during green season between male and female animals, and also between both cuts. P.E.R. of Egyptian Buffalo meat as 10% protein level ranged between 3.02 and 2.35 according to seasonal, cut and age variations. (Authors' abstract)

134. El-Nahry, F., Darwish, N. M., and Tharwat, S. "Effect of preparation and cooking on the nutritive value of local kidney bean." Qual. Plant-Pl. Fds. Hum. Nutr. 27(2), 1977, pp 141-150.

Nutritive value and protein quality of kidney bean before and after different methods of preparation and cooking was studied to evaluate the effect of soaking the seeds before boiling. Kidney bean seeds (var. Giza 3) were either boiled or soaked first and then boiled. Moisture, crude protein, fat, carbohydrate, ash, fiber, caloric value and minerals including calcium, phosphorus and iron were determined in both raw and prepared seeds.

Evaluation of the protein quality was done by determining the protein efficiency ratio, net protein ratio, and serum analysis of rats fed diets containing either raw or prepared seeds. Serum analysis included the estimation of total serum proteins, albumin/globulin ratio and free, non-essential to essential amino acids ratio. The results showed that kidney bean is rich in carbohydrate and protein and is a reasonably good source of dietary iron, but a poor source of calcium. It was also clear that seeds boiled without soaking contained higher percentages of minerals than those boiled after soaking, but were lower in protein quality. This was proved by the results of all the methods used for protein quality evaluation. (Adapted from authors' abstract)

135. El-Nahry, F. I., Darwish, N. M., and Nada, E. "Effect of local methods of preparation on the amino acid constituents of broad beans." Qual. Plant.-Pl. Fds. Hum. Nutr. 27(2), 1977, pp 151-160.

Dried broad beans (Giza 1) were subjected to different methods of preparation commonly used in Egypt: 1) germination, 2) germination and boiling, the method commonly used to make 'nabet soup' and 3) stewing, to make 'medammes', the popular breakfast dish in Egypt and Middle East.

Paper chromatography was used to separate and identify amino acids in dried and prepared broad beans. The amino acid analysis data were subjected to analysis of variance, and the t-test was applied to contrasts of different amino acids. The results indicated 17 amino acids in the hydrolysates of both raw and germinated seeds. These amino acids were determined quantitatively exept proline. Cystine was destroyed completely by either boiling or stewing. The amino acids that showed significant loss by germination were aspartic acid and alanine. Both boiling and stewing of germinated seeds caused significant loss in lysine, arginine, aspartic acid, alanine, methionine and tryptophan. The higher temperature used in boiling germinated seeds had a more destructive effect on some amino acids than stewing. The amino acids scores showed sulfur-containing amino acids to be the first limiting amino acids in both hard and prepared broad beans. (Adapted from authors' abstract.)

136. El-Sawy, M., Mahmoud, S. A., Abdel-Hafez, A. M., and Ramadan, E. M. "Studies on protein production by yeasts. IV. Incremental feeding modulus." Zentralbl. Bakteriol. (Naturwiss) 132(7), 1977, pp 648-654.

Various hourly rates of incremental feeding of S. cerevisiae Gr. 104 was used to investigate the optimum incremental feeding modulus for protein production at the greatest economy. The rates ranged from 1.14 to 1.22, and the yeast yield for each rate was measured. Molasses, ammonium sulphate, and potassium dihydrogen phosphate were fed to the yeast at optimum pH, temperature, and effective aeration in a 5 liter laboratory fermentor container. 1.18 was the optimum incremental feeding rate. At this rate, the rate of molasses feeding corresponded to the exponential growth rate with the production of yield close to a theoretically calculated yield of protein.

137. Gabr, M. "Malnutrition and diarrheal disease". Practical Approaches to Combat Malnutrition with Special Reference to Mothers and Children Cairo, Egypt. Publication of Proceedings of IUNS Conference held May 25-29, 1977. pp 145-157.

Various factors involved in the synergism between malnutrition and diarrheal disease are presented, utilizing epidemiologic and demographic data from Egypt to illustrate the main points. Diarrheal disease is the most common disorder in Egyptian infants less than 2 years old. The relative absence of diarrheal disease in infants below 9 months of age is related to breastfeeding, which is protective because of inherent immune factors and minimization of environmental contamination of ingested food. Several structural, mechanical, immunological, and functional factors necessary for protection of the GI tract against infection are impaired in the malnourished child. Increased nutritional requirements and decreased ability to absorb and utilize nutrients accompany diarrheal disease. Results of some Egyptian studies on D-xylose, carbohydrate, fat, and folic acid absorption in children during protein energy malnutrition with and without diarrheal disease were noted, and suggestions on the treatments of malnourished children with diarrhea were given.

138. Gabr, M., El-Beheiry, F., Soliman, A. A., El-Mahdi, M., El-Mougy, M., and El-Akkad, N. "Lactose tolerance in normal Egyptian infants and children and in protein calorie malnutrition." Gaz. Egypt. Paediatr. Assoc. 26(1), 1977, pp 27-33.

Oral lactose tolerance test was performed on a total of 100 cases of normal Egyptian infants and children aged 6 months to 12 years. The same test was performed on 30 cases of protein calorie malnutrition (15 cases of marasmus and 15 cases of kwashiorkor). Detection of sugar and determination of pH were also carried out on all stools passed after the test. Lactose intolerance, as judged by a maximal blood glucose rise of 20 mg. or less and/or stools positive for sugar with a pH less than 6 following lactose ingestion, was observed as follows in normal cases: 12% in the age group 6 months to 2 years, 32% in the age group 2-5 years, 32% in the age group 5-9 years, and 80% in the age group 9-12 years. On the other hand, lactose intolerance was demonstrated in 73.3% of cases suffering from protein malnutrition. The aetiology and practical implications of the present findings of lactose intolerance on normal and malnourished children are discussed. (Authors' abstract)

139. Girgis, A. N., el-Sherif, S., Rofael, N., and Neshaim, S. "Aflatoxins in Egyptian foodstuffs." J. Assoc. Off. Anal. Chem. 60(3), May 1977, pp 746-747.

Six samples each of wheat, corn, lentils, beans, fenugreek, peanuts and cottonseed cake from various areas of Egypt were analyzed for aflatoxins, both at the time of collection and after 12 months' storage. Aflatoxin was found at low levels (3-12 ppb total aflatoxins in 14 of 42 samples) as follows: 1 sample each of corn, lentils, and beans; 2 peanut samples; 3 fenugreek samples; and 6 cottonseed cake samples. None of the samples contained aflatoxins above 11.7 ppb. (Authors' abstract)

140. Harfouche, J. K. "Analysis of methods of approach to combat malnutrition (Introductory Talk)" Practical Approaches to Combat Malnutrition with Special Reference to Mothers and Children Cairo, Egypt. Publication of Proceedings of IUNS Conference held May 25-29, 1977, pp 279-302.

The need for a combined approach to malnutrition, both direct and indirect, and suited to the unique needs of each country, was stressed. Nutrition education and public awareness of the importance of nutritional supports for the young, food and nutrition policies targeting especially vulnerable groups, an integrated, multisectorial developmental approach, emphasis on attainment of socio-economic well-being population wide, equalization of development efforts between the urban and ural sectors, and development of national nutritional policies on a cost/benefit ratio basis were delineated. Primary health care via workers offering MCH/FP/Nutrition care and other services was stressed. Use of the MCH centers for nutrition care, the employment of the risk approach to nutrition care, use of growth charts, promotion of breast feeding, use of immunizations, management of dehydration by oral rehydration therapy, and the judicious application of supplements were discussed.

141. Madwar, K. R., Arafa, M., Sherif, N., and el-Saadani, A. M. "Fat

distribution in obese Egyptians." J. Egypt Med. Assoc. 60(7-8), 1977, pp 639-650.

This study included 250 obese Egyptians. The diet showed a high carbohydrate intake in 74.3%. Anaemia was present in 71% of cases and impaired glucose tolerance was found in 28.4%. Skin fold thickness showed that maximum fat deposition was in abdominal wall, buttocks and subscapular region. Such fat distribution may be due to racial or environmental factors. (Authors' abstract)

142. Morcos, S. R., and Morcos, W. R. "Diets in ancient Egypt." Prog. Food Nutr. Sci. 2(10), 1977, pp 457-471.

This description of the diets of ancient Egyptians, spanning the first through the thirtieth dynasties, lists the various classes of cultivated and wild plant foods eaten, e.g., the grains wheat, barley, millet, the era of their introduction, and their methods of processing and preparation. The animals, e.g. cattle, lamb, and pork, and fish used for food, along with food products derived from them, such as milk, cheese, and eggs, are enumerated and described, as well as the ancient slaughtering and preparation techniques used. Ancient tomb pictures depicting various food preparation scenes are included with the text. Typical diets of the priests, aristocracy, and common people and food preferences and taboos related to status and religion are discussed. The making of fermented beverages such as mead, palm wine, and Egyptian beer is also explained.

143. Morsy, Soheir A. "Gender, power and illness in an Egyptian village". Ph.D. dissertaton, Department of Anthropology, Michigan State University, Ann Arbor, Michigan 48106, U.S.A.

This doctoral dissertation focuses on male-female gender roles and their reciprocal relation to illness behavior among rural Egyptian peasants. Gender roles, power differentials and the medical system in a Nile delta village are outlined as well as culturally prescribed behavior in response to illness. The medical system is presented as an example of the social organization and power structure. Local beliefs about the human body's formation, structure and function, as well as village medical taxonomy, selection and extension of illness explanations, and the prevalence, diagnosis, and treatment of culture bound illnesses are described.

144. Nawar, Isis A. "Effect of socio-economic factors on the maternal and child nutritional status in an Egyptian village. I-Nutritional status of pregnant women." In: Paper by Dr. Isis A. Nawar, Associate Professor, Division of Home Economics Department of Agricultural Extension, Faculty of Agriculture, Alexandria University, Alexandria, Egypt. (Unpublished)

Seventy pregnant women were chosen randomly from those who visit the Health Center in Garawan, Menofia. Each subject was interviewed and socioeconomic and biological data were obtained, including hemoglobin level, weight and presence of frank nutritional deficiency symptoms. The subjects were classified into three categories according to size of landholding.

The results revealed that women belonging to the lowest level of landholding were less adequately fed and more likely to be anemic than those belonging to the other levels of landholding. Also there was a gradual decrease in weight gain at intermediate stages of pregnancy as size of landholding decreased. (Adapted from author's abstract)

145. Nawar, Isis A. "Effects of socio-economic factors on the maternal and child nutritional status in an Egyptian village. II-Birth measurements." In: Paper by Dr. Isis A. Nawar, Associate Professor, Division of Home Economics Department of Agricultural Extension, Faculty of Agriculture, Alexandria University, Alexandria, Egypt. (Unpublished)

A sample of 70 pregnant women randomly chosen from those who visited the Garawan, Menofia village health center were studied. The weight, height, head circumference and chest circumference of their offspring were measured at birth. Socioeconomic, biologic, and dietary data for each woman were obtained from an interview. The study showed that there were significant differences in birth measurements of infants where females belonged to different landholding levels. Meal pattern and dietary habits of mothers during pregnancy caused significant differences in birth measurement of their infants. On the other hand, differences in birth measurements in relation to parity or maternal age were not significant. (Adapted from author's abstract)

146. Nawar, Isis A. "Effect of socio-economic factors on the maternal and child nutritional status in an Egyptian village. III-Child growth during the first year of life." In: Paper by Dr. Isis A. Nawar, Associate Professor, Division of Home Economics Department of Agricultural Extension, Faculty of Agriculture, Alexandria University, Alexandria, Egypt. (Unpublished)

In a continuation of earlier studies in Garawan, Menofia, sixty two children were measured monthly from birth through the first year of life for height, weight, head circumference, and chest circumference. Socioeconomic, biologic, and dietary data for each child were obtained during an interview with the mother of each.

Measurements, especially heights and weights, for both sexes showed a clear socio-economic gradient, as measured by landholding levels, with lowest holding families' infants at a disadvantage through the entire first year. Females had smaller body measurements than males at all ages. This difference was significant for chest circumference from the second through seventh month, and for head circumference for the first seven months. In most cases, infants receiving breast milk plus supplementation had the highest body measurements, followed by those who were breast fed only and those fed artificial formula.

147. Nawar, Isis A. "Food habits and beliefs during pregnancy and lactation" In: Paper by Dr. Isis A. Nawar, Associate Professor, Division of Home Economics Department of Agricultural Extension, Faculty of Agriculture, Alexandria University, Alexandria, Egypt. (Unpublished)

A random sample of 310 women was selected from those visiting the Maternal & Child Health Center in Moharran Bey & Shatby Maternity Hospital in Alexandria and they were interviewed for socioeconomic, biologic, and dietary information. A seven day food survey was done for food beliefs, pica habit, food avoidance, and foods especially liked during pregnancy and lactation. Mothers were grouped according to family income, educational level, age, and parity. Foods were grouped as energy-rich, milk and its products, meat and its substitutes, and vegetable and fruit groups.

A majority obtained a "good" intake grade for energy-rich food. The general appraisal for the other food groups was "fair". Income and age were the factors most associated with nutritional status, followed by parity and educational level. Seasonings, fruits, eggs, and fish were avoided, and liver, fried onions, and radishes were especially used in pregnancy. In both cases, differences due to education and parity were highly correlated with lactation likes and dislikes of foods. Garlic, mutton, seasonings, fruits, and eggs were avoided and fenugreek, milk, and radishes liked during lactation.

148. Shukry, A. S. "Analysis of different methods of approach to combat malnutrition". Practical Approaches to Combat Malnutrition with Special Reference to Mothers and Children Cairo, Egypt. Proceedings of IUNS Conference, May 25-29, 1977, pp 303-308.

General and specific control measures to combat childhood malnutrition in developing countries were presented. General measures consisted of community development, increasing food availability both nationally and as targeted to rural populations, emphasis on family planning, and use of mass media for purposes of health education. Improvement of services and education and training of health personnel comprised specific measures. Maternal and child health services, nutrition education and food demonstration, and treatment of infectious diseases were discussed.

149. Yehya, S. A., Said, A., el-Hawary, M. F., and Sakr, R. "Protein-calorie malnutrition (PCM) in Egypt: infants socio-economic parameters." J. Egypt Med. Assoc. 60(3-4), 1977, pp 217-229.

A survey of 232 infants with protein calorie malnutrition (PCM) included 51 kwashiorkor, 99 marasmic, 5 nutritional edema, and 77 marasmic kwashiorkor cases from 3 to 30 months of age. Study parameters included age, sex, weaning age, type of infant food, birth order, and developmental indicators such as teething, walking, and speech. Disease incidence was low below 6 months, 42.7% between 6 and 15 months, 17.7% at 16-23 months, and 26.3% above 24 months. PCM affected more male than female infants between 3 and 30 months of age. 46% of PCM cases above 24 months had prior measles, with respiratory disease and gastroenteritis also seen as precipitating factors. Marasmus occured in 42.7%, marasmic-kwashiorkor in 33.4%, and kwashiorkor in 22% of cases, with severe cases predominating for each type. 39% and 46% of cases received breastmilk for up to one year and for over one year, respectively. Supplementary foods given were of low nutritional value, including sugared extract fluids and carbohydrate foods. Delayed teething, speech, and, most prominently, walking were noted in PCM infants.

150. Aly, H. E., Abdallah, N. M., Morsi, M. K. S., Moussa, B. M., El-Hashimy, F. S. A., and Saddik, M. F. "Effect of processing on protein and vitamin contents of broad beans (Vicia Faba)." Bull. Nutr. Inst. 6(1), 1976, pp 93-104.

Broad bean was processed in the form of germinated (nabet), cooked nabet, and medamis in the usual Egyptian ways of preparation. The effect of such processing on vitamin, protein and amino acids contents were studied. Results showed that thiamine and riboflavin contents in germinated bean (nabet) increased by 27% and 22% respectively over that of raw bean. In cooked nabet B_1 and B_2 contents were reduced by 10% and 12.77% respectively. Ascorbic acid did not exist in raw bean, but it appeared during germination and reached 27.8mg/100gm dry weight on the fourth day of germination and disappeared again from cooked nabet. However, addition of acetic acid or lime juice during cooking caused retention of vitamin C by 36% and 32% respectively and reached 44% when pressure cooking was used. Results showed also that adult thiamine and riboflavin requirements could be achieved by consuming 60 to 1308gm of nabet beans or 857 to 1700gm of medamis beans respectively. Eighteen amino acids were detected in raw and germinated bean proteins, while cysteine disappeared in cooked nabet and medamis. Sulphur-containing amino acids, threonine and valine were the most limiting amino acids in raw bean protein. Germinated bean protein had the same deficiencies as well as limited tryptophan. Cooked nabet was deficient in all the essential amino acids except isoleucine and aromatic amino acids. Medamis was also deficient in essential amino acids except isoleucine, lysine and aromatic amino acids. (Adapted from authors' summary)

151. Aly, H. E., Aref, N. M., Hasanyn, S. A., and Hanna, N. M. "Evaluation of school lunch program at technical secondary schools of A.R.E. II-Further anthropometric studies." Bull. Nutr. Inst. 6(1), 1976, pp 145-160.

A sample of 3400 school boys and girls attending secondary technical schools in 6 governorates was surveyed to evaluate the nutritional effects of the school lunch program. Statistical analysis of the height and weight data is presented and the effect of the school lunch program on measurements of the triceps skinfold thickness and mid-arm circumference is given. Improved measurements were observed in the group of beneficiaries of the lunch program over those of the control group. (Adapted from authors' summary)

152. Aly, H. E., Hassanein, M., Mansour, A., Abdelhay, M. B. "I-Investigation of bladder stone disease of early childhood in Upper Egypt II-Oral health status of preschool children and their mothers in Edfou." Bull Nutr. Inst. 6(1), 1976, pp 28-35

The dental health of 199 children less than 6 years of age and of 131 mothers in a village in Upper Egypt (Edfou) was evaluated. They were divided into 2 groups of children with and without bladder stone disease.

While the dental health status of those affected with vesical stones was relatively better than for the non-affected children, the situation was the reverse with the mothers. (Adapted from authors' summary)

153. Aly, H. F., Saddik, M. F., Abdallah, N. M., El-Hashimy, M. S. A., and Morsi, M. K. S. "Effect of processing on protein and vitamin contents of beef meat." Bull. Nutr. Inst. 6(1), 1976, pp 114-127.

Baladi cow's meat was processed by boiling and roasting. The effect of such processing on the vitamin and amino acid content as well as protein fractions was studied. The results were as follows:

1. Vitamin content: Boiled meat lost 28.9% and 9.4% of B_1 and B_2 as compared with raw meat, while roasting decreased the B_1 content by 23.5% and B_2 by 6.1%.

2. Amino acids: Determinations in raw, boiled and roasted meat indicated that there were 18 amino acids in each. Raw meat was shown to contain all the essential amino acids, while boiled and roasted meats showed that sulphur- containing amino acids and threonine were the most limiting amino acids.

3. Protein fractions: Boiling of meat decreased the total soluble nitrogen from 62.89% to 14.81%, the soluble protein nitrogen from 50% to 4.5% and the actomyocin from 24.8% to 2.48%. Roasting also decreased the total soluble nitrogen, soluble protein nitrogen, and actomyosin to 17.66%, 6.26%, and 3.2% respectively from that in raw meat. (Adapted from authors' summary)

154. Aly, H. E., Said, A. K., Shaheen, F. M., Hussein, W. A., and Ibrahim, E. D. "Evaluation of school lunch program at technical secondary school of A.R.E.1: Effect on height, weight, and clinical picture." Bull. Nutr. Inst. 6(1), 1976, pp 1-16.

3400 students were surveyed as a trial to evaluate the school lunch programme. Positive effects of the programme were noticed from the difference in body measurements (weight & height) signs of deficiency between the beneficiaries & the control groups. The beneficiaries also showed a longer duration of acceptance of the meals. (Adapted from authors' summary)

155. Aly, H. E., Maksoud, A. A., Moussa, W. A., and Gharib, N. "Effect of supplementary feeding on health and growth of infants and young children of low socio-economic group in Egypt. 1-fish-protein concentrate." Bull. Nutr. Inst. 62(1), 1976, pp 37-58.

This study was conducted to evaluate Astra fish protein concentrate (FPC) in weaning foods. Acceptability and tolerance tests as well as effect on growth were carried out on a test group of 83 infants and young children of age 4-24 months fed FPC-formula. A control group of 55 children of the same age, sex distribution and similar nutritional status was fed WSB-formula. Each group consisted of breast fed subgroup and another one totally depending on either mixture for their protein requirements. The minimum test period was 6 months for each child.

Results revealed that FPC as well as WSB were highly acceptable and tolerated and could promote normal growth in children of various grades of protein calorie malnutrition and in normal children.

The effect of the supplementation with FPC on weight gain was found to be significantly higher than that of WSB. (Author's abstract)

156. Awaad, S., Mourad, K. A., Abdel-Fattah, S., El-Sokary, S., and Khalil, F. "Serum 5-nucleotidase in some rachitic and jaundiced Egyptian children." Gaz. Egypt Paediatr. Assoc. 24(1-2), January-April 1976, pp 69-71.

5-Nucleotidase (5-Nase) was determined in the serum of 67 Egyptian children: 15 cases as a control group, 10 cases with infantile rickets, 8 cases with the so-called physiological jaundice of the newborn, 4 cases with rhesus incompatibility and 30 cases with infective hepatitis. In rachitic cases and in cases with icterus neonatorum, 5-Nase was not increased, while in cases with infective hepatitis it showed a statistically significant elevation when compared with the control group. (Authors' abstract)

157. Behairy, F. E., Mougi, M. E., Mostafa, S., and Osman, N. H. "The nutritionally at risk child. Part I: Study of some socio-economic and cultural factors". Gaz. Egypt Paediatr. Assoc. 24(102), January-April 1976, pp 23-29.

Various socio-economic and cultural factors prevalent in the Al Hussein locality were studied, in an attempt to decide the groups of children that were nutritionally at risk. The study was carried out on 110 children suffering from energy protein malnutrition and 98 normal children. Their age ranged between 4 and 36 months. The per capita income was found to be inadequate to meet the minimum requirements and was considered to be the most important high risk factor for malnutrition. (Adapted from authors' abstract)

158. Dakroury, A. M., Amin, E. K., Aly, H. E., Moustafa, E. K., and Saddik, M. F. "The protein efficiency ratio of bolti fish protein." Bull. Nutr. Inst. 6(1), 1976, pp 71-78

The protein efficiency ratio (PER) of bolti fish protein was evaluated in the fresh, suspicious and rejected stages of acceptability where it was $3.26\pm$ .13, $2.28\pm.28$ and $2.76\pm$, .20 respectively.

There was a consistently greater growth response of animals fed on fresh fish protein compared with that of animals fed on protein from suspected or rejected fishes. The difference was statistically significant.

A comparison of the PER of fresh bolti fish with that of casein indicated the former's superiority as a sole source of protein in the diet. There was no significant difference between the PER of casein and that of protein of suspected or rejected fish. (Adapted from authors' summary)

159. Dakroury, A. M., Saddik, M. F., Moustafa, E. K., Amine, E. K., and Aly, H. E. "Hygienic and quality aspects of market morgan fish." Bull. Nutr. Inst. 6(1), 1976, pp 79-92.

The hygiene and quality of market morgan fish were investigated in 6 markets chosen at random in Cairo and Giza, representing the main sources of the fish. The quality of the fish was assessed through microbiological and chemical indices, in addition to a sensory evaluation and inspection of the fish for parasitic infestations.

The total viable count ranged from $16X10^6$ to $4.2X10^6$/gm. The coliforms were detected in 42 samples (32%) and Streptococcus faecalis in 40 samples (80%). Clostridi spp. were detected in 3 samples, two of which were judged by sensory evaluation as doubtfully acceptable. Salmonella were absent in all the inspected samples, whereas Staph aureus showed its presence in 10 samples.

The total volatile basic nitrogen ranged from 15.4mg to 47.6mg and the TMAQ content from 55.52 to 68.12mg/100gm. The precipitation test was negative in 48 of the samples, but was suspicious in two samples which were doubtfully acceptable.

Sensory evaluation revealed that in all the inspected markets, the fish were acceptable or doubtfully acceptable, but fresh or rejected fish were not available.

Only one sample was found infested with a larval stage of a cestode (a plero cercoid) which represents a public health problem, as it may be transmissible to man. (Adapted from authors' summary.)

160. Darwish, N. M., El-Nahry, F., and Tharwat, S. "Effect of preparation and cooking on the nutritive value of broad beans." Qual. Plant Pl. Fds. Hum. Nutr. 25(3,4) 1976, pp 331-341.

Nutritive value and protein quality of dried local broad beans (Giza 1) were studied before and after preparation and cooking, according to the methods commonly used in Egypt. Dried broad beans were: 1) germinated, 2) germinated and boiled, the method commonly used to make 'Nabet Soup' or, 3) stewed to make 'Medammes', the popular breakfast dish in Egypt and the Middle East.

Moisture, crude protein, fat, carbohydrate, ash, fiber, caloric value and minerals including calcium, phosphorus and iron, were determined in both dried and prepared seeds. To evaluate protein quality, the 'protein efficiency ratio' (P.E.R.) and 'net protein ratio' (N.P.R.) were determined using weanling albino rats. Analysis of serum of rats maintained on diets containing both dried and prepared beans, was done to evaluate the effect on total serum proteins, serum albumin/globulin ratio, and free non-essential/essential amino acids ratio.

Germination, boiling and stewing slightly improved the P.E.R. values of broad beans, with stewed beans having the highest value. It was also clear that using either germinated, boiled germinated or stewed beans instead of dried ones, caused a slight increase in both total serum proteins and albumin/globulin ratios and a decrease in the non-essential/essential amino acids ratios. The effect was more marked with boiled germinated beans than with other kinds of preparation. (Adapted from authors' abstract)

161. El-Behairy, F., El-Mougi, M., Osman, N. H., and Mostafa, S. "The nutritionally at-risk child. Part 2: Study of factors pertinent to the child, siblings or mother". Gaz. Egypt Paediatr. Assoc. 24(1-2), January-April 1976, pp 31-42.

Several high risk factors were evaluated in an attempt to determine the Egyptian children who are more prone to become malnourished. The study included 110 children with energy-protein malnutrition and 98 normal children with ages between 4 months and 3 years. Among the factors investigated, the 2nd 6 months of life was found to be the most critical for nutritional deficiency. Presence of previous siblings with malnutrition, presence of more than 2 sibling deaths and presence of history of severe diarrhea with dehydration were significantly related to the nutritional status of children. Twinning, birth order and birth interval showed some relation to malnutrition but were not statistically significant. The sex of the child and maternal weight did not influence the nutritional state of children. However, these low-social class children were found to be mostly (92.8%) breast fed. (Authors' abstract)

Nitrogen percentage on a wet basis increased from 3.866% to 4.474% and then to 5.442% for rabbits; for rats, it was 3.976% to 4.415% and then to 5.209%.

Water percentage dropped from 77.220% to 70.925% and then to 65.948% for rabbits; from 85.150% to 68.678% and then to 64.104% for rats.

It is obvious that bleeding and/or death affected the chemical composition of the skins of the rabbits and rats. Further study is needed to understand the changes which took place in the skins during the transition from life to death. (Adapted from author's summary)

162. Eltawil, E. A., Moukhtar, S. A., Galal, E. S., and Khishin, E. S. "Factors affecting the production and composition of Egyptian buffalo milk". Trop. Anim. Health Prod. 8(2), May 1976, pp 115-121.

The data comprise 254 first and 150 second 305-day lactation records of buffaloes and their dams at Mahalet Mousa Experimental Station. These records were used for evaluation of the effect of various factors upon 305-day milk yield. Average daily milk yield and percentage constituents were measured on 58 lactation records. Samples were taken on the seventh, fourteenth and thirtieth day post-partum and at 30 day intervals throughout lactation. The parameters studied were: age at first calving, 305-day milk yield and butter fat, protein and total solids contents percentages. Average age at first calving was 42.9 and 40.9 months for calves and their dams, respectively. Average 305-day milk yield was 1,004.3 kg and 1,552.7 for first and second lactations, respectively. The later age at which buffalo cows produce their first calf, the greater the milk production in first lactation. Buffaloes that calve in summer produce more milk than those which calve in winter months. Average fat, protein and total solids percentages were 6.59, 4.11 and 16.52 respectively in the first lactation and 6.63, 3.99 and 16.48 respectively in the second lactation. Phenotypic correlations between milk yield and yields of constituents were high and positive. Those among constituent percentages were positive and moderate. In general, correlations between milk yield and constituents content were negative. Milk yield increased after calving towards a peak ranging between 30 and 90 days for the first and second lactations, respectively. Constituent percentages were high at the beginning, declining thereafter as milk yield increased, followed by a gradual rise till the end of lactation. (Authors' abstract)

163. Fattah, M. A., Hamid, G. A., Nassar, A. M., and Khourshid, R. "Ultrastructure of the liver in marasmic Egyptian infants." J. Egypt Med. Assoc. 59(5-6), 1976, pp 427-437.

Three marasmic Egyptian infants (two males aged 5 and 14 months, and one female 18 months old) were studied for liver changes via electron microscope investigation of liver biopsy. Irregular and ill-defined cell boundaries with intermingled cells were seen. Most mitochondria were replaced by dense granular bodies. Those mitochondria which did exist were small, rounded, few in number, and had a dense matrix. Ribosomes, especially free ribosomes and rough endoplasmic reticulum, and glycogen particles were completely depleted in some cells. Also depleted was nuclear chromatin, the granules of which were pale and evenly distributed in the nucleoplasm. Reticulin fibrils which paralleled each other in the area of the nuclei were also seen. No kwashiorkor-typical fat lobules were found in the cytoplasm. The lack of necrotic-type changes and the presence of healthy, intact nuclei indicated that the histological changes were reversible.

164. Gabr, M. "Gastro-enteritis in Egypt: certain epidemiological aspects." Gaz. Egypt Paediatr. Assoc. 24(3-4), July-October 1976, pp 109-118.

This epidemiologic review reports that gastroenteritis was responsible for nearly 50% of mortality in Egyptian infants under two years of age. The causative agents include Salmonella, E. coli, Shigella (up to 22% in one study) and other bacterial or parasitic intestinal pathogens. Shigellosis-related diarrheal case-age distribution show the lowest incidence to be in the youngest age groups. A seasonal fluctuation is found in gastroenteritis, with higher incidence in the summer months. Preventive measures, clinical fluid therapy, nutritional and hygienic education and sanitary measures are reviewed.

165. Gabrial, G. N., El-Masry, G. H., Shenouda, M. S., Morcos, S. R. "Nutritive value of Geotricum candidum yeast prepared from decaying fruits in Egypt". Z. Ernaehrungswiss 15(2), June 1976, pp 164-167. Dr. Dietrich Steinkoff Verlag.

The yeast Geotricum candidum contains 32 g. crude protein, 12.7 g ethereal extract and 37.2 g. total carbohydrates per 100 g. dry weight. The amino acid pattern of this yeast was investigated and eighteen amino acids including all the essential ones were detected. Animal feeding experiments showed that the yeast has poor digestibility, which was attributed to the high amount of purine in the dried cells. Pathological examination of different organs did not reveal any morphological or pathological changes. (Authors' abstract)

166. Gabrial, G. N., and Morcos, S. R. "The use of Lupinus termis L. cultivated in Egypt, as a food protein supplement." Z. Ernaehrungswiss 15(4), December 1976, pp 333-339. Dr. Dietrich Steinkopff Verlag.

A general analysis of the seeds of lupinus termis for protein, fats, carbohydrates, fiber and ash contents was performed and the results were given in g/100 g dry seeds. Lupinus termis contained a high percentage of protein (40.36%), 290 mg calcium and 6.5 mg iron. All the essential amino acids were present in fair amounts, with the exception of sulphur-amino acids and lysine. Cooking the seeds resulted in a slight decrease in most of the amino acids, with the exception of tryptophan and lysine, which exhibited a slight increase after cooking. Some toxic substances were present in the seeds, such as trypsin inhibitor which was destroyed by heat treatment, and alkaloids which were removed by soaking the seeds three days in running tap water. Supplementing the debittered seeds with lysine and methionine resulted in an increase in its nutritive value. (Adapted from authors' abstract.)

167. Hartage, R. "The history of breast feeding." Fortschr. Med. 94(27), September 23, 1976, pp 1435-1438.

Ancient Egyptians, Greeks, Romans, Indians and other peoples of antiquity placed importance on breastfeeding; mothers who successfully breastfed their children were given great respect. Breastfeeding customs developed in these cultures, and are described in this essay. The importance accorded breastfeeding still exists today notwithstanding the decades' old trend toward bottle-feeding. This may be partially due to the economy of breastfeeding compared to feeding with commercial formulas. It is also due to the advantages that breastmilk has over other feeding modes in terms of hygiene, nutritional balance and appropriateness, and immunity-conferring properties. All these factors increase the survival rates and decrease morbidity rates for breastfed infants, and knowledgeable mothers in developed nations choose breastfeeding over bottlefeeding for these reasons.

168. Khattab, A. K., Fattah, A. S., Sokkary, S. E., and Mostafa, F. A. "Hepatic succinic dehydrogenase in marasmic Egyptian infants". Gaz. Egypt Paediatr. Assoc. 24(1-2), January-April, 1976, pp 43-49.

Liver function and histologic state of livers of 15 marasmic and 10 normal infants was measured, with the activity of the liver enzyme succinic dehydrogenase (SDH) assessed. All of the marasmic infants showed decreased SDH activity, two thirds of them showed abnormal liver functions, and one third of them showed histologic changes. The universal incidence of decreased SDH activity was probably reflected in the predominance of disturbed liver function incidence without a comparable incidence of histologic hepatic changes.

169. Lebshtein, A. K., and el-Bahay, A. M. "The extent of breast and bottle feeding of children in Cairo and its effect on their growth." J. Egypt Public Health Assoc. 51(5), 1976, pp 246-257.

The extent of breast-feeding and bottle feeding was studied on a random sample of 250 non-working and 174 working mothers in Cairo. Breast-feeding was practiced by 78.8% of non-working and only 5.8% of working mothers. Bottle feeding was adopted by 7.6% of non working and 78.2% of working mothers. Only 13.6% of non-working and 16% of working mothers supplemented the diet of their children. The mean body weights and heights were higher in the breast-fed than bottle fed children at all age intervals. But both groups were less than U.S.A. standards after the first six months of age. (Authors' abstract)

170. Loutfi, A. H., and Hamid, G. A. "Research report on idiopathic urinary bladder stone disease in Egypt." Idiopathic urinary bladder stone disease. Van Reen, R., ed. DHEW (NIH) 77-1063, Bethesda W3 F049 No. 37, 1976, pp 177-185.

The incidence and types of bladder stone disease in Egypt were reviewed. About 77.6% of urinary calculi in Egyptian children were idiopathic urinary bladder calculi. Most of the patients requiring surgery came from Cairo, with fewer from Upper Egypt, and a minority from Lower Egypt. Maximal incidence occurred from September to October. Patients generally belonged to large families, and were either the last born or next to last born. All were in the lower socioeconomic classes. Breast feeding was usually greatly prolonged, with supplements consisting mostly of starchy food and tea. Gastroenteritis was present in 70% of cases, with patients complaining of dysuria for months. Bilharziasis did not effect the preschool bladder stone incidence. Most crystals were of mixed types, such as calcium oxalate and uric acid.

171. Mahiar, F. F., El-Deen, E., Wasfy, H., and El-Samra, I. A. "New leaf diseases of barley in Egypt." Zentralbl. Bakteriol. (Naturwiss) 131(8), 1976, pp 757-759.

New leaf diseases of barley were observed in Egypt. From leaves of barley the following were isolated: *Halminthosporium teres*, *H. graminaum*, *Stemphylium vesicarium*, *Alternaria triticina*, *Ulocaldium* chartarum, Acremonium kiliense, and Stemphylium spec. accompanied with the Pleospora stage. Inoculations on both attached and detached leaves showed that all the tested fungi were pathogenic, except Acremonium kiliense and Ulocladium chartarum.

172. Prasad, A. S. "Zinc deficiency in man." Am. J. Dis. Child 130(4), April 1976, pp 359-361.

This review article of the history of discovery of zinc deficiency in man, and of the progress in knowledge concerning the treatment of zinc deficiency was written by a man was a prime mover in the process. The author described studies in Iran and Egypt which established a clinical syndrome of severe zinc deficiency in the 60's. Similar findings in Turkey, Portugal, and Morocco were noted. The discovery of the zinc deficiency cause of the genetic disease, Acrodermatitis Enteropathica, was also noted, and speculation that the malabsorption of zinc was the mechanism was put forth. Assessment of zinc status in man via plasma, RBCs, hair, and urine was listed, together with use of zinc balance studies and enzyme activity studies on serum alkaline phosphatase and ribonuclease. Specific response to zinc supplementation in growth, gonadal maturation, and hair growth and skin effects were cited. The need for zinc in DNA and RNA synthesis and cell division was described, including its essentiality in thymidine kinase, RNA polymerase, and DNA polymerase, and its inhibition of RNAse activity. The paper concluded with a call for greater awareness of zinc's in role in human metabolism.

173. Rashwan, S., Edress, Z., Sultan, E., Labib, B., and Abdel-Fattah, H. "Effect of dietary fat on the histochemical picture of the thyroid gland of the rabbit." Bull. Nutr. Inst. 6(1), 1976, pp 161-167.

The thyroid glands of 18 rabbits were examined histochemically to determine the effect of a high fat diet for 5 months. The index for the activity of the thyroid gland was the diameter of the thyroid follicles, height of the thyroid epithelium, R.N.A. content and phosphatase activity. At the end of the first and second months, there was increased enzyme activity and RNA content, with an even more marked increase during the third and fourth months. However, the activity decreased during the fifth month.

The above results may suggest that a high fat diet may have increased the requirements of thyroxine of the body to utilize the dietary fat. (Adapted from authors' summary.)

174. Saddik, M. F., Dakroury, A. M., Moustafa, E. K., and Amine, E. K. "Effect of chilling temperature on the keeping quality of wet bolti." Bull. Nutr. Inst. 6(1), 1976, pp 59-70

This study deals with the effect of chilling temperature on the chemical quality attributes and on the organoleptic properties of whole wet bolti fish. The fish was stored at -4, 0, +4 and at room temperature +15°C.

Values of 40(VBN) or 10mgN/100g (TMA) represented the borderline level of acceptance of chilled whole wet bolti fish. These values were reached after 28, 8, 6 and 2 days when chilling temperature was -4, 0, +4 and +15°C respectively. With increasing storage period, the quality degradation was more pronounced in the texture of the flesh, and the fish lost its natural appearance and pleasant odor. Fresh fish had a total score more than 21 out of 25 and an accepted level quality over 15, while fish with a score of less than 13 out of 25 were graded as rejected quality. (Adapted from authors' summary.)

175. Saddik, M. F., Moussa, B. M., El-Hashimy, F. S., Abdalla, N. M., and Morsi, M. K. S. "Biologial evaluation of broad bean protein." Bull. Nutr. Inst. 6(1), 1976, pp 17-27.

Biological evaluation of broad bean protein using the protein efficiency ratio (PER) method showed that cooked nabet bean protein had the highest value with nabet, medamis and raw bean proteins following in descending order.

The results of the BV, DC and NPU showed a similar trend, indicating that cooked nabet protein had the highest biological values, digestability and net protein utilization, followed by nabet, medamis and raw beans. (Adapted from authors' summary)

176. Said, A., el-Hawary, M. F., Sakr, R., Abdel-Khalek, M. K., Samuel, S, and Ibrahim, A. M. "Protein-calorie malnutriton in Egypt. Proteinuria in marasmus. A possible differentiating factor between acutely and chronically developed cases." J. Egypt Med. Assoc. 59(1-2), 1976, pp 23-28.

Forty-seven hospitalized marasmic children between two months and three and a half years of age, and 24 healthy controls were evaluated for serum and urine total proteins and protein fractions by gel electrophoresis. Twelve marasmic cases with a short duration of protein-calorie malnutrition (PCM) showed normal serum total proteins and a slight increase in urine proteins, mainly albumin. The remaining marasmic cases were of long duration and had low serum total proteins. The proteinuria was markedly increased, affecting both albumin and globulin fractions, and indicating renal involvement. Authors suggested such examination for proteinuria of PCM cases was of diagnostic value regarding severity and extent of derangements, and was of prognostic value in providing care.

177. Said, A., el-Hawary, M. F., Abdel-Khalek, M. K., Samuel, S., and Abdin, M. A. "Protein-calorie malnutrition (PCM) in Egypt. V--Serum enzymes as indices of liver involvement." J. Egypt Med. Assoc. 59(1-2), 1976, pp 29-38.

This study was done on 360 children 6 to 36 months old with protein calorie malnutrition (PCM) as follows: 196 were oedematous cases (group A) and 156 non-oedamatous cases (group B). Normal values for serum alkaline phosphatase were seen in most PCM cases, but were elevated in 28% of severe kwashiorkor and 17% and 29% of 2nd and 3rd grade marasmic cases respectively. Mild and moderate kwashiorkor cases showed a normal range of acid phosphatase, but many severe PCM cases showed elevated levels. Serum pseudocholinesterase was depressed in PCM, mildly with mild kwashiorkor, and markedly with more severe PCM. Serum glutamic, pyruvic, and oxaloacetic transaminases (SGPT & SGOT) were almost normal in mild PCM, but elevated in moderate and severe kwashiorkor and in marasmic-kwashiorkor with lever involvement. Marasmus did not affect SGOT and SGPT activity in most cases, indicating little liver involvement.

178. Storey, A. "The diet and dentition of New Kingdom pharaohs."

Mastication, Anderson, D.J., and Matthews, B., eds. Bristol, England, Wright, 1976 pp 5-15.

This symposium presentation related diet to nutrition in the New Kingdom of ancient Egypt from the XVIIth to XXth dynasty, or 1600 BC to 1160 BC. Radiographs of pharaonic mummies' dentition were taken and examined. They showed that few dental caries existed, but that dental wear, which correlated well with age, was a problem. This wear exceeding the deposition of secondary dentine often caused destructive changes such as pulp exposure, pulp infection, pulp death and periapical pathology in the ancient Nubian and Old Kingdom nobles at Gizah. Textual evidence in the forms of extant medical papyri and stele inscriptions documented the existence of dentistry in the ancient kingdom. Temple inventories, records of routine daily food offerings, tomb paintings, banquet orders, and remains of funerary repasts were used as sources of dietary information. Ancient diets included a great deal of coarse bread, much of which was of varying grittiness due to sand particles, possibly originating in the stone grinding mortars and pestles. This may have contributed greatly to the excessive dental wear in pharoahs. Small quantities of honey were consumed, a factor in the small caries incidence. Malocclusions were found in several pre-Rameseid pharoahs and their queens.

179. Waslien, C. I. "Human intake of trace elements" Trace Elements in Human Health and Disease Vol. II Essential and Toxic Elements, 1976, Academic Press, Inc., pp 347-370.

Iron, zinc, selenium, and chromium content were determined in 98 common foods and food composites in the diet of the lower socioeconomic segment of Egypt's population. The composites were duplicates of hospital diets of infants and toddlers recovering from acute kwashiorkor. Calorie and protein intakes were high, 1940 Kcal/day and 53 gm/day respectively, as expected for children recovering from PCM. Selenium, with a mean of 29.4 ug/day, and chromium with a mean of 129 ug/day, had extremely varied intake ranges of 10 and 15 fold respectively, possibly reflecting variation in heat treatment of the composite foods. Dietary chromium contents and protein level showed a high correlation.

The diets of 50 families of Egyptian children being treated for PCM were also studied by questionnaire regarding purchases, by 24 hour diet recall, and collection of recipes. Middle East food tables were consulted for calories and protein contents, and iron, zinc, selenium, and chromium were estimated by analysis of individual foods. Bread provided most calories, total calories were 1400 to 1500/day, and protein was considered adequate. Intakes of minerals were: 14mg iron/day, 8mg zinc/day, 21ug selenium/day, and chromium 1/3 that of hospitalized Egyptian children/day.

180. Aal, A., El-Basousy, M. M., Khasba, A. A., El-Tahan, H. M., El-Hawary, M. F., and El-Shobaki, F. A. "Dual significance of hepatic cholinesterase as an index of liver involvement and state of protein-calorie malnutrition." Gaz. Egypt Paediatr. Assoc. 23(2), April 1975, pp 133-138.

One-hundred-fifty-nine cases of PCM (kwashiorkor, marasmic kwashiorkor, marasmus & nutritional edema) together with 20 cases of normal healthy controls were selected. Serum, red blood cell and liver cholinesterase were estimated together with serum total protein and serum albumin. Pathological liver examination was done for every case. Serum and hepatic pseudo-cholinesterase activity parallelled directly the serum albumin (not the total protein) as well as the pathological changes in the liver. The diminution in enzymatic activity and serum protein coincides with the severity of the liver involvement in the various forms of PCM. Insignificant change in true cholinesterase was demonstrated in all cases studied. Follow-up studies in a number of cases to clinical recovery revealed the return to normal of enzymatic activity and serum albumin, concomitant with restoration of normal pathological liver findings. The significance of changes in serum and liver cholinesterase activities as indices of the extent of liver involvement, as well as their diagnostic and prognostic values, are discussed.

181. Abdel Salam, F. E., Aboul-Seoud, A. A., and El-Gamal, S. A. F. "The evaluation of dietary protein by different techniques with growing chicks." Egypt. J. Nutr. 1(1), January 1975, pp 89-98.

One hundred fifty-day-old unsexed Fayoumi chicks were used to check three techniques of dietary protein evaluation. Chicks of the first group were fed a nitrogen-free diet from one to four weeks old. These depleted chicks were then fed, for four weeks, the test protein diets of fish meal and sardine meal which provided about 10 percent of the 20 percent total dietary crude protein. The second treatment group had the dietary fish meal and sardine meal from one week up to 8-weeks old. The third treatment of carcass analysis method was used to determine the NPU values for both meals. The three techniques of depleted, normal growth, and carcass nitrogen retention showed no significant difference between the two animal proteins. The data favored use of the depleted chick technique for evaluating dietary proteins. (Adapted from authors' summary)

182. Abdel Kader, M. M., Adham, K., Eissa, M., Adel, M., and Hodhod, S. "Nutritive value of lentils" Egypt. J. Nutr. 1(1), January 1975, pp 99-110.

The nutritive value of lentils as a possible substitution for animal proteins was investigated by the determination of the nutritive components (ash, lipids, proteins, carbohydrates and crude fibers) and the mineral content (Ca, P and Cu). The amino acid content of the lentil proteins showed the S-containing amino acids and tryptophan to be the first and second limiting amino acids respectively). The chemical score calculated was found to be high (43.4); however, the biological determination of the PER's of the raw and roasted lentils were low (0.66 and 1.15 respectively). Roasting improved the PER and the digestibility of this legume, demonstrating the beneficial effect of heat.

Rats were fed diets using either 10% or 15% lentils protein and growth curves compared. Growth was better with raw or roasted 10% than with the 15% lentils protein diet. The histopathological examination of the sacrificed animals showed a definite fatty degeneration of the liver with fat infiltration. These changes were more advanced in rats fed the 15% lentils protein diet than those fed the 10% lentils protein diet. (Adapted from authors' summary)

183. Abdel Kader, M. M., Eissa, A. M., Adel, M., and Hodhod, S. "Nutritive value of lupinus seeds" Egypt. J. Nutr. 1(1), January 1975, pp 111-124.

The nutritive value of the Egyptian lupinus-terminis was investigated as a possible substitute for animal proteins. The nutritional components (ash, lipids, proteins, carbohydrates and crude fibers), the amino acid content of its proteins (the S-containing amino acids and tryptophan were the first and second limiting amino acids), the mineral contents (Ca, P and Cu) and the effect of germination on the vitamin content (using whole seeds, cotyledons, radicle and pulmules) were determined. The calculated chemical score was 52.7 and the biological determination of the PER was 0.91. Soaking the seeds in water for four days improved the PER to 1.25 without improvement in digestibility, denoting the removal of water-soluble toxins by the water.

Growth curves of rats fed 10% lupmus protein were slightly less than those of rats fed 15% lupinus protein. Histopathological examination showed distension in the large gut of rats fed unsoaked termisprotein, but other organs were normal. (Adapted from authors' summary)

184. Abdin, Z. "Heart disease. A risk factor among Egyptian children." At-Risk Factors and the Health and Nutrition of Young Children. Publication of the International Conference held in Cairo, June 23-27, 1975, pp 77-81. Printed by Al-Shaab Printing House.

This presentation focussed on a major pediatric problem among Egyptian children more than five years old. Rheumatic heart disease (R.H.D.) accounted for 38% of deaths and 48% of important chronic diseases in these children from 1968-1973. Streptococcal infection was the main cause of R.H.D., and most children with positive test results failed to manifest tonsillitis. This may have been related to cases presenting with arthritis and arthralgia in the benign form. A significant drop in the relative mortality incidence in Cairo children between 1965 and 1975 from 52% to 38%, with a drop in severe cases from more than 40% to less than 14%, was seen to be related to increasing health education and propaganda and health service, including nutritional services.

185. Abdou, I. A., Awadalla, M. Z., and Wassef, S. A. "A biochemical and histopathological study of the effect of high calcium intake prevailing in the oases on the thyroid gland of rats." Egypt. J. Nutr. 1(1), January 1975, pp 1-16.

An experimental study was performed to assess the goitrogenic effect of excess calcium in drinking water (0.5 gm calcium carbonate/1 litre water) on rats kept on normal and 75% of their requirement of iodine for a period of three months.

Studies included:

a) Biochemical studies for thyroid weight, percentage of dried matter and iodine content, as well as thyroxine level of blood and rate of growth.

b) Histopathological examination of the thyroid gland.

Results suggested the possible goitrogenic effect of excess calcium. Maximum effect was observed in animals receiving excess calcium in the presence of 75% of their requirements of iodine. (Adapted from authors' summary)

186. Abdou, I. A., and Moussa, W. A. "Study of dietary factors causing growth retardation of boys in Egyptian villages." Egypt. J. Nutr. 1(1), January 1975, pp 43-57.

Some previous studies revealed that zinc deficiency is one of the factors causing growth retardation in Egypt. Thus in the present study of the factors contributing to this growth retardation, a sample of 90 school-boys (11-18 Y.) of Sindion Preparatory School with heights 2-S.D. below Iowa and 1 S.D. below Cairo Standards was selected for detailed a socio-economic, medical and quantitative dietary survey in different seasons with chemical analysis of composite food samples.

Results of the socio-economic study showed that the average monthly per- capita income in families of physically retarded group is L.E. 3.65 while it is L.E. 7 in the control group.

The diet of the retarded group was found to be inadequate in calories, calcium, iron, vit. A, riboflavin and ascorbic acid, while in the taller group the diet was only slightly below recommended daily allowances of vit. A and calcium. The diet of the taller group was better in quality, and all nutrients were significantly higher in amounts than the diet of the physically retarded. However, there was no difference in the amount of zinc in the diet of both groups which was found to be normal for both diets.

We can thus conclude that growth retardation in the Egyptian village is not a matter of genetic difference [and]...is rather a matter of social, economic, environmental and nutritional difference between upper and lower classes compatible with chronic under-nutrition and malnutrition. (Authors' summary)

187. Abdou, I. A., Shukry, A. S., Labib, F. M., and Moussa, W. A. "Nitrogen balance studies on protein-rich food mixtures for preschool children in Egypt". Gaz. Egypt. Paediatr. Assoc. 23(2), April 1975.

Nitrogen balance measurements were performed on children aged 5 to 30 months fed diets supplemented by PRFMs (protein-rich food mixtures) or by SMA milk powder as the sole source of dietary protein. Sesamena (or SLW-II) was fed to a group of 8 children, Arabeana to another group of 9 and Supramine to a third group of 8 children. The same children were measured when given SMA milk powder as a reference protein. Therefore, each subject acted as his own control. The technique used was that of Fomon et al with certain modifications.

All three mixtures maintained positive nitrogen balance. Sesamena gave the best mean NPU value (69 ± 5.9) which is 9% of reference. Supramine gave the highest mean digestibility (87 ± 6.8) which is 102% of reference. Sesamena proved a suitable weaning food satisfying all the standards of PRFMs recommended by the PAG (Protein Advisory Group). It contains a good quality protein, is cheap and easily prepared at th family level after appropriate education of mothers. This mixture can be also manufactured at the national level. (Authors' abstract)

188. Aly, H. E., Dakroury, A. M., Hamed, S., Abdel Hay, M. B., Mansour, A. G., and Hafiz, M. I. "Investigations on bladder stone disease of early childhood in Upper Egypt V. Biochemical investigation on mothers' milk in Edfou". Bull. Nutr. Inst. 5(1),

1975, pp 39-44.

The biochemical content of breast milk was studied in the Edfou region, where primary vesicle calculi were reportedly common in early childhood. Milk samples were randomly collected from nursing mothers in subject families, who were all clinically examined. Total protein content; Ca,#P and Mg content; and vitamin A content of milks were determined and were compared with values of milk from nursing mothers in Sanhour Beheira, a region of low calculi incidence. Mg levels were deficient in 77% of Edfou samples. Mean Ca content of Edfou milk was 32.9mg%, about normal value. Edfou P was 12.9mg% and Beheira P 12.7mg%, all below the norm of 15mg%. Average Edfou protein was .9gm% with a range of .5 to 1.1gm%, while that from Beheira was 1gm%. Therefore, all Edfou protein was below the 1.2g%, which is considered normal; 80% of Beheira's was deficient. Edfou's average vitamin A was 233 I.U.%, with a range of 178 to 288 I.U.% considered in the normal range. All nutrients except vitamin A were considered low. Mg was much lower in Edfou than in Beheira, and protein was comparatively lower. These factors may play an etiological role in formation of vesicle calculi.

189. Aly, H. E., Dakroury, A. M., Mansour, A. M., Agdelhay, M. B., and Ghoneme, F. "Investigations on bladder stone disease of early childhood in Upper Egypt I. The nutritional status of preschool children in Edfou." Bull. Nutr. Inst. 5(1), 1975, pp 13-25.

The nutritional status of preschool children in a randomly chosen sample of families in the Edfou region was studied and compared with that of preschool children in a randomly chosen sample of families in the same region having children with primary vesical calculi.

The nutritional status of preschool children in both groups of families was assessed by their anthropometric measurements. The data obtained for weight-age, height-age and mid-arm circumference-age all point to a high prevalence of mild and moderate cases of protein calorie malnutrition. The so called nutritional dwarfing, characterized by low-weight and short stature, was found among the preschool children of both groups of families, with a peak of stunting during the second year of life. A higher prevalance of PCM was found among the preschool children in the families having children with primary vesical calculi. (Adapted from authors' summary.)

190. Aly, H. E., Dakroury, A., Ghoneme, F., Abelhay, M. B., Mansour, A. G. and Diab, A. Sh. "Investigations on bladder stone disease of early childhood in Upper Egypt II. Nutritional deficiency signs and anaemia among preschool children in Edfou." Bull. Nutr. Inst. 5(1), 1975, pp 27-32.

A clinical examination for nutritional deficiency signs and the determination of blood haemoglobin concentration were carried out on preschool children in a randomly chosen sample of families in the Edfou region. The results were compared with those for preschool children in a randomly chosen sample of families living in the same region and having children with primary vesical calculi history.

The data obtained show that clinical signs suggestive of vit. B complex, vit. D and iron deficiencies are prevalent among Edfou preschool children in both groups of families, with a higher incidence among those in the families having children with primary vesical calculi. The latter also show a higher prevalence of aneamia of moderate and severe degrees during their first two years of life. (Authors' summary)

191. Aly, H. E., Dakroury, A. M., El-Ghorab, M. I., and Hafez, M. I. "Effect of oral contraceptive agents and intrauterine devices on hemoglobin and serum iron of Egyptian women." Bull. Nutr. Inst. 5(1), 1975, pp 1-6.

The effect of oral contraceptive agents and intrauterine devices on hemoglobin, hematocrit, serum iron and iron binding capacity was studied in women of lower socioeconomic status attending maternal and child health centers.

All values were found to be higher among women taking oral contraceptive pills. Among women using the intrauterine device (IUD), the hemoglobin level was lower than the control and the pill taker groups. Serum iron and iron binding capacity were higher for the pill takers than for those using IUD. (Adapted from authors' summary)

192. Aly, H. E., Dakroury, A. M., Ghoneme, F., Adbel Hay, M. B., Mansour, A. G., and Hafez, M. I. "Investigations on Bladder Stone Disease of Early Childhood in Upper Egypt IV. Urine studies and crystalluria among preschool children in Edfou." Bull. Nutr. Inst. 5(1), 1975, pp 33-37.

Urine samples from both Edfou and Beheira children were examined for crystals and oxalate content. Oxalate content was higher in urine collected from Beheira, with a range of 50-8000 mg/litre, than in urine of Edfou children, which showed a range of 31.25 to 6250 mg/litre. Ca oxalate crystals were not detected in most samples showing a high oxalate concentration. On the other hand, Ca oxalate crystals were found in most urine samples obtained from Edfou, including those with a low oxalate content.

Urine was examined also for parasites, red blood cells and white cells. Specimens of drinking water were analysed and were found to be within the acceptable standards. The underlying factors related to the prevalence of crystalluria in Edfou were discussed. (Authors' summary)

193. Anonymous "Guidelines on the at-risk concept and the health and nutrition of young children". At-Risk Factors and the Health and Nutrition of Young Children. Publication of the International Conference held in Cairo, June 23-27, 1975, pp 265-280. Printed by Al-Shaab Printing House. Also published in pamphlet form by Al-Ahram Press, 23 pages.

These guidelines, based on papers and reports presented at a Working Conference on "At-Risk Factors and the Health and Nutrition of Young Children" held in Cairo, Egypt, were discussed and approved by the participants to the conference. At-risk factors for the mother and for the young child, as well as cultural, socio-economic, geographic-climatic, and miscellaneous other factors were listed and discussed. In addition, the dietary and non-dietary factors in the various biological stages of life from fetus through toddlerhood were listed, as were the locally predominant and geographically relevant preventable conditions.

Use of at-risk factors in training health personnel to recognize at-risk populations and in national planning programs was covered.

194. Awwaad, S. "At-risk factors and the health of young children, factors affecting fetal life" At-Risk Factors and the Health and Nutrition of Young Children. Publication of the International Conference held in Cairo, June 23-27, 1975, pp 53-56. Printed by Al-Shaab Printing House.

This presentation focussed on risk factors affecting fetal life. The list discussed consisted of both physical and mental health-related factors. Malnutrition and severe anemia were found to affect the fetal growth, pregnancy outcome, and birth weight. Demographic risk factors included past obstetric history, genetic anomalies and chromosomal aberrations, maternal medical diseases, secondary obstetric factors, acute infectious diseases, and early adverse influence such as drugs, radiation, and work while pregnant. Suggested measures to decrease risk factors included both preconceptual preparations such as marriage, genetic, and birth planning counseling, and maternal care during pregnancy and labor, including prenatal care and management of specific clinical problems.

195. Awwaad, S., Khalifa, A. S., Naga, M. A., Tolba, K. A., Fares, R., Gaballa, A. S., Hayeg, O. E., and Wahhab, S. A. "A field survey on child health in a rural community in Egypt." J. Trop. Med. Hyg. 78(1), January 1975, pp 20-25.

Results of a field survey in the rural village of Bani Shebl in Sharkieh Province are reported. Two hundred fifty-six children 1 1/2 months to 12 years of age were assessed by clinical exam, vaccination history, height, weight, left arm circumference, hemoglobin level and examination of urine, stool and blood for parasites. The vaccination program was found to be inadequate as officially required vaccinations against smallpox, diphtheria, polio and TB were found in 61.2, 46.5, 34.4, and 29.2% chldren, respectively. Parasitic infestation was found to be higher than urban areas, but significantly lower than 1959. The latter is attributed to a safer water supply. Growth and development lagged behind the whole national standards, particularly during the 1-6 years age period. Twenty seven percent were below 3rd percentile for weight and 37% for height. Twelve point nine percent had rickets and 15.1% had vitamin A deficiency. Health care for the preschool age, taking advantage of cooperation from medical faculties and local health authorities, is recommended. The value of health education is stressed. (Adapted from authors' abstract)

196. Awwaad, S., Mourad, K. A., El Fattah, S. A., El Sokkary, S., and Mostafa, F. A. "Histopathology and histochemistry of the kidney in marasmic Egyptian children." Gaz. Egypt Paediatr. Assoc. 23(2), April 1975, pp 151-159.

Percutaneous renal biopsy was done in 15 infants and children with third degree marasmus and in five normal controls. All cases were free from infection. Histopathological changes as shown in sections stained with hematoxylin and eosin included patchy areas of colloid degeneration and thickening of the walls of some blood vessels in 10 out of 15 marasmic cases. Some proximal convoluted tubules appeared small or atrophic, others were somewhat dilated with decreased thickness of their walls, and still others showed necrotic changes. The distal convoluted tubules in the medulla appeared vacuolated and distorted. The activity of the enzyme succinic dehydrogenase was markedly inhibited especially in the distal convoluted tubules in all the patients studies. (Authors' abstract)

197. Dakroury, A. M., Aly, H. E., and Saddik, M. F. "Effect of cooking on the nutritive value and the microbiological quality of kishk (Upper Egypt variety)." Bull. Nutr. Inst. 5(1), 1975, pp 7-12.

The nutritive value of kishk, a fermented, grain-based food particularly popular in Upper Egypt, was assessed through a determination of its chemical composition. It was characterized by a high carbohydrate content (79.468g%), protein (10.108%), fat (1.927g%), fiber (0.00768g%), calcium (248mg%) and iron (1.6mg%). The thiamine content was 69.866 ugm% and riboflavin 81.707 ugm%, while ascorbic acid was undetectable.

The cooking process caused little or no effect on the chemical ingredients except the vitamin content, which was markedly affected. The microbial load which was $12X10^6$/gm in the raw food was considerably reduced in the cooked state. Coliforms were not detected in the raw or the cooked product. (Adapted from authors' summary)

198. Darwish, N. M., El-Nahry, F., and Souba, A. S. "The nutritive value of local roasted sunflower seeds." Ann. Agric. Science (Egypt) 20(1), June 1975, pp 101-109.

The effect of the local roasting method on the varieties 1 - Giza 12 - Miak 3 - Dahr El-Haia was investigated.

The decorticated seeds of both raw and roasted varieties were subjected to biochemical analysis. All the investigated varieties of sunflower seeds contained high amounts of protein and fats, while their carbohydrate contents were low, making them good sources of energy and protein.

Fat provided the highest percentage of calories in the investigated varieties. Roasting the seeds slightly increased protein and fat contents, and decreased water and carbohydrate contents. Both raw and roasted varieties were shown to contain appreciable amounts of phosphorus and iron. (Adapted from authors' abstract)

199. El-Attar, A. F., Fahmy, A. H., and Abdou, A. I. "Income and food expenditure relationship." Egypt. J. Nutr. 1(1), January 1975, pp 59-65.

By estimating income demand elasticity, this study determined that changes in income of the average Egyptian consumer were accompanied by only slight changes in food expenditure. The only exceptions were semi-necessary foods like meats, fruits, oil and legumes, especially in rural regions. The results are attributed to the low income level of the Egyptian consumer which encourages the consumption of relatively expensive foods like meat and fruits with increased income.

200. El-Bebeidi, M. A., and Gomas, E. A. "The effect of 2,4-D and Dicamba on the growth and yield of garden broad bean (Vicia faba L. var. major)." Beitr, Trop. Landwirtsch. Veterinaermed. 13(2), 1975, pp 185-193. Article in German with English abstract.

Two experiments were conducted in Egypt to investigate the effect of sublethal concentrations of 2,4-D and Dicamba on the growth and yield of garden broad bean. It was found that: (1) As compared to the effects of Dicamba, 2,4-D had a better stimulating effect on the growth characters, the yield, and the yield components of the beans; (2) The application at the flowering stage was superior to the earlier application in every respect; (3) The optimum rate of 2,4-D and Dicamba that gave the highest increase of the growth, yield, and yield components was 2-5 ppm. (Authors' abstract)

201. El-Gindy, M. M., Abdou, I. A., Alian, A., and Mohamed, T. M. "Effect of some preparation processes on the amino acids content of lentils, kishk, and fereek." Egypt. J. Nutr. 1(1), January 1975, pp 77-88.

The protein, crude fiber, fat, moisture, carbohydrates, calcium and phosphorus contents of lentils, Kishk and Fereek were determined. Fourteen amino acids were identified and determined quantitatively in the proteins with the use of a paper chromatographic technique. Two developments with butanol: acetic acid: water (4:1:5) separated lysine, cystine, histidine, arginine, phenylalanine, and tyrosine. Using phenol solvent with phosphate buffer (pH 12) (1:1), the amino acids aspartic acid, glutamic acid, serine, glycine, threonine and alanine were separated. The third solvent was butanol: benzyl alcohol 1:1 in borate buffer (pH 8.4) to separate leucine and isoleucine. Ninhydrin acetone was used alone for spraying with the first solvent, with 4% acetic acid for the second solvent and with 2% acetic acid for the third solvent. (Authors' summary)

202. El-Hassan, A. A. "Schistosomiasis in the New Valley and the reclaimed northern coastal zone in Egypt." Egypt J. Bilharz. 2(2), 1975, pp 191-212.

A field survey of wells and drainage channels indicate the prior existence of the snail intermediate hosts of schistosomiasis in the New Valley area, as well as the present existence of Bulinus truncatus in some wells in Bahariya. Repeated treatment with mollusicides has resulted in the disappearance of B. truncatus from Dakhla and Kharga Oasis, although Lynnaea truncatula and Lymnaea cailliaudi are still found in some wells. In a few uncovered wells surveyed in Farafra Oasis, L. truncatula, L. cailliaudi and Melanoides tuberculata were detected.

In the northern coastal area, no snails were detected in the surveyed wells and the main drainage channels.

203. El-Hawary, M. F., El-Shobaki, F. A., Kholeif, T., Sakr, R., El-Bassousy, E. M., Abdel-Khalek, K., and Khashaba, A. "Ascorbic acid effect on intestinal iron absorption in different types of anaemias." Gaz. Egypt Paediatr. Assoc. 23(3), April 1975, pp 145-149.

The effect of ascorbic acid on the rate of intestinal iron absorption was investigated in anaemia due to iron or protein-calorie deficiency and that associated with acute glomerulonephritis, nephrosis and schistosoma haematobium. The basic rate of intestinal iron absorption was enhanced in pure iron deficiency anemia, acute glomerulonephritis and infection with Schistosoma haematobium and retarded in kwashiorkor, marasmus and nephrosis. Ascorbic acid markedly promoted iron absorption in normal subjects, but only slightly in pure iron deficiency anaemia. It improved iron absorption in acute glomerulonephritis and Schistosoma haematobium infection, but not in kwashiorkor, marasmus and nephrosis. Ascorbic acid supplementation is of beneficial effect in alleviating anemia when intestinal iron absorption is not impaired. It may also be of value when given with protein rehabilitation in anaemias associated with protein deficiency.

204. El-Nahry, F. I., Darwish, N., and Souba, A. S. "The biological value of local roasted sunflower seeds." Ann. Agric. Science (Egypt 20(1) June 1975, pp 119-128.

Protein quality of some local sunflower seeds--Giza 1, Miak and Dahr El-Haia, and the effect of local roasting techniques were studied.

The protein quality of both raw and roasted seeds was evaluated by determining the protein efficiency ratio, net protein ratio and a serum analysis of rats maintained on diets containing either raw or roasted sunflower seed proteins. The serum analysis included the determinations of total serum proteins, serum albumin/globulin ratio and free nonessential to essential amino acids ratio.

All the investigated varieties were of high biological values and roasting the seeds improved their protein quality. The best protein quality was that of Dahr El-Haia, followed by Miak and then Giza 1. This was shown also by serum analysis results. (Adapted from authors' abstract)

205. El-Nahry, F. I., Darwish, N., and Zahran, E. "Comparative studies on the biological value of local linseed and lettuce seed cakes." Annals Agric. Sci. (Ain Shams Univ.) 20(1), June 1975, pp 111-118.

Local linseed and lettuce seed cakes were subjected to nutritional evaluation by chemical and biological methods. Moisture, protein, fat, ash, fiber and carbohydrate contents were determined. The protein quality of the cakes were evaluated by determining the protein efficiency ratio, net protein ratio and serum analysis of rats maintained on diets containing the investigated cakes. The serum analysis covered the determinations of total serum proteins, serum albumin/globulin ratio and free nonessential to essential amino acids. Both cakes were found to be of high protein quality, but lettuce cake was superior to linseed cake and also contained a higher percentage of protein. Addition of seed oil to seed cake in diets of rats raised the biological value of seed cake proteins. (Adapted from authors' abstract)

206. Gabr, M. "At-risk factors and the health of young children." At-Risk Factors and the Health and Nutrition of Young Children. Publication of the International Conference held in Cairo, June 23-27, 1975, pp 99-111. Printed by Al-Shaab Printing House.

Sociocultural and economic factors, infections, accidents, and genetic, racial and nutritional factors affecting the health of young children in Egypt were described. An important nutritional factor in early life, particularly for those less than 2 years of age, was breastfeeding, which protected the infant from protein calorie malnutrition (PCM) and related diarrheal disease. More than 60% of preschoolers suffered from PCM according to urban and rural surveys, with the highest incidence before 2 years of age. Iron deficiency was prevalent in Egyptian children, particularly those with PCM. Deficiency of vitamin D was prevalent due to cultural overdressing of children. Vitamin A deficiency was rarely seen, but occurred in children with severe PCM, with 8% showing xerosis cornea or keratomalacia. Cultural factors influencing nutrition were late and inadequate introduction of supplementary foods, abrupt weaning, and starvation following infections such as measles and gastroenteritis. Frequent pregnancies and close birth spacing contributed to poor nutritional state of mothers and therefore fetuses and infants. Infection, particularly gastroenteritis, and parasitic infestations, particularly Giardia lamblia, Entamoeba histolytica, and Schistosomiasis were contributors to malnutrition. Relative prevalence of consanguinitiy increased incidence of metabolic defects and genetically determined diseases such as G-6-PD deficiency, intestinal lactase deficiency, and thalassemia.

207. George, Y., and Soliman, M. M. "A standard diet for the nutrition of the laboratory rats and mice." Egypt Dent. J. 21(4), October 1975, pp 1-6.

Three types of rat diets with different constituents were studied. 72 albino rats divided into three groups with equal males and females were fed the diets from 21 days of age for three months. Growth and health were recorded. The first diet, registered under item No. 114 with the Ministry of Agriculture, was optimal in producing growth and contained 20% protein, 3.5% fat and 5% fiber. The second diet was cariogenic, consisting of 25% sugar, 25% dried powdered milk and 50% barley. The rats fed this diet gained less and were less healthy than the first group. Rats fed the third diet of 25% dried powdered milk and 75% barley exhibited poor growth.

208. Hanafi, A., Lebshtein, A., and Hassan, H. A. "Growth and diet of children with congenital heart disease." Bull. Nutr. Inst. 5(1), 1975, pp 81-92.

The growth pattern and dietary intake of children with congenital heart disease was studied in 70 cases of both sexes compared to a control group of 415 apparently normal children. All growth indices studied (body weight, height, chest circumference and skin fold thickness) were significantly lower in the diseased than the control group. The effect of congenital heart disease on growth appears early in life. The amount of food intake seems not to play a role in growth retardation associated with this congenital malformation. (Authors' abstract)

209. Helmy, Z. A., Abd-el-Malek, Y., and Mahmound, A. A. "Incidence of coagulase-positive staphylococci in Damietta cheese." In Zentralbl. Bakteriol. (Naturwiss) 130(5), 1975, pp 461-467.

Three selective media: Mannitol Salt Agar, Staphylococcus Medium 110, and Ludlam's Medium, were used to study 40 samples of Damietta cheese for the presence and count of coagulase-positive staphylococci. 10 samples were from the Ministry of Public Health laboratories, and 30 were retail market samples purchased throughout one year. Ludlam's Medium inhibited the growth of the staphylococci in the samples, and so was not recommended for culturing purposes. Mannitol Salt Agar produced the highest percentage of recovery of staphylococcus, and Staphylococcus Medium 110 also produced a good percentage of recovery. Results showed all the laboratory samples to have coagulase-positive staphylococci, and 30% (9 of 30 samples) of the market samples also contained it. In these cases the numbers ranged from 1,000 to several million per gm. Depending on the cheese sample's age, the count correlated with acidity and salt content.

210. Hussein, L. A., and El-Naggar, B. M. "Normal ranges and diagnostic value of serum albumin and leucine aminopeptidase activity in Egyptian children." J. Trop. Pediatr. 21(6), December 1975, pp 301-306. (Environ. Child Health)

One-hundred-four children of low socioeconomic background were clinically classified as healthy (24), malnourished (41), or ill with respiratory disease (11), infectious disease (16), renal, malignant and other diseases (12). Serum albumin and leucine aminopeptidase activity (LNA) were determined in the various groups. Mean serum albumin levels in all diseases were invariably lower than the mean control values, which were at least 4.9 g/100 ml. Serum albumin mean level in PCM was 1.75 g/100 ml, in nephrotic syndrome was 2.45 g/100 ml, and with hepatitis was 3.7 g/100 ml. Two categories of PCM children were distinguishable on the basis of serum LNA activities, the first with activity of 50 U/L or less and the second with activity above 80 U/L. Authors concluded that serum LNA activity in PCM children could be used as an early predictor of liver damage prior to rise in serum bilirubin, and that the electrophoretic pattern of all the studied diseases were distinguishable from one another and of diagnostic value.

211. Lebshtein, A. K., Hanafi, A., and Hassan, H. A. "Study of physical development of school children with rheumatic heart disease." Bull. Nutr. Inst. 5(1), 1975, pp 93-106.

A study of the physical development of school children with rheumatic heart disease was performed on 616 children and 415 controls of both sexes between the ages of 6 and 20 years. All growth indices studied (weight, height, chest circumference and skin fold thickness) were lower in the rheumatic heart boys and girls than the controls. There was also delayed pubescence in both sexes compared to the matched controls. (Authors' abstract)

212. Lebshtein A. K., Hanafi, A., and Hassan, H. A. "A study of the dietary pattern of rheumatic heart children." Bull. Nutr. Inst. 5(1), 1975, pp 73-79.

The dietary pattern and average daily intake of protein and calories were studied in 616 rheumatic heart cases between 6-20 years age and 415 matched controls. The diet falls within the pattern characteristic of the Egyptian diet. The intake of protein and calories increased with advancement of age in the diseased and control groups but the rheumatic heart cases were always at a lower level. The only exceptions were the age group below 10 years enrolled in school and the boys of age group 10 years not educated, where the intake was higher than the corresponding controls.

It appears that diet is involved in growth retardation associated with rheumatic heart disease, but it is not the sole factor playing. (Adapted from authors' abstract).

213. Metwalli, O. M. "Effect of protein depletion on the rate of some transamination processes." Egypt. J. Nutr. 1(1), January 1975, pp 68-75.

The rate of the transamination process in liver and muscle tissues of animals suffering from protein depletion was compared with animals receiving an adequate quantity of proteins. Tissue transaminases seem to behave differently in different organs as well as in response to the protein content of the diet. (Author's summary)

214. Miladi, S. "Food availability". At-Risk Factors and the Health and Nutrition of Young Children Publication of the Internationl Conference held in Cairo, June 23-27, 1975, pp 7-17. Printed by Al-Shaab Printing House.

Global statistics quoted in this presentation indicated no world-wide food shortage. Rather, distribution of available supplies within some regions and countries was seen as not equitable. In 1969/71, Far East, African, and Asian centrally planned economies experienced a 6 - 8% deficit in per capita energy supplies. In 1973/74 the rapid rise in world food prices contributed to lower socioeconomic and childhood populations experiencing a deterioration in nutrition. Ecologic, technologic, and financial factors affected distribution patterns of available food in geographic areas. Traditional emphasis on nutritional repletion of the adults within the family unit contributed to the presence of malnutrition within the young child population. Statistically, family size was inversely proportional to caloric intake from total protein and animal protein. Seasonal fluctuations affected nutritional state, pre-harvest periods being particularly lean times. A sexual differentiation in nutritional state in pre-school children occurred in some areas. This was related to cultural preference of male children, with significantly more females suffering malnutrition than males.

215. Peipp, V. L. "Possibilities for improved production of meat and milk in state agricultural plants in Egypt". Bietr. Trop. Landwirtsch. Veterinaermed. 13(3), 1975, pp 251-257. (Article in German, abstract in English.)

Starting in August 1973, the test station for agricultural machinery of the GDR VVA Land-und Nahrungsg utertechnik at El Ghasair has investigated the problems connected with a continuous daily supply of fresh feed-stuff to large livestock (cattle) and with preservation methods suited to this aim. First results are reported of applying an advanced technology - and partly GDR farm machinery - in cultivating and harvesting green fodder and hay, using Alexandrian clover and lucern. (Adapted from author's abstract.)

216. Saddik, M. F., Moustafa, E. K., Dadroury, A. M., and Amine, E. K. "Objective and subjective quality indices of fish stored in insufficient and in sufficient amounts of ice." Bull. Nutr. Inst. 5(1), 1975, pp 45-61.

Sufficient icing of morgan and bolti fishes (ice:fish ratio 10:1) resulted in a considerable improvement of the storage quality of the fish in comparison to insufficient icing (ice:fish ratio 2:1). This led to a prolongation of shelf life from 4 to 12 days for morgan fish and from 6 to 14 days for bolti fish. Quality of fish during ice storage was evaluated by objective methods (bacteriological and chemical) and by subjective methods (sensory evaluation). Bacteriological indices of quality included the determination of total viable count, psychrophiles, coliforms,

Streptococcus faecalis and Clostridia sp. Chemical quality attributes included the determination of total volatile bases, trimethylamine and its oxide, and the protein precipitation test. Sensory evaluation included appearance, odor and texture of raw fish as well as odor, taste and texture of cooked fish. (Adapted from authors' abstract)

217. Saddik, M. F., Moustafa, E. K., Dakroury, A. M., and Amine, E. K. "Effect of lowering the storage temperature on retarding the microbial growth in the fish of wet bolti." Bull. Nutr. Inst. 5(1), 1975, pp 64-71.

The effect of storage temperature on the microbial growth in the flesh of Tilapia nilotica (Bolti fish) was evaluated. The fish were stored at -4°C, 0°C, +4°C and +15°C (room temperature).

Total viable count and number of psychophiles both rapidly increased with increasing storage temperature. The magnitude of their accumulation proved to be a reliable index of spoilage. The amount of coliforms in the fish flesh increased with temperature, but their detection was seen as a sanitary index, Streptococcus faecalis proved to be storage temperature dependent and was considered a reliable index of quality as well as sanitary condition of the fish.

218. Said, A., El-Hawary, M. D., Sakr, R., Khalek, M. K., El-Shobaki, F. A., and Noseir, M. B. "Biochemical and haematological aspects of anaemia associating protein energy malnutrition (PEM)." Gaz. Egypt Paediatr. Assoc. 23(2), April 1975, pp 139-144.

Biochemical and haematological aspects of anaemia were studied in relation to protein energy malnutrition (PEM). Control subjects studied have had relatively lower Hb, Ht, and R.B.C.S. count than European standards. Hypochromic anaemia was predominant in 83.3% of children with moderate kwashiorkor (KWO), with normocytic in 50% and microcytic in 33.3%. In severe KWO, anaemia was normocytic in 42% and microcytic in 19.2%. Normochromia was found in 9.7% and hypochromia in 29%. Macrocytosis was found in 38.8% with severe KWO. In 2nd degree marasmus, normocytic anaemia was revealed in 74%, normochromic in 82% and hypochromic in 40%. Macrocytic anaemia was detected in 26%. In 3rd degree marasmus, normocytic normochromic anaemia occurred in 70% of the cases and macrocytosis was encountered among 30% of the cases. Serum iron and transferrin level dropped in both KWO and marasmus, with the extent of decrease greater in the former. (Authors' abstract)

219. Salem, S. A. "Changes in carbohydrates and amino acids during baking of Vicia faba." J. Sci. Food Agric. 26(3), March 1975, pp 251-253.

Chemical changes in carbohydrates, proteins and amino acids of the broad bean Vicia faba which occur during the production of the baked beans "foul midamis" were studied. During baking, part of the sugars and amino acids of the beans were involved in discolouration reactions with subsequent decrease of the components studied. (Authors' abstract)

220. Shukry, A. S., and Kamel, L. M. "Nutrition rehabilitation." At-Risk Factors and the Health and Nutrition of Young Children.

Publication of the International Conference held in Cairo, June 23-27, 1975, pp 235-239. Printed by Al-Shaab Printing House.

In this presentation, the Egyptian methods of reaching at-risk babies and young children and of treating them effectively were discussed. The use of Maternal and Child Health Centers' (M.C.H.) services was stressed, and the use of day care centers and nurseries was also mentioned. Suggested nutrition rehabilitation programs were based on staging the service according to the baby's condition and available resources. For children with increasing degrees of malnutrition and related problems, the following treatments were suggested: Nutrition Rehabilitation Clinics with health education classes and a demonstration kitchen; Nutrition Rehabilitation Centers including child nourishment and maternal education programs; and Residentation Rehabilitation Centers where children and mothers are admitted as patients with nutritional and medical care provided.

221. Wahba, S. A., Galal, O., Kamel, L. M., Morsi, K. S., and El-Wakeil, F. A. "Improved feeding patterns in the prevention of childhood malnutrition". Gaz. Egypt Paediatr. Assoc. 23(2), April 1975, pp 97-109.

Simple assessment of the nutritional status and evaluation of the dietary, economic, and social conditions were done for a sample of urban and rural infants and young children. Home-made diets supplying the recommended dietary allowances for proteins and calories were suggested. These diets cost the same amount of money originally spent on foods for the baby. A follow-up study for three months showed that babies reached growth standards better than the original diet for the same group at similar ages. (Authors' abstract)

222. Wishahy, A., El-Ella, W. M., and El-Sokkary, S. A. "Effect of preservation and skimming on the nutritional value of raw milks under house conditions." Gaz. Egypt Paediatr. Assoc. 23(2), April 1975, pp 129-132.

Raw cow's and buffalo's milk are frequently used in infant feeding in Egypt. The milk may be stored either fresh or after boiling and it is common practice to skim the milk and dilute it before feeding. An analysis of the resulting decrease in fat content produced the following: a) raw cow's milk-52.48%, b) raw buffalo's milk - 33.61%, c) boiled cow's milk - 34.1%, and d) boiled buffalo's milk - 26.14%.

Clostridia sp. were detected only in decomposing fish and so were not considered useful as an index of sanitation.

223. el-Fattah, M. A., Gabrial, G. N., and Morcos, S. R. "A need for nutrition education in Egypt; studies on some obesity-producing preparations present in the local market (Cow-pearl jams)." J. Egypt Public Health Assoc. 49(4-5), 1974, pp 225-230.

A stock control rat diet and 3 commercially sold "obesity-producing" preparations, termed Cow-Pearl Jams, were compared for biochemical composition, nutritional values, and their effect on rats' body composition. Twenty percent of each jam by weight was incorporated into the stock rat diet. Jam-containing diets resulted in less weight gain, lower food and protein efficiency ratios and lower body nitrogen contents in rats compared to the straight stock diet's results. All groups of rats showed the same body water and fat contents. Nutrition education, governmental licensing control, and mass media advertisement supervision were recommended for such expensive preparations which failed to produce claimed results.

224. El-Hassan, A. A. "The importance of the effect of the chemical composition of water on the population of snails--intermediate hosts of schistosomes in Egypt". Folia Parasitol (Praha) 21(2), 1974, pp 169-179.

The study elucidates the effect of the chemical composition of water on the distribution of Bulinus truncatus truncatus (Audouin) and Biomphalaria alexandrina alexandrina (Ehrenberg), the two snail intermediate hosts of schistosomes in the A.R.E. The lethal concentration of common ions present in fresh water for different stages of the snails was obtained. The least tolerant stages are newly hatched snails of both species. Biomphalaria snails are more tolerant than Bulinus snails to the examined ions. In the field, the concentration of various ions seldom reaches these lethal extremes. The restricted distribution of Biomphalaria snails in the Delta and its absence from Upper Egypt cannot be attributed to variations in the chemical constituents of water. Both the Delta and Upper Egypt contain microhabitats suitable for the establishment of both snail species. The chemical composition of water may indirectly influence the distribution of snail intermediate hosts by influencing the types and growth of microflora which is essential as food for the snails. (Author's abstract)

225. el-Naka, N. M. "A study of the family diet in a district in Cairo." J. Egypt Public Health Assoc. 49(1), July 26, 1974, pp 49-59.

The general food consumption pattern in a traditional Cairo district was surveyed by analyzing one week's daily food intake in 550 households. Information on family composition, heights, weights, and economic status, and a seven-day daily menu was gathered. Six economic levels of family income/person/month were used in data organization and analysis. Twenty-four percent of the people were in the poorest income class of less than 3 L.E./person/month and fifty-two percent had income less than 5 L.E./person/month. Animal protein in the form of meat, fish, and eggs was low. Legume and fruit consumption were also low. Meat and fruit consumption differed noticeably according to income group. Nutrition education might encourage increased consumption of skim milk cheese for protein, green and yellow vegetables and fruits for vitamin A, and legumes with the cereals for high quality plant protein intake.

226. Farid, Z., el-Masry, N. A., Young, S. W., Bassily, S., Sparks, H. A., and Hassan, A. "Treatment of schistosomal polyposis of the colon with niridazole (Ambilhar)." J. Trop. Med. Hyg. 77(3), March 1974, pp 65-67.

Seventeen male farmers aged 16 to 45 years with multiple schistosomal polyposis of the colon, acute bloody diarrhoea, severe anaemia, and hypo-albuminaemia were treated with niridazole 25 mg/kg/day for 10 days.

Immediate results of treatment were excellent. Symptomatic

improvement was rapid and blooody diarrhoea ceased in 11 patients within one to two weeks of completing treatment. Three to six months after parasitic cure, sigmoidoscopic and air contrast barium enema examinations showed complete disappearance of polyps in 12 patients and marked improvement in the remaining five with a few polyps restricted only to the rectosigmoid colon.

Two to three years later, 15 of the 17 patients had become re-infected with Schistosoma mansoni, and in 10 of these, sigmoidoscopic and barium enema examinations showed a recurrence of multiple inflamed infected polyps of the colon. (Authors' abstract)

227. Fattah, M. A. "Dietary faults in health and disease leading to protein-calorie malnutrition." Gaz. Egypt Paediatr. Assoc. 22(1), January 1974, pp 31-37.

A dietary questionnaire given to mothers of 102 infants and young children suffering from PCM showed that failure of breast feeding was common among infants and that this may be an important cause of PCM in the first year of life. Supplementary feeding was seldom practiced and when given was markedly deficient in all the nutrients. Foods given after weaning were also deficient in every respect. Foods given during 24 hours were found severely deficient in proteins and calories and to a greater extent in minerals and vitamins. The most deficient nutrients were iron, vit A, thiamine and ascorbic acid. The subjects were suffering from PCM as well as such nutritional deficiency diseases as anaemia, vit. C deficiency, rickets and others. Food intake during disease was restricted for unduly prolonged periods, thus worsening the already lowered nutritional status of the children. A comprehensive nutrition education program is recommended. (Author's abstract)

228. Hamdi, Y. A., Abd-el-Samea, M. E., and Lofti, M. "Nodulation of soybean under field condition". Zentralbl. Bakteriol. (Naturwiss) 129(6), 1974, pp 574-578.

Seeds of the soybean variety Clark were inoculated at the rate of 28 x 106.28 x 10^5 and 28 x 10^4 cells/seed. Inoculated seeds were planted in field plots and pots containing the same soil, and kept under greenhouse conditions.

Nodulation was frequent within 3 weeks in the pot experiments, where the seeds were inoculated with 28 x 10^6 cells/seed. At three weeks, nodulates were observed under field conditions or in plants receiving 28 x 10^4 cells/seed in the greenhouse.

After 37 days in the field, nodulation was between 87 to 92% when rhizobia were at the rate of 28 x 10^6 cells/seed. Nodulation dropped to 19% when the rate of rhizobia was 28 x 10^4 cells/seed. 100% nodulation was noticed in plants receiving 28 x 10^6 cells/seed in pot cultures and decreased to 50% in those inoculated with 28 x 10^4 cells/seed.

At 102 days, nodulation frequency, fresh weight of nodules, dry weight of stems and pods were increased with the increase in the number of rhizobia seed, applied at the time of planting. (Authors' abstract)

229. Hussein, L., Gabriel, G. N., and Morcos, S. R. "Nutritional value of mixtures of baladi bread and broad beans". J. Sci. Food Agric.

25(12), December 1974, pp 1433-1440.

Several supplementation mixtures to the local Egyptian bread were designed and tested for their p.e.r and n.p.u. values using weanling rats. In the first experiment, broad beans var. baladi) were subjected to five different methods of preparation and each of the products was added to bread-based diets at 50:50 nitrogen ratio. When the p.e.r. (1.78) and n.p.u. (53) values of the raw beans were set at 100 and 100, the respective following values were obtained: 94, 98 for soaked; 94, 87 for germinated followed by boiling; and 59, 79 for autoclaved beans (1 h). In the second experiment, 11 different protein mixtures were tested for their p.e.r. values. The tested protein mixture with the lowest p.e.r. value is that from bread + 0.5% Dl-Met (p.e.r = 1.3). The most favourable mixture found is bread + Met + Lys + Thr (p.e.r. = 3.3) to bring it to level furnished by whole egg, followed by the mixtures bread N and raw broad bean N 40:60 (p.e.r. = 3.0); bread N and stewed broad bean N 70:30 (p.e.r. = 2.8). Upon supplementation with 0.5% DL-Met, mean p.e.r. values of 3.0 and 2.7 were obtained for raw and stewed broad beans diets, respectively. The amino acid analysis showed losses of 10% and 35% in the lysine and S-containing amino acids, respectively, after autoclaving the beans for 1 h. (Authors' abstract)

230. Loutfi, A., Waslien, C., and Van Reen, R. "Studies on bladder stone disease in Egyptian children. IV. Evaluation of vitamin A status." J. Egypt Med. Assoc. 57(3-4), 1974, pp 116-123.

Vitamin A deficiency was proven to cause urinary calculi in experimental animals. Therefore, fifty patients with bladder stone disease were studied to determine whether vitamin A deficiency occurred in those patients. Clinical and histological examinations failed to reveal evidence of vitamin A deficiency. Serum values for retinol were considered acceptable in 68% of the cases, low in 32% and deficient in none, conforming to the pattern of serum vitamin A in Egyptian children noted in several other surveys. Collectively, our data provide evidence that vitamin A is not involved in the etiology of bladder stone disease. Total serum proteins and albumin levels were also normal indicating that severe protein deficiency was also not an etiological agent. (Authors' abstract)

231. Nassar, A. M., Abd-El Hamid, J., Sabour, M. S., Awwaad, S. A., and Mahran, Z. Y. "Ultrastructure of skeletal muscles in protein deficiency." J. Trop. Pediatr. 20(2), April 1974, pp 77-81. (Environ. Child. Health).

Four patients with advanced marasmus from 4 months to 2 years of age were studied via muscle biopsy for ultrastructural changes. Electron microscopic examination of the fibers showed that contractile actin and myosin filaments were most affected. Many irregular fibers with localized swellings were seen. Irregular sarcomeres and resultant irregular Z lines occurred, as did short, dense sarcomeres without I bands and long, pale sarcomeres without A bands or with several interrupted narrow A bands. In some segments intermyofibrillar spaces disappeared and they and sarcomeres were replaced by narrow dense and pale bands across the fiber's breadth. Irregular filaments also intermingled, and the area became electron dense. Irregular nuclear outlines, fragmented nuclei, and increased nucleoplasm granularity and chromosomes occurred. Mitochrondria aggregated, and lost regularity of arrangement and striations. Sarcoplasm showed large irregular granular vacuoles. Irregular sarcolemma with elevations and depressions inside muscle fiber were seen.

232. Nofal, M. A., Kamel, K., Mahran, A. E., el-Ramly, Z., and Hashem, N. "Plasma volume and hemoglobin changes in children recovering from kwashiorkor." J. Egypt Med. Assoc. 57(9-10), 1974, pp 397-405.

Nine kwashiorkoric children from 11 to 28 months of age were studied for plasma volume, hemoglobin concentration, hematocrit value, total serum protein, serum albumin concentration, and bone marrow examination during the disease and the initial stage of clinical recovery. Treatment consisted of a diet containing reconstituted milk and supplemented biscuits supplying a total of 5 gm protein and 150 calories/kg body weight per day. Results showed a definite increase in both plasma and total blood volume early in the period of clinical recovery, and a simultaneous correction of the protein deficiency. Hemoglobin concentration in children with hypoplastic marrow changes dropped from 7.4 gm/100 ml on admission to 5.1 gm/100 ml during recovery. Total serum protein and albumin significantly increased during recovery from an average 4.1 gm/100 ml and 2.1 gm/100 ml respectively on admission to 6.9 gm/100 ml and 3.0 gm/100 ml after treatment. A non-significant increase in hemoglobin occurred with the start of recovery in children without hypoplastic bone marrow changes. The increase in plasma volume was 28.2%, which was larger than the increase in blood volume, 24.2%. Authors suggested that caution be used in giving blood transfusions to kwashiorkor patients to avoid overloading the circulation and inducing heart failure.

233. Samson, R. A., and Mouchacca, J. "Some interesting species of Emericella and Aspergillus from Egyptian desert soil." Antonie van Leeuwenhoek 40(1), 1974, pp 121-131.

Emericella desertorum Samson et Mouchacca spec. nov. is described and illustrated. It differs from the other Emericella species by the large ascospores with low crests. An Aspergillus conidial state was not observed. Additional information on the morphology and physiology of Emericella fruticulosa (Raper et Fennell) Malloch et Cain and Aspergillus egyptiacus Moubasher et Moustafa is given. The osmophilic and halophilic properties occurring within the genus Aspergillus are discussed. (Author's abstract)

234. Shousha, S., Kamel, K., and Admad, K. K. "Cytochemistry of polymorphonuclear neutrophil leukocytes in kwashiorkor." J. Egypt Med. Assoc. 57(7-8), 1974, pp 298-308.

Cytochemical studies were performed on the neutrophils of 37 children with active kwashiorkor, 20 with apparent recovery from it, 8 on follow-up a few months later and 18 normal control children. High activities of alkaline phosphatase, acid phosphatase, myeloperoxidase, glucose-6-phosphate dehydrogenase, lactic dehydrogenase and ribonucleic acid were noticed in the neutrophils from the kwashiorkor children at the height of the disease. The glycogen content in these cells was reduced. All cytologic activity estimations were normal on clinical cure. Lipids were within the normal ranges in all cases studied. (Authors' abstract)

235. Shukry, A. S., and Kamel, L. M. "Classification and epidemiology of protein-calorie malnutrition." Gaz. Egypt Paediatr. Assoc. 22(1), January 1974, pp 1-5.

Methods for assessment and classification of protein-calorie malnutrition are reviewed. Classifications included those depending on weight--Gomez, Wellcome, and Garrow methods--and those depending on length--Jelliffe, McLaren, and Waterlow methods. Other anthropometric measurements and ratios discussed are weight/head circumference; arm circumference/ age, / height, / head circumference; and chest/head circumference ratio. Clinical signs classification by Jelliffe and McLaren are also mentioned. Weight, length, and age are considered important for field surveys, with divisions into percentages of 10, whereas all physical signs are considered necessary in hospital cases. Surveys of PCM in preschool Egyptian children showed prevalence in 61.1-71% of urban and rural areas studied, with severe forms prevalent in 1.3-5.4% of children 0-6 years old.

236. Abdel-Kader, M. M., Abdel Salam, E., Massoud, S., and Ishaac, S. "Blood serum vitamin A and beta-carotene in marasmic Egyptian infants." Gaz. Egypt Paediatr. Assoc. 21(3), July 1973, pp 77-81.

Blood serum vitamin A, beta-carotene and proteins were estimated in 20 marasmic infants as well as 17 age matched normal controls. There was a significant reduction in the mean value of vitamin A and beta-carotene in the marasmic infants. Beta-carotene was completely absent in 75% of cases. The diminution of the vitamin A correlated with the duration of undernutrition, more than with the severity. Correlation coefficient with blood proteins showed the highest level with $alpha_2$ globulin. (Authors' abstract)

237. Abdel Salam, A. A. A., Ahmed, K. K., and Waslien, C. I. "Zinc and iron levels and their effect on growth in male subjects in an Egyptian oasis." Ain Shams Med. J. 24(6), November 1973, pp 449-451.

Serum iron and zinc, and heights and weights were measured in a group of male students from Kharga Oasis who were free of parasitic infestation. Correlations average serum iron to be 91.8 $\pm$ 1.74 ug/dl, serum zinc to average 78.11 $\pm$ 3.89 ug/dl, Hb. to average 14.08 $\pm$ 0.27 gm/dl, Hct. to average 41.75 $\pm$ 0.57 %, height to average 156.21 $\pm$ 1.28 cm, and average weight to be 46.99 $\pm$ 1.47 Kg. Iron, Hb, and Hct showed no significant correlation with growth, but serum Zinc showed a significant correlation with both height and weight at the 0.0001 level of significance.

238. Abd El-Salam, M. H., Hofi, A. A., Mahran, G. A., and Abdel-Hamid, L. B. "The use of spray-dried Buffalo milk as a potential infant food". J. Sci. Fd. Agric. 24, 1973, pp 1163-1170.

Four different formulae were used to modify buffalo's milk. These formulae shared the basic modifications of dilution with rennet whey, addition of sucrose and starch and fortifying with vitamins. Formula B differed from A by replacement of butter fat with liquid butter fat at 23°C; formula C one-third of its fat content was replaced with corn oil, while formula D was acidified with citric acid to pH 5.7 before processing. The chemical properties of formula A, B and C were nearly the same, while formula D differed considerably. The rate of peptic and tryptic digestion of the different formulae were comparable to spray-dried buffalo milk.

Milk powder with different formulae were stored under nitrogen for 6 months at room temperature. The samples were analysed every month for moisture, free fat, pH, solubility and wettability. Changes in these properties were slight, being in the same order in formula A, B and C; formula D showed slightly greater changes. Formula A and D showed good oxidative stability; formula B and C became oxidised in the fifth month. (Authors' abstract)

239. el-Naka, N. M. "A longitudinal study of the weaning of children in a rural community." J. Egypt Public Health Assoc. 48(5), 1973, pp 387-394.

This study was done in the village of Minshat El-Bakari on 100 children from age 1 year to time of complete weaning. Weaning practices and diets fed to children during early childhood were studied by monthly interviews with the mothers. Results showed 21.7% weaned between 12 and 15 months, 36.7% weaned between 15 and 18 months, 13.2% weaned from 18 to 21 months, and 16% weaned between 21 and 24 months, for a total of 88.6% of the children weaned at or by 24 months.

From age 0 to 6 months only sugared fluids were given to supplement breast milk. From 6 to 12 months, orange and tomato juice, vegetable soup, cooked legumes (medamis), sugared starch gruel (balouza), and milk pudding (mehalabia) were also given to some children. From 12 to 24 months, other starchy foods similar to the adult diet were added, but very few or no eggs or meat were given. Owning a milk animal did not mean that the family would use it's milk for the child's consumption because of the local belief that animal foods led to putrefaction in young children's abdomens.

240. Farghaly, A. M., Ezzat, A. A., and Shabana, M. B. "Effect of temperature and salinity changes on the blood characteristics of Tilapia zilli G. in Egyptian littoral lakes."

Several characteristics of the blood of Tilapi zilli G., which are fish found in Egyptian littoral lakes, were measured for the effects of temperature and salinity changes. Hemoglobin, creatinine, globulins, erythrocyte count, total leukocyte count, and agranular and granular leukocyte counts were among the characteristics studied. Results showed that increased water temperature increased most of the measured parameters. The exception was the agranular leucocyte count. Decreased water temperature depressed most parameters, and totally eliminated gamma globulins. High salinity produced increased concentrations of most parameters. Exceptions were alpha and beta globulins. High salinity also decreased blood coagulation time. Low salinity affected hemoglobin slightly, as well as total leucocyte count and erythrocyte count. Creatinine was stable under various conditions of temperature and salinity.

241. Gibriel, A. Y., and Abd-el Al, A. T. "Measurement of heat resistance parameters for spores isolated from canned products." J. Appl. Bacteriol. 36(2), June 1973, pp 321-327.

Spores of Bacillus subtilis, B. cereus, B. megaterium and B. pumilus were isolated from canned products. Heat resistance parameters were determined for these spores in distilled water and in different juices and brines. D values for B. subtilis, B.

cereus, B. megaterium and B. pumilus suspended in distilled water were 1.5, 0.8, 1.6, and 1.5 min at 212°F. The D value for B. stearothermophilus in water was 3.4 min at 248°F. Both D and Z values were reduced when spores of B. metaterium were heated in orange and mango juices. Similarly, spores of B. stearothermophilus were destroyed in okra brine faster than in water. Sodium chloride increased the thermal resistance of B. megaterium spores and this effect was independent of NaCl concentration of 2-15%. Pectin also conferred some protection against heat inactivation of spores of B. megaterium but sucrose had no effect. (Authors' abstract)

242. Hussein, L., Gabrial, G. N., and Morcos, S. R. "A possibility to improve the protein quality of Baladi bread by enrichment with synthetic amino acids." Z Ernaehrungswiss 12(3), September 1973, pp 201-208. Article and abstract in German. Dr. Dietrich Steinkopff Verlag.

The amino acid content of Baladi bread was established to determine the lack of certain essential amino acids. Measured by the "provisional pattern" of the FAO, the bread protein has an FAO protein score of 61.

The limited essential amino acids Lysine and Threonine were then added in free form to the Baladi bread diets where Baladi bread protein made up 10% of the total diet. The supplementation of the Baladi bread with .24% L-Lysinhydrochloride, 0.088% DL-Threonine and .50% DL-Methionine proved to be the best and increased the "protein efficiency ratio" of the protein to a value of 3.31 compared with a value of 1.28 for Baladi bread with methionine addition only. (Authors' abstract translated by Brigette Woolsey.)

243. Mahmoud, S. A., Abdel-Hafez, A. M., el-Sawy, M., and Hanafy, E. A. "Ribonucleic acid and lecithin-hydrolyzing bacteria in soil and rhizosphere of wheat and broad bean, cultivated in Egypt". Zentralbl. Bakteriol. (Naturwiss) 128(3), 1973, pp 196-202.

Ribonucleic acid and lecithin-hydolyzing bacteria found in Egyptian soils and in wheat and broad bean rhizosphere at different stages of growth were studied. RNA and lecithin decomposers showed higher densities at all stages of plant development in rhizosphere compared to soil. The seedling stage showed the highest stimulatory effect of rhizosphere on RNA hydrolysis, but this stimulatory effect existed at all plant growth stages. Broad bean rhizosphere produced higher densities of RNA hydrolysers than wheat rhizosphere, and densities in both rhizospheres increased at heading and flowering stages. Broad bean rhizosphere during seedling and flowering stages, and wheat rhizosphere during seedling stage, stimulated induction of lecithin-hydrolyzing bacteria.

244. Mahmoud, S. A., Abdel-Hafex, A. M., el-Sawy, M., and Hanafy, E. A. "Phytin hydrolyzing bacteria in soil and rhizosphere of wheat and broad bean in soils of Egypt". Zentralbl. Bakteriol. (Naturwiss) 128(5), pp 538-531.

Phytin decomposing bacteria found in Egyptian soils and in wheat and broad bean rhizosphere at different stages of growth were studied. Rhizosphere soil contained higher numbers of phytin decomposers than did non-rhizosphere soil of both plants and at all stages of growth, as indicated by high R/S ratios. Flowering and seed formation stages produced the greatest density of phytin hydrolyzers in both plant rhizospheres. The authors hypothesized that since these periods coincided with maximum phosphorus uptake by the plants, the phytin decomposers might have a role in supplying available phosphorus to the plants. Streptomyces and sporeformers were the predominant phytin hydrolyzers in both rhizospheres and at all stages of growth, particularly at maturity stage. This may be due to their ability to withstand unfavorable conditions such as those the Egyptian soils experience in summer.

245. Mahmoud, S. A., Abdel-Hafez, A. M., el-Sawy, M., and Hanafy, E. A. "Phenolphthalein diphosphate splitting bacteria in soil and rhizosphere of wheat and broad bean in soils of Egypt. Zentralbl. Bakteriol. (Naturwiss) 128(5), 1973, pp 524-527.

Phosphatase producing bacteria found in rhizosphere of Egyptian-grown wheat and of broad bean during different stages of growth and found in Egyptian soils were studied. Phosphatase producers have the ability to split phenolpthalein disphosphate by hydrolysis. Many organisms isolated from all the samples examined were phosphatase producers, but the densities of these bacteria were much higher at later stages of growth in broad bean rhizosphere than in wheat rhizophsere. Seedling, seed formation, and maturity stages showed a particularly high positive rhizosphere effect on the phosphatase producers, with G + ve rods and pleomorphic organisms prevailing among them in both plant rhizospheres during almost all stages of growth. Streptomyces and sporeformers were the predominant phosphatase producers only during the maturity stage of broad bean growth. Authors suggested that high densities of phosphatase producers possibly played a role in supplying plants with available phosphorus.

246. Mikhail, M. M., Patwardhan, V. N., and Waslien, C. I. "Plasma and red blood cell amino acids of Egyptian children suffering from protein-calorie malnutrition." Am. J. Clin. Nutr. 26(4), April 1973, pp 387-392.

Changes in plasma and RBC nonessential and essential amino acids and their ratios were studied in kwashiorkor patients 6 to 36 months old compared to controls to identify the best index to clinical status during recovery from protein-calorie malnutrition (PCM). A high protein diet was given to the patients. Fasting blood samples were taken on admission and during recovery 4 to 6 weeks later. The plasma glycine/valine and leucine (G/VL) ratio and the alanine/leucine (A/L) ratio in PCM patients were more than 2 times that of apparently healthy control children. However, one month into treatment, most values had returned to normal. Individual spot values for PCM patients showed normal G but significantly reduced A,V, and L values on admission, with increases to control values on recovery. PCM patients' mean admission RBC amino acid spot concentrations were significantly lower than controls. All amino acid spots were normal 6 to 17 months after discharge. Combining plasma and RBC amino acid values as a ratio may produce a good index of PCM and complete recovery from it.

247. Molleson, A. L., Moses, M. J., and Hackel, D. B. "Protein synthesis in pancreatic beta cells of the normal and diabetic Egyptian sand rat (Psammomys obesus). An autoradiographic study with the electron microscope." Am. J. Pathol. 73(2), November

1973, pp 495-512.

The pattern of protein synthesis was studied in pancreatic beta cells of Egyptian sand rats (Psammomys obesus). When fed a standard Purina Laboratory Chow diet instead of a leafy vegetable diet, these animals develop the characteristic signs of diabetes mellitus. Tritiated leucine was injected intravenously into pairs of sand rats (one on a vegetable diet and one on a Purina Laboratory Chow diet). Two pairs of animals were sacrificed at 5-, 20-, and 60-minute intervals, and pancreatic tissue was studied by electron microscopic autoradiography. At 5 minutes, the relative grain density was greater over the rough endoplasmic reticulum; at 20 minutes it was greatest over the Golgi complex and at 60 minutes, over the granules. There were no statistically significant differences in the relative grain densities over the rough endoplasmic reticulum, over the Golgi complex or over the secretion granules between the sand rats on the vegetable diet and Chow diet. These results show that in the early phase of the development of diabetes mellitus, the pattern of protein synthesis in the beta cells of the normal and diabetic sand rat comares with that of other endocrine glands. The tritiated leucine was apparently incorporated into the newly synthesized secretory product in the rough endoplasmic reticulum during the first 5 minutes. The formed product migrated to the Golgi complex at 20 minutes, and at 1 hour was seen mainly over the light granules. In addition, there was no obvious difference in this pattern of protein synthesis between the normal and diabetic sand rats. This suggests that the secretory product, considered to be mainly insulin, is produced in the usual or in increased amounts, but it is not fully utilized by the diabetic animal and remains in circulation, thus increasing the plasma insulin level. (Authors' abstract)

248. Morcos, S. R., Hegazi, S. M., and el-Damhougy, S. T. "Fermented foods in common use in Egypt. I. The nutritive value of kishk". J. Sci. Food Agric. 24(10), October 1973, pp 1153-1156.

Kishk in Egypt is a soup of meat and yoghurt with or without a small amount of rice and flour to thicken. It is served cooled with garnish of fried chopped onion. The nutrient contents as well as the amino acid pattern of kishk samples were determined. The level of most of the amino acids were also estimated. High figures for digestibility, biological value and net protein utilization of kishk were obtained. The use of kishk in school feeding programmes and in military canteens as a high protein food is discussed. (Authors' abstract)

249. Morcos, S. R., Hegazi, S. M., and el-Dumhougy, S. T. "Fermented foods of common use in Egypt. IV. The chemical composition of bouza and its ingredients". J. Sci. Food Agric. 24(10), October 1973, pp 1157-1161.

Bouza in Egypt is a drink made by fermenting balady bread with a little sugar in water for a week or ten days. The nutrient content of different samples of bouza, either prepared in the laboratory or brought from the local market, were determined and compared with the individual ingredients.

Changes that occur in the pH values, diastatic power, alcohol and nutrient content of bouza when fermented for 24, 48 and 72 h were also studied. (Authors' abstract)

250. Rifaat, M. A., Wishahy, A. G., Sadek, M. S., el-Khalek, K. A., and Munir, A. M. "A case of congenital toxoplasmosis in Egypt." J. Trop. Med. Hyg. 76(10), October 1973, pp 255-256.

A male child one and a half years old was seen who was microcephalic, mentally retarded, and severely marasmic. Liver function tests showed reduction in the total serum proteins with a reversed albumin/globulin ratio. The fundus had an extensive punched out central chorioretinal lesion with a band of fibrous tissue in the vitreous. The chorioretinal lesion was typical of toxoplasmosis, but the vitreous fibrous band was not common. Treatment was given to the mother and child for six weeks, and a multivitamin preparation was given to the child for the marasmus. General improvement and weight gain occurred after two weeks, but the child died three weeks later from severe gastroenteritis.

251. Said, A., el-Hawary, F. S., Sakr, R., Abdel Khalek, M. K., and Ibrahim, A. M. "Protein-calorie malnutrition in Egypt. I. Immunoelectrophoretic studies on urinary proteins." Am. J. Clin. Nutr. 26(12), December 1973, pp 1355-1359.

The pattern of urine proteins in 170 malnourished young children were studied by immunoelectrophoresis. Three clinical groups were formed: Group A, 40 cases of edematous malnutrition; Group B, 104 marasmic cases; Group C, 26 marasmic kwashiorkor cases. 24 healthy infants were controls, and their urine showed 0-30 mg total proteins/100 ml urine with occasional traces of albumin. Results obtained in mild kwashiorkor showed a faint albumin arc; with moderate cases, albuminuria was accompanied by other proteins including alpha-1 antitrypsin, ceruloplasmin, transferrin, and/or IgG. With severe kwashiorkor a much larger number of protein components were found in urine, almost matching in quantity that of serum. Nutritional edema cases showed only a faint albuminuria. Second grade marasmus showed faint areas of mainly albumin with transferrin and IgG. In 3rd grade marasmus, a variable pattern ranging from albumin and IgG arcs only, to arcs of several proteins was found. Marasmic kwashiorkor patients showed a large number of protein components in urine. Overall, early disease stages selectively affected mainly albumin, with nonselectivity increasing with severity. With recovery from protein-calorie malnutrition, proteinuria was reversible.

252. Shukry, A. S., Labib, F. M., and Kamel, L. M. "Assessment of the health and nutritional standards of infants and preschool children in high density Cairo community." Gaz. Egypt Paediatr. Assoc. 21(3), July 1973, pp 47-56.

A field survey was carried out in a high density Cairo community to assess the health and nutrition status of preschool children through a randomly selected sample of 695 children aged 0 - 6 years. The children were subjected to a full clinical examination, including anthropometric measurements, haemoglobin determination, examination of urine and stools for parasites and a thorough medical history. The results obtained pointed to the high prevalence of preventable infectious diseases and deficiency states. (Adapted from authors' abstract)

253. Smith, F. R., Goodman, D. S., Zaklama, M. S., Gavr, M. K., el-Maraghy, S., and Patwardhan, V. N. "Serum vitamin A, retinol-binding protein, and prealbumin concentrations in protein-calorie malnutrition. I. A functional defect in hepatic retinol release." Am. J. Clin. Nutr. 26(9), September 1973, pp 973-981.

Thirty-three children with varying degrees of PCM were compared with fifteen healthy children from the same socioeconomic background for serum retinol-binding protein (RBP), prealbumin (PA), serum vitamin A and carotenoids, as well as total serum protein and albumin concentrations, and renal status by way of urine osmolarity. Pretreatment concentrations of vitamin A, RBP, and PA in PCM patients were generally significantly lower than mean values of the control group. All serum bilirubin concentrations were within normal limits. Kwashiorkor patients showed a mean hepatic vitamin A level of 21 ug/g liver tissue compared to marasmic kwashiorkor patients with 14 ug/g, and one marasmic patient with 108 ug/g. All patients except the kwashiorkor children who died (3 children) or did poorly (1 child) showed an increase in vitamin A, RBP, and PA concentration with therapy. The three concentrations were highly correlated. Nutritional status regarding dietary protein and calories may strongly influence vitamin A metabolism via that of RBP and PA.

254. Waslien, C. I., Farid, Z., and Darby, W. J. "The malnutrition of parasitism in Egypt." South Med. J. 66(1), January 1973, pp 47-50.

Blood and nutrient losses in Egyptian patients infested with hookworm and/or Bilharzia, as well as complications from Salmonella infections, are presented. Ancylostoma duodenale was identified as the probable main cause of iron deficiency anemia in Egyptian farmers, losses averaging 29 ml of blood/day, or 6 mg iron/day. The complications from Schistosoma mansoni infections included a mean colonic daily blood loss of 13 ml, or 4 mg iron/day. Schistosoma hematobium infection resulted in a mean daily urinary loss of 23 ml blood and 7 mg. iron. In addition, bilharzial polyposis of the colon produced hypo-proteinemia; patients lost up to 110 ml plasma, equal to 2.2 gm albumin daily. Proteinuria also accounted for great loss of albumin. Trace elements or vitamins, such as zinc and vitamin A, which are tightly bound to albumin, were also lost. Absorptive functions were relatively intact. Home diets of patients were low in calcium and vitamin A, but not in calories, protein, iron, B vitamins, and vitamin C. Iron and vitamin A supplementation may be advisable; iron because of low bioavailability due to high phytate intake.

255. Zakhra, M. K. "Alteration of the economic coefficient as a result of aerobic cultivation of baker's yeast on Egyptian cane molasses." Prikl. Biokhim. Mikrobiol. 9(2), March-April 1973, pp 169-173. (Article in Russian)

Variations of the economic coefficient of the growth of yeast Saccharomyces cerevisiae during aerobic cultivation on the nutrient medium with Egyptian cane molasses were investigated in eleven successive generations. The economic coefficient of the yeast growth averaged 82.33% in the first two generations, 85.40% in the next five generations, and 96.32% in the final four generations, ranging from 87.62 to 106.97%. Following the main growth period during 2 hour after-fermentation without an addition of molasses and salts, the yeast yield increased by 8.4 g and the consumption of dry substances from the medium reached 6.4g. The economic coefficient of the growth during this after-fermentation was 131%. The yeast showed an invariably stable and high baking strength of 42 to 50 min. upon an increase of the economic coefficient of the yeast growth and the number of successive generations on the nutrient medium with Egyptian cane molasses. (Author's abstract)

256. Zaklama, M. S., Gabr, M. K., el-Maraghy, S., and Patwardhan, V. N. "Serum vitamin A in protein-calorie malnutrition." Am. J. Clin. Nutr. 26(11), November 1973, pp 1202-1206.

Preschool Cairo children from a low socioeconomic background were tested for serum retinol, carotenoids, total protein, and albumin before and during treatment with a high protein diet which contained no vitamin A or its precursors. A control group of 75 apparently healthy children matched for age and background were compared with 111 cases of kwashiorkor and 26 cases of marasmus.

The average serum protein levels before treatment were lower in kwashiorkor than those of marasmic children, which were lower than those of apparently healthy children. Average pretreatment serum retinol level was lower in kwashiorkor than in marasmus, which averaged similar to that in controls. Treatment increased serum retinol significantly in kwashiorkor in two weeks and maintained the level at 21 ug/dl thereafter; treatment of marasmic cases did not result in significant changes in serum retinol, total protein or albumin. The authors suggest serum carrier protein amounts may determine retinol levels in protein-calorie malnutrition.

257. Zawahry, M. E. "Pellagra: notes and comments." Int. J. Dermatol. 12(3), May-June 1973, pp 158-162.

The etiology, symptoms, clinical signs and histopathology of pellagra (nicotinic acid deficiency) are reviewed. The incidence in Egyptian patients in Cairo was reported at 1.66% in all ages, 1.25% in adults, and 2.5% in children. A study of pellagra in 50 Egyptian patients with varying degrees of malnutrition from a population of 3000 people with different skin diseases revealed four patients with pellagra, an incidence of 0.2%. Secondary GI tract inflammation produced diarrhea. Pellagra was the most common dermatosis found among people suffering from parasites. Daily doses of 500 mg of nicotinic acid until symptoms subsided were recommended, to be followed by a maintenance dose.

258. Abdin, Z. H., Lutfi, S. H., Miniawa, L., el-Fil, S., Abbsas, A., and Zaki, A. "Field studies on school children in rural and urban areas in Egypt." J. Egypt Med. Assoc. 55(7), 1972, pp 542-550.

Five-hundred school children between 6 and 12 years of age were measured in Ein el Sera urban district and in Kafrit Nassar rural village as follows: 1) growth and nutrition were measured by height, weight, and hemoglobin; 2) streptococcal disease incidence was assessed by throat swab and culture and grouping of beta hemolytic strains and A.S.O.T. measures; 3) history and clinical exams gauged incidence of other ailments; 4) urine and stool examinations were used to measure parasite incidence. Both areas were of moderate socio-economic status.

Results showed that mean weight and height were lower in rural children. Higher frequency and severity of anemia, higher icidence of intestinal and urinary parasites, and more diarrheal episodes

(36%) occurred in rural children. Urban children experienced much more common streptococcal disease with 60% of them having repeated sore throats. Both groups ate diets high in bread and beans and low in meat, with meat even more scarce in the rural population.

259. El-Hawary, M. F., Sakr, R., Abdel-Hkalek, Samuel, S., and Abdin, M. A. "Studies on serum and liver proteins and enzymes in kwashiorkor in Egypt." J. Egypt Med. Assoc. 55(2), 1972, pp 121-136.

Eleven kwashiorkor patients, 27 to 40 months of age, were studied with mild, moderate, or severe PEM. Five control children aged 6 to 36 months were also evaluated. Measurements included serum and liver total proteins and the essential enzymes aldolase, lactic dehydrogenase, and alkaline and acid phosphatases. Differential results were analyzed in view of the clinical picture and disease duration. Serum total proteins in kwashiorkor patients ranged from 3 to 6 gm%, representing a reduction of from 15 to 57% compared to controls. Total liver protein were even more reduced, at 4.5 to 16.2 gm%, a 24 to 78% reduction compared to controls. Liver aldholase activity was reduced below lowest-normal range in 72.7% of cases, and serum aldolase activity was elevated higher than the highest-normal range in 63.6% of cases. Serum lactic dehydrogenase activity was variable but liver lactic dehydrogenase was low in 90.0% of kwashiorkor subjects. Serum alkaline phosphatase showed no gross variation from normal, and liver alkaline phosphatase in kwashiorkor was normal with mild, higher with moderate, and low with severe kwashiorkor. Serum acid phosphatase varied, but liver acid phosphatase was low in 82% of cases with kwashiorkor.

260. El-Shobaki, F. A., El-Hawary, M. F., Morcos, S. R., Abdelkhalek, M. K., El-Zawahry, K., and Sakr, R. "Iron metabolism in Egyptian infants with protein-calorie deficiency". Br. J. Nutr. 28(1), July 1972, pp 81-89.

1. Studies were made of iron absorption in 85 infants suffering from protein-calorie deficiency (kwashiorkor and marasmus) and in 8 infants suffering from Fe-deficiency anaemia; 21 healthy infants were controls. Factors affecting absorption--concentration of serum total protein and its fractions; serum Fe; transferrin (as indicated by total Fe-binding capacity) and its percentage saturation; blood haemoglobin; total blood Fe; and the state of Fe stores in the liver--were also investigated. Four infants suffering from severe kwashiorkor were selected for follow-up and were given a high-protein diet and blood transfusions.
2. Alimentary iron absorption was retarded in infants with protein-calorie deficiency. Total serum proteins and its fractions were reduced. Blood haemoglobin, total blood Fe, serum Fe and total Fe-binding capacity were also decreased but the percentage of transferrin saturation was increased. Liver protein per g wet weight of liver were decreased, whereas liver non-haem Fe was increased. The extent of these changes varied according to the clinical condition.
3. Infants with Fe-deficiency anaemia had no change in liver protein concentrations or total serum proteins, except for a slight increase in the B-globulin fraction of the latter. Blood haemoglobin and total Fe were reduced, whereas serum Fe-binding capacity was raised and percentage of transferrin saturation was lowered. A fall in liver non-haem Fe concentration was observed.

4. After giving a high-protein diet to infants with severe kwashiorkor, the characteristic anaemia associated with protein-calorie deficiency changed and the general manifestation of Fe-deficiency anaemia emerged. After blood transfusion, these infants showed a marked clinical improvement. (Authors' abstract)

261. Ghoniem, N., Abdel-Hafiz, Y. Z., Abdel-Hady, H. "Occurrence of pathogenic microorganisms in Egyptian domestic rabbits." Dtsch. Tieraerztl. Wochenschr. 79(15), August 1, 1972, pp 370-371. Article in German, Schaper Verlag Hannover, Frg.

One-hundred slaughtered, apparently healthy rabbits were bacteriologically examined for pathogenic microorganisms. From lung samples, Diplococcus pneumoniae and Streptococcus pyogenes were the most frequent organisms while Pseudomonas aeruginosa, Escherichia coli and Corynebacterium pyogenes were less frequent. Corynebacterium pyogenes was isolated from both heart blood and liver samples. Salmonella typhimurium was isolated from the gall-bladder in a percentage of 3%. (Authors' abstract in English)

262. Hamada, G., and Rida, A. "Orthopaedics and orthopaedic diseases in ancient and modern Egypt." Clin. Orthop. 89, 1972, pp 253-268.

Mummies, and ancient iconography and papyri were used as sources for ancient information. Imhotep was credited with the first actual practice of medicine. Houses of life, attached to temples, were centers of medical learning. Skeletons revealed that fractures were extremely common, particularly in the left ulna and the forearm in general. Spinal trauma, possibly from falls at construction sites, were common. Splints and casts were used to fix fractures. Reduction for dislocated shoulders were used. Surgical instruments were used. The Edwin-Smith medical test papyrus was extensively quoated and discussed, with several cases described in the paper. These cases included a mandibular dislocation, dislocation, crushing, and sprain of cervical vertebrae, and a clavicle fracture. Advanced equinus of the left foot in Pharoah Siptah, tuberculous kyphotic hunchback from Pott's disease, achondroplastic dwarfism, pyogenic and osteo-arthritis and osteomyelitis, syphilis, gout, rickets, and bone tumors were all discussed.

263. Hanafy, M. M., Morsey, M. R., Seddick, Y., Habib, Y. A., and el-Lozy, M. "Maternal nutrition and lactation performance: a study in urban Alexandria." J. Trop. Pediatr. 18(3), September 1972, pp 187-191.

In a cross-sectional study of infants aged from birth to 12 months, the authors compared breast milk quantity and quality between 24 apparently healthy and 17 malnourished mothers, and correlated these parameters with the mothers' and childrens' nutritional status. Maternal nutritional status was measured according to a NSIM (Nutritional State Index of Mother), including 4 features: arm circumference, weight, serum albumin, and urea N/creatinine N. Similarly, an NSII (Nutritional State Index of the Infant) took into account weight, arm circumference, and serum albumin. Infants of apparently healthy mothers grew well through 4 months when growth plateaued, similar to the pattern found in developed countries. Malnourished mothers' milk contained 15% less protein, and 7% less calories, than that of healthy mothers. In addition, malnourished mothers produced an average 22% lower volume of milk.

NSIM correlated closely with the amount of milk and its proximate constituents produced per day. Most infants exhibited a suboptimal nutritional state. A high correlation was seen between amount of milk and proximate constituents per day, and NSII, but not between NSII and the concentration of constituents. NSII and NSIM correlated highly. Authors thought test feeding a relatively valuable method of assessing maternal lactational performance.

264. Hegazi, S. M., and Salem, S. A. "Amino acid pattern of the Egyptian apricot fruits (Hamawy)". J. Sci. Food Agric. 23(4), April 1972, pp 497-499.

Apricot fruits were subjected to acid hydrolysis and the amino acids were separated and quantitatively determined by paper chromatography. The analysis revealed the presence of 19 amino acids, predominantly glutamic acid, aspartic acid, histidine, arginine and tyrosine. The results also demonstrated that the concentrations of cystine, methionine and hydroxyproline were relatively small. (Authors' abstract)

265. Moubasher, A. H., Elnaghy, M. A., and Abdel-Hafez, S. I. "Studies on the fungus flora of three grains in Egypt". Mycopathol. Mycol. Appl. 47(3), August 7, 1972, pp 261-274.

In wheat, corn and sorghum grains, 26 genera and 77 species including 16 of Aspergillus and 21 of Penicillium were identified. In grain samples adjusted to various moisture levels (up to 18.8% on a dry-weight basis) and stored 4 months at 8, 20 and 30°C, seed-borne fungi were monthly identified and counted, and the germinability of the grains was tested. In control samples (moisture content 7.1-8.2%) temperature had no effect on fungal counts and on percentage germination. With the rise of temperature and moisture content fungal counts markedly increased and germinability declined. Fungi dominant in one or more of the experiments, included 8 species of Asperigillus, 6 of Penicillium, 2 of Fusarium and 1 each of Alternaria and Curvularia. The order of dominance of these fungi varied according to type of grain, length of storage and treatment. A. niger was the dominant organism in the control samples of the three grains. It could grow successfully at high moisture contents, but above 15%, it was usually overgrown by other fungi. In wheat P. citrinum and A. sydowii, in corn P. citronum and A. terreus, and in sorghum A. Terreus and A. niger were the dominant fungi at moisture contents above 15% after 4 months storage at 30°C. When stored at 80°C, Penicillium species tended to predominante over other fungi in grains with high moisture contents. In surface-sterilized grains adjusted to 15% moisture content, innoculated with 6 dominant fungi separately and incubated at 30°C, A. niger, P. citrinum and P. variabile caused severe deterioration in the three grains: A. ochraceus in wheat only and E. moniliforme in wheat and corn; C. spicifer was slightly injurious to the three grains. (Authors' abstract)

266. Naguib, K., and Shouman, M. T. "Identification and typing of clostridia in raw milk in Egypt." J. Appl. Bacteriol. 35(4), December 1972, pp 525-530.

Three spp. of clostridia were isolated from samples of raw cow and buffalo milk obtained near Cairo. Of 150 isolates of anaerobes, 108 were Clostridium perfringens, 30 were Cl. butyricum, and 12 were Cl. sporogenes. The Cl. perfringens isolates comprised 100 nonhaemolytic and 8 pathogenic haemolytic strains. The latter strains typed by neutralization tests were of type A. Fifteen of the nonhaemolytic strains were also of type A; of these, 6 strains produced heat resistant spores nd 9 strains produced heat susceptible spores. Feeding mice with these 15 nonhaemolytic strains caused marked reduction in intestinal passage time. (Authors' abstract)

267. Shukry, A. S., Eisa, E. A., Fayad, I. M., and Salem, S. I. "Phosphorylase activity in liver and muscle tissue in protein calorie malnutrition." J. Trop. Med. Hyg. 75(12), December 1972, pp 240-245.

Biopsy specimens were used to study activity of the phosphorylase enzyme in 105 subjects' livers and in 5 subjects' muscle tissue. All subjects were children suffering from varying grades of PEM. Protein concentration of both tissues was decreased, particularly with severe PEM; intensity and duration of calorie restriction were seen as determining factors in extent of loss of liver protein, and the level of liver protein was thus used as an index of severity of PEM. Liver glycogen showed a significant increase paralleling the degree of severity of kwashiorkor. Half of the marasmic cases had decreased liver glycogen. The 5 muscle biopsy specimens showed almost normal levels of glycogen. Reduction of liver phosphorylase activity in kwashiorkor cases paralleled the severity of PEM, but in marasmus the reduction was evident only when expressed as units/g tissue. The muscle phosphorylase activity was also significantly reduced in PEM children. In PEM, the inactive form of phosphorylase may be present in liver and muscle, causing glycogen buildup in liver and low fasting blood sugar.

268. Abd-Rabbo, H., Hillal, G., and El-Gohary "Chemotherapy of acute intestinal and extra-intestinal amoebiasis with nitro-imidazole." J. Trop. Med. Hyg. 74(3), March 1971, pp 62-65.

Thirty-five patients with acute amoebiasis ranging in age from three to 60 years of age were studied for their response to a new nitro-imidazole derivative known as BT 985. Patients were given medicine orally. Stool examinations, blood haemograms, skiagrams, and liver function tests were done before and after treatment. Four subgroups were formed on the basis of magnitude, frequency, and duration of treatment with tablets. Patients showed rapid clinical improvement in urgent symptoms, such as colic and abdominal pains. In cases with hepatic involvement, swelling, local pain and tenderness diminished, showing good response to the nitro-imidazole. Only minor side effects were noted: nausea and vomiting in two cases; and skin rash, headache, and abdominal colic in one case each. Authors concluded that a 10 to 14 days treatment seemed the most effective schedule in adults dosed at 250 mg 2 to 3 times per day. The amoeba disappeared from the stools by the third to the seventh day of treatment, with cessation of the blood and mucous passage also.

269. Coble, F. D., Bardin, C. W., Ross, G. T., and Darby, W. T. "Studies of endocrine function in boys with retarded growth, delayed sexual maturation and zinc deficiency." J. Clin. Endocr. 32, 1971, pp 361-367.

Eighteen boys with retarded growth and delayed sexual maturation and 8 normally developed boys from the rural Nile Valley were studied for pituitary and gonadal function. Both groups of boys had iron and zinc deficiencies, hepatosplenomegaly, and various parasites. Hypogonadotropism was indicated in the "retarded" boys by lowered plasma LH levels. Both groups had a normal increment in plasma testosterone during HCG treatment in only 75% of their members, and both groups were insulin sensitive. An appropriate rise in plasma growth hormone during insulin hypoglycemia occured in only half of the "normal" boys and in less than one quarter of the "retarded" boys. The authors concluded that the boys' delayed development could not be attributed solely to zinc deficiency in light of the results and associated socioeconomic conditions.

270. El-Shabrawy, Ali M. "Effects of nutrition education on the dietary patterns of two socio-economic groups of pregnant females in Dakahlia Governorate (Egypt)." J. Egypt Med. Assoc. 54(11), 1971, pp 829-840.

583 pregnant women either under obstetric care at University Hospital or the Maternal and Child Welfare Centre at Mansoura were given interviews concerning habitual diets during pregnancy as well as serving size, food types, meal and snack frequency, and cooking methods. Two socio-economic levels were studied: satisfactory and non-satisfactory. Each level was divided into a nutrition education group or a non-education group. Results indicated faulty dietary habits of a large segment of subjects. Nutrition education resulted in improving intakes of calcium, animal protein, iron (all were satisfactory for iron intake), riboflavin, ascorbic acid (all were still below recommended allowances for vitamin C) and vitamin A. Adding milk, skimmed cheese, or low-cost dry milk solids can remedy the low intakes of all above but for vitamin C. Special efforts in nutrition education are necessary for improving vitamin C intake.

271. Guirgis, S. S. "The subgenus Persicargas (Ixodoidea, Argasidae, Argas). II Ecology and seasonal dynamics of A. (P.) arboreus Kaiser, Hoogstraal & Kohls in Egypt." J. Med. Entomol. 8(4), October 30, 1971, pp 407-414.

Argas (Persicargas) arboreus Kaiser, Hoogstraal & Kohls forms dense populations on trees supporting rookeries of the Cattle Egret, Bubulcus i. ibis (Linnaeus) in the Nile Delta and Valley and nearby oases. Ticks bred in spring and summer during the egret nesting season. At this time, larvae and nymphs were the most abundant stages. When birds abandoned the rookery in autumn, larvae and first-instar nymphs disappeared. Later nymphal instars survived the winter. Adults constituted the major part of the winter population, but no oviposition occurred. The life cycle of ticks reared experimentally under outdoor conditions took 2-3 months in Cairo area summer weather. In winter oviposition ceased, fed larvae failed to molt, and nymphal premolting periods increased significantly. There were 2-4 nymphal instars. Males passed through fewer instars than females before the final molt. Survival periods for each developmental stage were determined. Survival of the tick population depends on the prompt return of host birds to their regular breeding colony in the spring. (Author's abstract)

272. Hedayat, S., Ani, P. A., and Kamali, P. "Influences of economic status and certain maternal factors on birth heights." J. Trop.

Pediatr. 17(4), December 1971, pp 163-167. (Environ. Child Health)

Serum vitamin A of 36 Egyptian women at delivery and in their respective foetuses was determined. 24 non-pregnant women attending the same hospital at the time of investigation were used as controls. Foetal serum vitamin A was always lower than the maternal values, but the difference was not statistically significant.

No sex-difference existed between male and female foetuses. No significant difference in serum vitamin A level in mothers and non-pregnant women was observed. The extent of transfer of vitamin A across the placenta seems to depend on the vitamin content of maternal blood, as there was a highly significant correlation between maternal serum vitamin A and their corresponding foetal values. The results were discussed and compared with those of other workers. (Authors' abstract)

273. Karawya, M. S., Balbaa, S. I., and Hifnawy, M. S. "Peel oils of different types of Citrus sinesis L. and C. aurantium L. growing in Egypt". J. Pharm. Sci. 60(3), March 1971, pp 381-386.

A comparative chromatographic study including column chromatography, TLC and GLC was carried out on the peel essential oils (cold-pressed and steam-distilled) of different types and varieties of Citrus sinensis L. and C. aurantium L. growing in Egypt. A mineral oil capillary column was successfully employed in the GLC analysis of these cells. IR patterns of the oils were used in the differentiation between the cold-pressed and steam-distilled oils. (Authors' abstract)

274. Khalifa, A. S., Mourad, K. A., Khattab, A. K., Sallam, M. S., and Hosny, S. "Repeated doses of vitamin D in rickets." J. Trop. Med. Hyg. 74(3), March 1971, pp 66-69.

Twenty male and 14 female cases of active rickets between six months and three years of age were studied clinically and various serum laboratory tests were done before and after therapy. Therapy included 600,000 units of vitamin D given in three doses, 15 days apart, along with a good diet and antibiotics when required. All cases were underweight, with delayed dentition and delayed walking present in 84% of cases. Other signs of active rickets were present in varying percentages of cases. Serum sodium, potassium and calcium did not vary significantly from normal. Sodium decreased temporarily after the second dose, and calcium decreased temporarily after the first dose of vitamin D. Serum phosphorus, which was initially low, decreased during therapy and returned to within normal values after the final dose of vitamin D. Potassium level did not vary significantly during treatment, but alkaline phosphatase, which was significantly elevated prior to treatment, increased more during treatment and gradually decreased to normal. Although within normal limits prior to and at the start of vitamin therapy, total serum proteins experienced a component change with treatment, with albumin rising and gamma globulin falling, as well as a drop in total protein levels.

275. Moawad, H. "Occurrence of yeasts in U.A.R. soils". Zentralbl. Bakteriol. (Naturwiss) 126(3), 1971, pp 280-285.

The quantitative and qualitative distribution of soil yeasts has been investigated in 65 soil samples, collected from different parts of Egypt.

Yeasts were found in 31 (47.7%) of the samples. The Lower Egypt soils contained the highest number of yeasts (66--4660/g soil), whereas in Upper Egypt soils they were rare. In the soils of the Oases and the north Coast and desert soils, yeasts were detected in 61.1 and 41.2% of the samples, respectively, though in lower number (20-4000/g) than in Lower Egypt.

From the samples, 72 strains were isolated and identified. Asparagenous yeasts were the most common, representing 79.3% of the total isolates. They were identified as Rhodotorula glutinis (30.6%), Cryplococcus allidus (26.4%), Crypt difflucus (8.3%), Torulopsis aeria (7.0%), and Torulopsis famala (7.0%).

15.1% of the isolates were spore-forming yeasts, over half of them were Dygolipmyers tetrasporus; Sacharamyers and Dehryomyers sp. were rare, represented only by one isolated from the Lower Egypt and Oases soils, respectively. Only 5.5% of the isolates were yeast-like fungi of which three were Pullularia pullulans and one was Endomyers sp. (Author's abstract)

276. Rihan, Z. E., and Lebshtein, A. K. "Control of diabetes in different socio-economic groups." J. Egypt Public Health Assoc. 46(4), 1971, pp 265-272.

Control of diabetes was studied in two different socio-economic groups of patients. The first group included patients who were treated at Maadi Armed Forces Hospital and consisted of officers, their families and citizens who could afford an expensive line of treatment. The second group included an industrial population, mainly laborers who were treated freely at an outpatient diabetes clinic of the Insurance Health Organization.

More successful control of diabetes was achieved in the former group although the medical care, laboratory, therapeutic tools and health education were the same for both groups.

A study of the dietary pattern and one day diet by the questionnaire method was done for both groups. The results showed that success in the control of diabetes depends on the co-operation of the patient in following the prescribed diet rather than supplying him with drugs.

The work presented emphasizes the value and the need for an extensive program of nutrition and health education specially for paricuts of low socio-economic standard. (Authors' abstract)

277. Sakr, A. H., el-Hawary, M. F., Zawahry, K., Abul-Hassan, A. M., and Ibrahim, A. M. "Biochemical studies on early and late vitamin D - deficiency rickets in Egyptian infants and children." J. Egypt Med. Assoc. 54(1), 1971, pp 1-16.

50 children with vitamin D deficiency rickets were studied for serum total proteins and their fractions, selected serum and urine minerals and enzymes, and fasting blood sugar. Two clinical groups were formed: Group A, 20 patients, 7 months to 2 years old, with infantile vit. D deficiency rickets, and Group B, 30 patients, 3 to 5 years old, with late infantile rickets. Serum proteins and their electrophoretically separated fractions in Group A showed no

striking variations from controls, but in Group B showed certain changes. These included a 26.7% reduction in serum total proteins, a 46.4% reduction in serum albumin, and a resulting derease in the albumin/globulin ratio. Vit. D therapy resulted in clinical cure in 8 - 10 weeks with subsequent protein pattern normalization. Serum and urine mineral deviations included variable pattern decrements in sodium, potassium, and calcium, with a lowered serum and raised urine phosphorous. Calcium urinary output was low. Normal values for serum iron and iron binding capacity was shown in 70% of cases. Some selected serum enzymes which were normal for Group A were increased for Group B. Reduced glutathione in blood was lowered in many long duration cases but not glucose utilization.

278. Zayed, M. N., Saber, M. S., Abd-e; -Malek, Y., and Monib, M. "Antibacterial substances in dry residues of certain higher Egyptian plants". Zentralbl. Bakteriol. (Naturwiss) 126(6), 1971, pp 615-629.

Aqueous, alcohol and ether extracts of the dry residues of 27 Egyptian higher plants were prepared and bio-assayed by the hole method for the presence of antibacterial substances against 40 soil test micro-organisms.

Of the aqueous extracts, only those of tomato tops, eggplant tops and guava leaves showed antibacterial activity. Of the alcohol extracts, 81% exerted inhibitory activity--the non-active extracts being those of dry leaves of mango, watermelon, sugar-cane, banana and clover. Ether appears to be the best solvent, since all ether extracts, except that of sugar-cane, contained antibacterial agents.

Gram-positive bacteria were more sensitive to the antibacterial effect of the plant extracts than gram-negative ones. Strains of Lihizobium, Azolobacter, Staphylococcus, Bacillus and Mycobacterium were susceptible to the antibacterial action of the plant extracts, while E. coli was resistant to them.

The antibacterial agent tomatin was separated only from dry tomato tops, while quereitin was found in onion peels, as well as in dry apple and guava leaves. Phloretin was separated from apple leaves and was present in the other plants of Rosaceae tested, i.e., peach, almond, apricot and pear. (Authors' abstract)

279. Hanfy, M. M., Seddik, Y., and Aref, M. K. "Formulation of a protein-rich vegetable mixture for prevention of protein-calorie malnutrition". J. Sci. Food Agric. 21(1), January 1970, pp 9-12.

Several mixtures of crushed decorticated groundnuts (Arachis hypogaea), line-roasted chickpea (Cicer arietinum) and the white dregs of sesame (Sesamum indicum) are quantitatively and qualitatively compared with 'standard' proteins.

Using a selection of both children and adults, a blend ratio 3:2:1 (groundnut-chickpea-sesame) was selected as being fully palatable and readily acceptable to Egyptian adults and children. (Authors' abstract)

280. Labib, M. A., Moussa, A. H., Shalash, B. A., and el-Antably "Assessment of the relation between soft cataract and deficiency of vitamins in U.A.R." Bull. Ophthalmol. Soc. Egypt 63(67), 1970, pp 305-314.

Of 115 Egyptian patients having different vitamin deficiency disorders, 90% of cases were males, from 7 to 16 years of age. An assessment of the relation between soft cataract and the main vitamin deficiency disorders in U.A.R. suggested a real association between cataract production and ariboflavinosis, pellagra, and vitamin D deficiency. However, a similar relation between vitamin A deficiency and cataract production was not seen.

281. Oparin, I. A., and Oparina, N. V. "Relationship between the natural content of cobalt in food products and incidence of parapernicious anemia among the population of the Aswan Basin." Gig. Sanit. 35(3), March 1970, pp 111-113. (Article in Russian).

595 samples of major grain and other food crops from all economic and geographic zones of Egypt were analyzed for cobalt content. The average food cobalt concentrations in the Awan Plain regions were 3 to 4 times lower than that in foods from other areas of Egypt. Average concentrations for each food analyzed in the other regions were close to one another. The Aswan valley also has the greatest incidence of pernicious anemia, with a rate from 1952 to 1962 of 1:1288 population vs. that in villages in Northern areas of 1:34,700 people. An inverse relationship was calculated between the cobalt content in food products and incidence of megaloblastic (parapernicious) anemia in the Aswan Basin.

282. White, H. S. "Man and his diet." Arch. Environ. Health 20(1), January 1970, pp 84-87.

Man's diet throughout history has been dependent on his environment. The early civilizations of Egypt and Mesopotamia were dependent on irrigated agriculture, and trade developed between areas with disparate food-producing ability. Wheat and bread were essential to the Roman empire, and the breakdown in that empire was a result of the breakdown in the food supply due to usage of Italian land as pasture land. The search for spices played a major role in European exploration and colonization. The eastern American cities were populated by Irish fleeing the 1822 potato famine. Adequate nutrition potentiates the growth of populations. Scientific advances have taken place in nutritional treatment of inborn errors of metabolism, and there has been an increase in the incidence of degenerative diseases which are linked to bad nutritional habits. Future directions of food production research, including agriculture and food production from petroleum and protein derived from human waste, are mentioned.

283. Zaki, O. A., and Ghoniem, N. A. "The yeast flora of Egyptian butter." Mykosen 13(2), February 1970, pp 97-101.

200 samples of cooking butter randomly obtained from Egyptian markets were examined within one hour of collection for yeast flora. Morphological and physiological characters of yeast formed the basis of categorization, with rice agar used for studying morphological characters. Yeasts were found in all the butter samples. Authors speculated that the high incidence found might be related to the use of antibiotics in cattle. Transmittance of mycotic infection by unclean workers to cow's teats when milking was also cited as a cause. Saprophytic yeasts comprised the majority of the isolated yeast strains. Of the facultative pathogenic yeasts seen in the sample, Candida albicans which infects fingernails was found.

Iran

1. Froozani, M. D. "Serum zinc, copper, calcium and phosphorous in pregnant women and their newborns." J. Trop. Pediatr., 29, June 1983, pp 190-192.

   Serum zinc, copper, calcium and phosphorus in 194 women hospitalized for delivery at Mottahedin (Public) and Misaghirdeh (Private) Maternity Hospitals before delivery and from cord at the delivery of the placenta were determined. No significant differences were found in the serum zinc, copper, calcium and phosphorus levels between the two groups of pregnant women. However, the serum zinc and copper levels in cord blood in the case of the private group were significantly higher (p less than 0.01) compared to the public group. No significant differences were found between the serum calcium and phosphorus levels in these two groups. (Authors' abstract)

2. Munoz, N., Crespi, M., Grassi, A., Qing, W. G., Quiong, S., and Cai, L. Z. "Precursor lesions of oesophageal cancer in high-risk populations in Iran and China." Lancet 1(8277) April 17, 1982, pp 876-879.

   To determine the prevalence of precursor lesions of oesophageal cancer in Linxian, People's Republic of China, which has an extremely high incidence of oesophageal cancer, 527 subjects were interviewed by a questionnaire about exposure to suspected risk factors. They also underwent oesophagoscopy, cytology, and biopsy. 84% had a chronic oesophagitis which had similar endoscopic and histological characteristics to that reported in Iran. The oesophagitis was accompanied by atrophy of the epithelium in 10% of these subjects and by dysplasia in 8%. Re-examination of 20 selected subjects one year later showed progression of the oesophagitis to atrophy and dysplasia in 4 individuals and to cancer in 4 others. The surveys in Iran and China suggest that the natural history of oesophageal cancer starts with an oesophagitis which, in a few individuals, progresses to atrophy and dysplasia of the epithelium and finally to cancer. Thermal injury resulting from the drinking of very hot beverages, physical injury caused by ingesting very coarse food, and deficiencies of riboflavin, vitamin A, and zinc are proposed as risk factors for these precursor lesions. (Authors' abstract)

3. Salimpour, R., Vossough, P., and Youssefi, S. "Some aspects of malnutrition in Tehran." J. Trop. Pediatr. 28(1), February 1982, pp 29-34.

   A prospective study was made of 139 malnournished children in Shahrazad Children's Hospital in Tehran. Malnutrition was not sex related in the studies and had a peak incidence at 3 months of age in marasmus and 12 months in kwashiorkor. Marasmus was common during the warm season when diarrhea was common in Tehran, and carried higher mortality than kwashiorkor. The presence of hepatomegaly and/or purpura increased the risk of death. Infections were very common in both groups, particularly respiratory infections. Serum total protein and gamma globulins were lower and hypokalemia was marked in kwashiorkor. The weight was higher in children who were breastfed for a longer time, and lower in children who belonged to large families. (Authors' abstract)

4. Geissler, C. A., Brun, T. A., Mirbagheri, I., Soheli, A.,

Naghibi, A., and Hedayat, H. "The energy expenditure of female carpet weavers and rural women in Iran." Am. J. Clin. Nutr. 34(12), December 1981, pp 2776-2783.

The energy expenditure of rural females in the village of Gorg Tapeh and Deh Namak were compared with that of town females in Isfahan. The village women were measured during summer when most of their time was spent in domestic duties. The 22 Isfahan females were urban workers in light and domestic industry, particularly carpet weaving. Indirect calorimetry using Max-Planck respirometers was used to measure the energy cost of the subjects' typical activities. Together with a 24-hour activity diary, these measurements constituted the daily energy expenditure, which averaged 2000 kcal/day for both groups. This average was close to, but below the FAO recommendations. Since the rural women were not assessed at the time of year when they would be doing agricultural work, the FAO recommendations would be valid for winter and summer, but not necessarily for spring and fall when agricultural work is done.

5. Dabestani, A., Aliabadi, P., Shah-Rookh, F. D, and Borhanmanesh, F. A. "Prevalence of colonic diverticular disease in southern Iran." Dis. Colon Rectum 24(5), July-August 1981, pp 385-387.

Barium enemas were performed on 556 men and women over 20 years old. Overall frequency of diverticulosis was 1.6%. It was more common in people over 50 years of age (2.4%) than in people under 50 years of age (1.2%). This compares with an incidence of about 20% in Western countries. The high fiber intake of most Iranians may be the cause of this low incidence of diverticulosis.

6. Page, L. B., Vandevert, D. E., Nader, K., Lubin, N. K., and Page, J. R. "Blood pressure of Qash'qai pastoral nomads in Iran in relation to culture, diet, and body form." Am. J. Clin. Nutr. 34(4), April 1981, pp 527-538.

Blood pressure, diet, urinary electrolyte excretion, and body form were studied in 264 traditional nomadic herdsmen of the Quash'qai tribe, southern Iran. The population sample included male and female members over 14 yr of age at six winter campsites. Interviews established biological age, any experience of nonnomadic living, and 24-h dietary recall. Height, weight, triceps skinfolds, and blood pressure were measured. Overnight urine samples were analyzed for sodium, potassium, and creatinine. Samples of dietary staples were analyzed for selected nutrients and electrolyte content. Urinary sodium excretion averaged 186 mEq/24 h in males, and 141 mEq/24 h in females. Urinary Na/K ratios were 3.64 and 3.24 in males and females, respectively. Systolic, diastolic, and mean blood pressure in both males and females increased significantly with age. Blood pressure greater than or equal to 140/90 was found in 12% of males and 18% of females age 30 yr or over. Body weight showed no tendency to increase with age in either sex. Systolic and mean blood pressure correlated with urinary sodium excretion in males and with urinary Na/K ratio in females. From cultural observations, the population sample was considered to be at a low level of acculturation. The data suggest that blood pressure trends in this population are related to habitual dietary electrolyte intake. (Authors' abstract)

Sadre, M., and Ghassemi, H. "Milk intolerance among Iranian school children." J. Trop. Pediatr. 27(6), December 1981, pp 312-314.

The ability of 101 healthy children, ranging in age from 7 to 12 years, to tolerate milk, was investigated with regular lactose-containing and lactose-hydrolyzed milk in a double blind study. Twenty-five children, 12 milk intolerant and 13 tolerant, were tested for lactose tolerance (LTT) after ingestion of 40-50 g of lactose. Fourteen (14%) of the subjects developed symptoms suggestive of milk intolerance after drinking regular milk, but none of the children complained of symptoms after consumption of lactose-hydrolyzed milk. Fifteen (60%) of 25 children tested for lactose tolerance (LTT) manifested clinical symptoms after ingestion of a test dose of lactose. Twenty (80%) of 25 subjects did not absorb lactose and had a flat blood glucose curve. However, the rate of lactose malabsorption in 7 to 10 and 11 to 12 year olds was 64% vs. 100% respectively. (Authors' abstract)

8. Froozani, M. D., Malekafzali, H., and Bahrini, B. "Growth of a group of low income infants in the first year of life." J. Trop. Pediatr. 26(3), June 1980, pp 96-98.

Six hundred forty infants aged 1 to 12 months were studied for relation of low income to growth. Children were from the Isfahan area. Weight and height data were compared with Boston standards, and arm circumference was compared with Wolanski's standard. All three measurements, particularly arm-circumference, were lower in both sexes of study infants than the standards. Mid-arm circumference of Isfahan females was significantly lower than that of Isfahan males. Approximately 96% of the mothers breastfed their babies at birth, 65% at age 3 months, and 41% at age 6 months.

9. Mahboubi, E. O., Aramesh, B. "Epidemiology of esophageal cancer in Iran, with special reference to nutritional and cultural aspects." Prev. Med. 9(5), September 1980, pp 613-621. Academic Press.

For several hundred years, the high incidence of esophageal cancer in the Caspian Littoral of Iran, particularly among the Turkoman population, has been recognized. It is now recognized to be among the highest in the world. The distinctive geographical distribution of esophageal cancer was studied as to possible etiologic agents in a multidisciplinary epidemiological investigation. The findings showed that alcohol and tobacco were not significant factors in Iran, although they have been found to be causative in certain Western areas of the world. The use of opium was not seen as significant in causation either. Occupational factors such as felt and carpet making were not seen to affect the rate. Dietary factors were seen to be significant, with high incidence occurring in the lower socioeconomic classes, and the diets of the high risk populations to be highly restricted to homemade bread and tea. Lack of essential nutrients, vitamins, and minerals was commonplace in the high esophageal cancer incidence areas. Green vegetable and fresh fruit intakes were very low in the high-incidence area, and the intake of vitamins A and C and riboflavin were also low. The ingestion of very hot tea in large amounts also distinguished the high-incidence areas. Further investigation of environmental factors was suggested.

10. O'Neill, C. H., Hodges, G. M., Riddle, P. N., Jordan, P. W., Newman, R. H., Flood, R. J., and Toulson, E. C. "A fine fibrous silica contaminant of flour in the high oesophageal cancer area of

north-east Iran." Int. J. Cancer 26(5) November 1980, pp 617-628.

The Caspian littoral of Iran and several other areas of south-central Asia have long been noted for the unusually high incidence of esophageal cancer. A fibrous mineral contaminant in the milled wheat flour used in this area of Iran was discovered and characterized. The fibre, which is between 50 and 150 micrometers long and has a smoothly tapering shape, consisted of almost pure silica. The fibre was found to originate from seeds of the common Mediterranean grass Phalaris minor, and up to 3,000 fibres per gram of wheat flour were found after milling. Commercially grown related species of grass produced fibres of similar size and composition. A semi-solid suspension culture of these fibres and cells of the 3T3 mouse fibroblast line stimulated cell proliferation more than 100-fold. The plant mineral fibres were suspected of being etiologically involved in the local high esophageal cancer incidence.

11. Brun, T. A., Geissler, C. A., Mirbagheri, I., Hormozdiary, H., Bastani, J., and Hedayat, H. "The energy expenditure of Iranian agricultural workers." Am. J. Clin. Nutr. 32(10), October 1979, pp 2154-2161.

The energy cost of agricultural and standard activities and the daily energy expenditure of male agricultural workers were measured during different seasons in Iranian villages to assess the validity of past and present Food and Agricultural Organization recommended energy allowances for that population. Studies included low income farmers in a village representative of those around the central desert where harvesting takes place under conditions of extreme summer heat. Measurements were also made during the Moslem fasting period when no food may be eaten between dawn and dusk. Energy cost of typical activities was measured by indirect calorimetry using the Max-Planck respirometer and daily energy expenditure was assessed using these figures combined with a diary of activities throughout the 24-hr period. Results of individual activity values are compared with other published figures. Comparison of daily energy expenditure of fasting subjects and nonfasting after Ramadan showed no significant difference. No significant difference was found between values of standardized activities at high summer temperatures and moderate temperatures. Mean values of daily energy expenditure during winter when activity is low are around 2600 kcal/day and for the other seasons of high activity 3400 kcal/day. These figures suggest that past and present Food and Agricultural Organization standards are low for this population. (Authors' abstract)

12. Cook-Mozaffari, P. J., Azordegan, F., Day, N.E., Ressicaud, A., Sabai, C., and Aramesh, B. "Oesophageal cancer studies in the Caspian Littoral of Iran: Results of a case-control study." Br. J. Cancer 39(3), March 1979, pp 293-309.

The results are presented of a case-control study conducted in the north of Iran. The main aim was to study factors identified in a previous study as potentially causally related to cancer of the oesophagus. Other tumors (lung, stomach, breast, large bowel, larynx and pharynx) were included to distinguish findings specific for oesophageal cancer from general characteristics of cancer patients, due for example to ascertainment bias, and to verify that expected associations, such as between lung cancer and cigarette smoking, would emerge under the prevailing field conditions. Two controls were chosen per case, matched for village of residence, age, sex and language group. Reinterviewing was performed to a limited extent to assess the accuracy of replies to questionnaires. The following were found not to be associated with oesophageal cancer: consumption of sheep's milk and yogurt, sesame oil, chewing of nass, making of carpets, use of pregnancy diets, salting and sun-drying of meat, and use of wild spinach. The use of opium, bread and tea could not be assessed in the retrospective framework. Strongly associated with risk of oesophageal cancer were low socio-economic status and low intake of fresh fruit and vegetables. The two factors each had an independent effect, and were more marked for oesophageal cancer than for the other tumors. (Authors' abstract)

13. Geissler, C., Margen, S., and Calloway, D. H. "Lactation and pregnancy in Iran. III. Hormonal factors." _Am. J. Clin. Nutr._ 32(5), May 1979, pp 1097-1111.

The study was undertaken to investigate the serum levels of some hormones other than prolactin that have been shown in animal studies to play a role in lactation, and to examine their relationship to adequacy of lactation and to nutritional and socioeconomic status in urban Iranian women. Serum levels of placental lactogen, growth hormone, cortisol, and thyroid hormones were measured under standard conditions in two groups of pregnant women from low and low middle socioeconomic areas of Teheran, 1 or 2 weeks before parturition and again the 3rd month postpartum. Significant differences were found in the biochemical parameters between socioeconomic groups. Hemoglobin and serum albumin values were lower, and all the globulin fractions (except alpha 2 globulin during pregnancy), growth hormone and cortisol were higher in the low than the middle socioeconomic subjects, both during pregnancy and postpartum. The discrepancies between the socioeconomic groups were greater postpartum. Growth hormone and cortisol levels were significantly lower in subjects with adequate lactation. No correlations were found between the measured parameters of nutritional status or free thyroxine values and lactation adequacy. In view of the role of growth hormone and cortisol in stress and malnutrition, and some evidence of a reciprocal relationship between growth hormone and prolactin, these hormones may be a link in the chain between the urban environment, malnutrition and lactation failure.

14. Mojtahedi, H., Rabie, C. J., L"ubben, A., Steyn, M., and Danesh, D. "Toxic aspergilli from pistachio nuts." _Mycopathologia_ 67(2), May 1979, pp 123-127.

Pistachio nut samples, taken during various states of development from orchards in Iran, showed that contamination with fungi occurred mainly during the later stages of nut development. Members of the genera Aspergillus and Penicillium occurred most frequently. Of the Aspergilli, the species _A. niger_, _A. flavus_ and _A. fischeri var. spinosus_ occurred most frequently, followed by _A. terreus_, _A. tamarii_ and _A. nidulans_. Twenty-two isolates comprising 13 species were tested for toxicity to ducklings. Isolates of known toxic fungi included _A. flavus_, _A. niger_, _A. parasiticus_ produced aflatoxin B1, the isolates of _A. versicolor_ and _A. nidulans_ produced sterigmatocystin, while the toxic isolate of _A. ochraceus_ did not produce ochratoxins. (Authors' abstract)

15. Parvaneh, V. "An investigation on the mercury contamination of

Persian Gulf fish." Bull. Environ. Contam. Toxicol. 23(3), October 1979, pp 357-359.

Mercury content on random samples of the four most important species of Persian Gulf fish and on samples of canned tuna fish was determined by flame AAS. The level of mercury in fish samples ranged from .04 to .56 mg/kg. The mean value of mercury was .17, .14, .19, and .15 mg/kg in Cybium comersonii, Cybium guttatum, Lutjanus cocineus, and Psettodes erumei, respectively. Mean mercury content in tuna fish (Euthynnus offinis) was .30 mg/kg, with a range of .20 to .44 mg/kg. Authors concluded that currently mercury contamination was not a problem for Persian Gulf fish and sea foods, but suggested that environmental health control be instituted to prevent any future pollution in the area.

16. Tuyns, A. J., P'equignot, G., and Jensen, D. M. "Role of diet, alcohol and tobacco in oesophageal cancer, as illustrated by two contrasting high-incidence areas in the North of Iran and West of France." Front. Gastrointest. Res. 4, 1979, pp 101-110. S. Karger, A.G. Basel.

This paper reviews various hypotheses on the relationship of nutritional factors to oesophageal cancer, and highlights two sets of studies conducted in Iran and France by the IARC. The Iranian study showed that a very high incidence area in the Caspian littoral had a population consuming a higher amount of daily bread and tea than other areas. In addition, there was a lower riboflavin intake. Widespread opium use was also indicated by urine studies of morphine metabolites.

The western France study showed only minor differences between low and high cancer incidence groups, with the average pyridoxine intake about two times higher in cancer cases. In addition, the alcohol intake was double in the cancer cases, and the resulting total calorie intake was also higher among them; fewer cancer cases consumed mineral water, and they ate less meat, more offals, more salted butter, less fatty foods other than butter and oil, and more vegetables, potatoes, and smoked fish.

17. Abbassioun, K., Aarabi, B., and Zarabi, M. "A comparative study of physiologic intracranial calcifications." Pahlavi Med. J. 9(2), April 1978, pp 152-166. (Pahlavi Med. J. is now Iranian J. of Medical Sciences.)

It has been the impression of clinicians that pineal calcification is infrequent in Shiraz, Iran. In order to evaluate this clinical impression, 2000 consecutive skull X-rays taken at Saadi Hospital, Shiraz, Iran, were reviewed for the presence of physiologic intracranial calcifications. The incidence of these calcifications in males and females, in consecutive age groups of 10 years from 0 to over 70 years of age, were assessed and compared with previous reports from other countries. The average incidence of pineal calcification for those over 20 years of age was 18.29% in this study compared with 55% in the U.S.A. The incidence of calcification in the choroid plexus and the falx cerebri was also considerably less than previously reported. The literature is reviewed and the possible causes for the geographical differences in the reported frequency of physiologic intracranial calcifications is discussed. It is possible that racial and dietary factors may be significant in the variation in the incidence of pineal and other cranial calcification noted in different countries. Within a population group, age and sex are additional factors. (Authors' abstract)

18. Bodaghi, E., Sadre, M., and Ziai, M. "Bacteriuria in malnourished Iranian children." J. Trop. Pediatr. 24(2), April 1978, pp 77-79. (Trop. Peds. & Environ. Child Health)

347 malnourished children, 205 males and 143 females between 2 and 24 months of age, were studied for occurrence of urinary infection. A control group of 319 well-nourished children, 174 boys and 140 girls, were compared with the malnourished children. Positive urine culture was noted in 30 malnourished children compared to only 5 cases in the control. Marasmic children ranging from 2 to 18 months of age showed significant bacteriuria. Most malnourished patients had hemoglobin below 12 gm/100 ml. Hemoglobin concentration and white blood cell count of malnourished children with or without bacteriuria showed no significant difference. The significant bacteriuria incidence was 8.6% in malnourished and 1.56% in well-nourished children.

19. Doll, R. "Geographical variation in cancer incidence: a clue to causation." World J. Surg. 2(5), September 1978, pp 595-602.

This paper, based on a lecture given by the author in September 1977, discusses the great variation in incidence of cancers of various types in different communities, a variation not usually due to genetics. Esophageal cancer is particularly representative in this respect, since its incidence varies 500-fold around the world, and the high and low incidence areas are often quite close to each other geographically. Soviet Central Asia, parts of Africa and China, and northern Iran are noted as areas of high incidence. The association with tobacco smoking and alcoholic drinking are seen as important in Europe and America, but not in the other high incidence areas. Iranian high incidence areas occur where semi-nomadic people eat a traditional diet of wheat bread, sheep's milk, yogurt, tea, and very small amounts of fruit, vegetables, or meat. Nutritional deficiencies, carcinogenic agents in wheat seeds in the fields, mycotoxins formed during storage, or carcinogens in tar swallowed from opium pipes are some future areas of research. Other cancers are mentioned, such as Burkitt's lymphoma, facial basal cell carcinoma, and melanoma on the sole of the foot. The possible connections between diet and cancer are discussed, such as the connection between gastric cancer and consumption of salted and pickled fish and vegetables in Japan.

20. Feiz, J., Sabbaghian, H., and Miralai, M. "Brucellosis due to B. melitensis in children. Clinical and epidemiologic observations on 95 patients studied in central Iran." Clin. Pediatr. (Phila) 17(12), December 1978, pp 904-907.

An epidemiologic survey of brucellosis in Renan village and a report of clinical features in patients of the Isfahan Medical School health station is presented. In 14 months 766 suspicious brucellosis cases were seen, with 283 children under 14 years of age. Of all patients, 170 showed acute brucellosis by clinical and laboratory evidence; 95 of these were children under 14 years old. No significant sex difference was seen. Median age in children was 9.7 years, indicating more active children were more likely to acquire the infection. 58% of cases occurred from April through August, the period of highest milk production, parturition, and abortion among goats and sheep. Most of the patients consumed dairy products locally prepared from unpasteurized milk. Fresh cheese, raw milk, and cream were considered to be major sources of childhood brucellosis. Arthralgia was the most frequent symptom seen.

21. Froozani, M. D. "Weight, height and arm circumference of a group of low income Esfahan children." J. Trop. Pediatr. 24(3) June 1978, pp 117-119. (Trop. Peds. & Environ. Child Health)

Weight, height and arm circumference of 400 Esfahan children aged 1-24 months attending Pahlavi Public Health Center were measured. It was found that 240 (60%) of children had a weight for age and 58 (14.5%) had a height for age less than Boston standards.

Comparing the 80% weight for age as an upper limit for protein-calorie malnutrition with the arm for age and the age-constant arm standards in the children aged 13-24 months gives similar results for both. Also, the number of infants aged 13-24 months classified as malnourished in arm circumference criteria was found to be similar to the total number in the 1st, 2nd and 3rd degree malnutrition groups by weight. Thus, arm circumference measurement can be used for detection of malnutrition in crisis situations.

The values of correlation coefficient (r) between mid-upper-arm circumference (MAC) for age and weight, length, head, and chest circumferences show that the correlation of MAC for age is better with weight-for-age than other parameters. (Author's abstract)

22. Geissler, C., Calloway, D. H., and Margen, S. "Lactation and pregnancy in Iran. I. Social and economic aspects." Am. J. Clin. Nutr. 31(1), January 1978, pp 160-168.

A study of lactation failure and its consequences in Tehrean was conducted. 52 low socioeconomic (LSE) status women from the patient register of Farah Maternity Hospital, and 36 middle socioeconomic (MSE) status women from the Firuzgar Hospital were followed from 2 weeks prepartum to 3 months postpartum. Socioeconomic characteristics, food beliefs relating to lactation, and infant mortality rates and reasons were documented. MSE mothers' food supplementation beliefs reflected Western nutritional beliefs and knowledge, whereas LSE mothers did not reflect Western knowledge in the food supplementation beliefs and practices. Subsequently, LSE mothers fed only sugary liquids to their infants betweeen breast feedings. MSE mothers ate a greater variety of foods during lactation than their LSE counterparts. 15 to 30% of LSE mothers and 40 to 55% of MSE mothers retained a fully adequate milk supply in the third month postpartum. Mortality indicated by the data suggested that LSE infants sustained 250 deaths per 1000 live births compared to 100 deaths per 1000 live births in MSE infants. Early onset of lactation failure in both urban groups compared to rural women indicated that environmentally-related health or social factors were impacting on the time of lactation failure. Hormonal data collected during this study was published in a separate report. Authors had collected hormonal data in an effort to determine whether there was a linkage of nutrition, hormonal status, and lactation adequacy.

23. Geissler, C., Calloway, D. H., and Margen, S. "Lactation and pregnancy in Iran. II. Diet and nutritional status." Am. J. Clin. Nutr. 31(2), February 1978, pp 341-354.

Thirty-six low socioeconomic (LSE) status and 52 middle socioeconomic (MSE) status pregnant women close to term from the out-patient population of two Teheran hospitals were studied through the 3rd month postpartum for nutritional status and dietary intake. This was done as part of a study investigating hormonal status, nutrition, and lactation because lactation failure is a serious problem locally. 24 hour recall assessed dietary intake. Hematologic and anthropometric assessed the infants' growth. Postpartum weight and % of standard weight for height in LSE infants, and hematocrit in the MSE mothers were significantly correlated with lactation adequacy. No significant differences between socioeconomic groups was seen in weight or height. However, significant differences between LSE and MSE were seen for total serum protein, serum albumin and globulin fractions, hemoglobin, and hematocrit values. Nutrient intakes less than or equal to 80% of RDA in both groups included energy, vitamin B_6, folacin, calcium, iron, and zinc. Only vitamin C, thiamin, and protein intakes met recommended standards in the LSE group.

24. Nadim, A., Barzegar, M. A., and Daneshpajooh, M. "Comparison of the prevalence of hypertension in the rural and urban areas of Guilan Province, Northern Iran." Acta Cardiol. (Brux.) 33(1), 1978, pp 31-42.

Blood pressure levels of three groups of people 35 years and older in the Guilan province, Northern Iran were compared. One group was from the city of Bandar Pahlavi (550), another group from the coastal villages near the city (510), and the third from the mountain villages, less than 100 km far from the city (272). This study showed that in both sexes, both systolic and diastolic blood pressures were lowest in the mountain villages, highest in the city and intermediate in the coastal villages. The possible causes of the observed differences are discussed. (Authors' abstract)

25. S'odergren, A., Djirsarai, R., Gharibzadeh, M., and Moinpour, A. "Organochlorine residues in aquatic environemtns in Iran, 1974." Pestic. Monit. J. 12(2), September 1978, pp 81-86.

Organochlorine pesticide residues in various organisms from different aquatic ecosystems in Iran were investigated in spring 1974. DDT levels were high in fish taken from two rivers in southern Iran, whereas low levels were detected in samples obtained from a freshwater lake in the same area. Fish from two of the reservoirs supplying Tehran with potable water contained moderate levels of DDT. The low residue level in pike collected in the Bandar-Pahlavi Mordab in northwest Iran indicates that only a small amount of organochlorine pesticides used in this area enters the pelagic food chain. Sturseon collected at different places in the Caspian Sea showed similar accumulations of DDT in the muscles and in the eggs. Polychlorinated biphenyls (PCBs) were detected only in samples of sediment from the drainage systems in Tehran. (Authors' abstract)

26. Tuyns, A. J., P'equignot, G., and Jensen, O. M. "Nutrition, alcohol and oesophageal cancer." (author's translation) Bull. Cancer (Paris) 65(1), 1978, pp 58-64.

Nutritional factors are suspected to cause oesophageal cancer as well as other cancers of the digestive tract. Sideropenia, lack of molybdenum and tannins have been reported to be associated with the disease. Polycyclic hydrocarbons and nitrosamines have been found in alcoholic beverages from high incidence regions; the significance of the small amounts detected remains to be assessed. A recent survey in Iran points out the role of poor and monotonous diet. In Brittany, no major deficiencies were found, either in quantity or quality, in the diet of 200 male cases of oesophageal cancer when compared with a population control group. Differences in consumption were detected for a few items; the most obvious discrepancies concerned the various alcoholic beverages for which the proportion of heavy consumers was systematically greater among cases. Alcohol and tobacco are both independently associated with the disease; there is a dose-response relationship for both and their effects are multiplicative. The mechanism of action of alcohol in oesophageal cancer is briefly discussed. (Authors' abstract)

27. Vaezzadeh, K., and Dutz, W. "Diet and intestinal diseases." Am. J. Proctol. Gastroenterol. Colon Rectal Surg. 78(2), March-April 1978, pp 22-23, 25.

The influence of diet in Iran on the incidence of intestinal diseases such colon and rectal cancer and volvulus of the intestine is discussed. The records of all patients with large intestinal conditions who were treated at hospital attached to Pahlavi University and other data from other publications was reviewed. Adenomatous polyps were found in only 1.5% of autopsies performed in Shiraz in 1973. No diverticulosis was found in 247 Barium enema records. Twenty years of data revealed only 157 colo-rectal cancers, and no colon cancer due to familial polyposis or ulcerative colitis. However, from 1962 to 1967, 209 cases of intestinal obstruction were found, of which 10.6% were due to small intestinal volvulus, 16.7% due to sigmoid volvulus, and only 2.8% due to malignancy. In the traditional diet of Iran, 85% of the total protein intake is provided by cereals, and only 12% by animal food. The authors suggested that small intestinal volvulus was linked to the high fiber diets.

28. Wise, A., Boroumand, M., and Farivar, H. "Nutritional value of multivitamin preparations." Lancet 1(8078), June 24, 1978, pp 1353-1354.

Twenty-four multi-vitamin preparations from a large pharmacy in the city of Isfahan, Iran were surveyed. The vitamin preparations were compared with accepted requirements for women, pregnant women, lactating women, and infants. The authors found that the amounts of vitamins provided by manufacturers was the opposite of the recommended requirements for these groups. They noted that all the studied products were formulated outside Iran in major drug-producing countries, and suggested they be reformulated to provide the best overall nutritional balance, or to specifically provide the vitamins which may be missing from the local diet of the ultimate consumer population.

29. Anomymous "Esophageal cancer studies in the Caspian littoral of Iran: results of populaton studies--a prodrome. Joint Iran-International Agency for Research on Cancer Study Group." U.S. Natl. Cancer Inst. J. 59(4), October 1977, pp 1127-1138.

Epidemiologic studies were undertaken on the Caspian littoral of Iran to investigate the geographic distribution of factors that might underlie the signal differences in incidence of cancer of the esophagus. In zones of contrasting incidence and sex ratio, information was obtained on food intake, smoking and drinking patterns (including tea), other personal habits, occupation, economic and agricultural practices, and methods of food storage preservation, and preparation. The diet in the highest incidence area was markedly restricted to bread and tea. The poor quality of the diet itself was thought to have a role in the increased risk of developing esophageal cancer. The use of opium and sesame oil, consumption of sheep's milk and yogurt, the chewing of nass (confined to men), and the use of dyes (confined to women) were also more prevalent in the high incidence areas. Typical dietary items were analyzed for the polycyclic aromatic hydrocarbons, volatile nitrosamines, aflatoxins, nitrates, and nitrites. The results showed no unusual levels of any of the carcinogens tested or geographic differences. (Author's abstract)

30. Ismail-Beigi, F., Reinhold, J. G., Faraji, B., and Abadi, P. "Effects of cellulose added to diets of low and high fiber content upon the metabolism of calcium, magnesium, zinc and phosphorus by man." J. Nutr. 107(4), April 1977, pp 510-518.

Three adult male Iranian volunteers were measured for fecal calcium and zinc excretion when given a low fiber content diet for 20 days with an additional daily intake of 10 gm of cellulose via 150 gm of apple compote. Balance of both metals bebame negative, plasma levels decreased, and fecal excretion increased significantly in all three men. Magnesium balances also became negative in 2 subjects, and phosphorus balance became negative in 1. A second study was conducted in which the same amount of cellulose was added to a high fiber content diet for 20 days. In 2 men, calcium and zinc fecal excretions increased significantly, and magnesium excretion increased in 1. Plasma calcium and zinc levels fell, and negative balances became more negative in all men. Fecal dry weight depended on fecal fiber content, as measured by acid-detergent assay. Fecal fiber and zinc correlated significantly in 1 man, and fecal fiber and calcium correlated significantly in 2 men. This was not true for the subject who apparently digested fiber most effectively. When fecal fiber concentrations were high, less increments of dry matter per gm of fiber were seen. High fiber intakes in the diets of rural Iranians can impair zinc, calcium, and magnesium utilization.

31. Rouhbakhsh-Khaleghdoust, A., and Pourtaghva, M. "A large outbreak of type E botulism in Iran." Trans. R. Soc. Trop. Med. Hyg. 71(5), 1977, p 444.

This report describes an outbreak of type E botulism affecting 75 persons in Rasht, Iran during April and May 1976. These people had a history of eating uncooked salt-cured fish eggs, known locally as "ashbal". Symptoms are described. 288 samples of salt-cured and smoked fish eggs obtained from shops and homes, including uneaten parts of nine incriminated meals of carp fish eggs were analyzed for type E botulinum toxin. The toxin was found in 137 of 208 samples of salt-cured eggs, in 10 of 54 samples of smoked carp eggs, and in 8 of 26 samples of salt-cured white fish eggs. In addition, the toxin was demonstrated in 8 of 11 sera and 12 of 21 stomach contents samples from victims. Authors speculated that the use of carp eggs in place of traditional salmon eggs which had become rare was a causative factor, since carp inhabit muddy coastal areas of the Caspian Sea which are heavily contaminated with Cl. botulinum. In addition, rising costs of the fish food have resulted in people re-using leftovers instead of discarding them. This may also have contributed to the epidemic's occurence.

32. Russell, R. M., and Ismail-Beigi, F. "A review of the pathogenesis of folic acid deficiency: a problem in Iran?" Pahlavi Med. J. 8(2), April 1977, pp 255-270. (Pahlav Med. J. is now Iranian Journal of Medical Sciences.)

This review article discusses the geographical distribution of folic acid deficiency among rice and corn-eating populations of the world, its high age distribution among the elderly, and the history of folate research. The clinical signs of folate deficiency, the human requirement for folate in PGA form, absorption of folate, and the possible causes of folate deficiency are outlined. Folic acid deficiency incidence in the Middle East is highlighted, emphasizing a 1974-75 survey conducted in Shiraz, Iran and in villages surrounding Marvdasht. Survey results showed good folate nutriture in Iran. Consumption of large amounts of unrefined wheat wholemeal bread staples with a short cooking time was considered the major factor in the observed adequate folate nutriture in Iran.

33. Sadeghy, A., Bahmard, S., Shafiepoor, H. I., and Zeoghmani, E. "Cancer of the esophagus in southern Iran." Cancer (40)2, August 1977, pp 841-845.

A study of hospital records in the capital city of Fars Province in Southern Iran established the annual esophageal cancer incidence among the local population. The minimal annual rate was 5 to 10 times higher than that of the Conneticut, U.S.A. 15 to 44 years age group population. The true cancer rate was thought to be much higher due to commonly unreported and untreated cases. The upper third of the esophagus was affected in 32% of the cases, a high proportion of cases. Tumor location was strongly related to age. It was not related to sex, however, once age was accounted for. The proportion of female esophageal cancer cases was much higher than the female cancer cases for other GI tract areas.

34. Tavasolian, B. "Native Iranian peanut resistance to seed infection by Aspergillus". (letter). J. Agric. Food Chem. 25(6), November-December 1977, pp 1422-1423.

The presence of aflatoxin in three varieties of peanuts currently cultivated in Iran was examined by two methods. The results indicated that two varieties of the peanuts were contaminated with this toxin, but the native Iranian seed, Local Gilan Iran, in comparison with standard, showed no contamination. The finding of this peanut which resists seed infection by Aspergillus is important from nutritional and economical points of view. (Author's abstract)

35. Auda, H., Al-Wandawi, H., and Al-Adhami, L. "Protein and amino acid composition of three varieties of Iraqi dates at different stages of development". J. Agric. Food Chem. 24(2), March-April 1976, pp 365-367.

Protein contents and amino acid composition of date fruits were determined in three Iraqi varieties (Khastawi, Khadhrawi and Zahdi) at different stages of development. Protein concentration for the three varieties was highest at the green stage. Seventeen total amino acids were detected and determined; their concentrations (dry basis) varied. Khastawi and Khadhrawi showed a higher concentration than the Zahdi variety. At the green stage, concentrations of glutamic acid, aspartic acid, lysine, leucine, alanine and serine were highest. At the yellow and ripe stages, glutamic acid, aspartic acid, lysine, leucine, proline and glycine were present at a high concentration. For most amino acids, the concentration was higher at the yellow stage than at the ripe stage. (Authors' abstract)

36. Campbell, B. J., Reinhold, J. G., Cannell, J. J., Nourmand, I. "The effects of prolonged consumption of wholemeal bread upon metabolism of calcium, magnesium, zinc and phosphorus of two young American adults". Pahlavi Med. J. 7(1), January 1976, pp 1-17. (Pahlavi Med. J. is now Iranian Journal of Medical Sciences.)

The ability to adapt to a large daily intake of unleavened bread made from wheaten wholemeals of high extraction rate was examined in two young Americans who had not previously consumed fiber, phytate-, and phosphate-rich bread of this type. Adaptation was evaluated by comparing balances of zinc, calcium, magnesium and phosphorus for a 12-day period after ten days of bread consumption with those during a similar period after 50 days, and also by observing changes in blood composition during this period of bread consumption. Significantly negative balances of zinc, magnesium and phosphorus were observed in the initial period. However, all had become positive or nearly so after 5 days. By contrast, calcium balances which were also negative during the initial period remained negative at the end of the study. Plasma calcium and zinc concentrations had declined to low normal or subnormal values at this time. The failure to overcome the disturbing effects of consumption of wholemeal bread upon calcium metabolism occurred despite daily exposure to sunshine for many hours under conditions favorable for Vitamin D biosynthesis. (Authors' abstract)

37. Daneshbod, G. "Amino acid screening in Tehran." J. Trop. Pediatr. 22(1), February 1976, pp 7-8.

Amino acid screening of 308 randomly selected patients in the Pediatric Department of Tehran Medical School and John F. Kennedy Center Institute of Mentally Retarded Children was performed by chromatography using prepared thin layer of cellulose on aluminum foil.

Among 154 patients with mental retardation, there were 8 cases of phenylketonuria, one case of maple syrup urine disease and one case of histidinemia. There were 30 patients with nutritional rickets, of which 26 had severe and 4 mild generalized aminoaciduria. Four patients with resistant rickets and 2 patients with myopathy showed generalized aminoaciduria. High excretion of hydroxyproline was found in two patients with Marfan Syndrome. (Author's abstract)

38. Dutz, W., Post, C., Vessal, K., and Kohour, E. "Endemic infantile Pneumocystis carinii infection: the Shiraz study." Natl. Cancer Inst. Monogr. 43, October 1976, pp 31-40.

Orphanage epidemics of interstitial plasma cell pneumonia (IPCP) occur among premature infants whose passive immunity due to maternally transferred antibodies has lost its effectiveness before the infants' humoral immune systems have reached sufficient maturity to respond effectively to Pneumocystis carinii. IPCP occurs also among mature newborns receiving substandard care in understaffed and crowded orphanages. Infantile diarrhea in these institutions leads to marasmus and deficient immune response in infants 3-4 months after birth. The P. carinii organisms in the alveoli elicit a plasma cell response in the interstitial tissues of the lung, which may be so massive that it interferes with respiration and leads to death by asphyxiation. Such observations at the Shiraz Orphanage are discussed. (Authors' abstract)

39. Muir, C. S., and P'eron, Y. "Special demographic situations." Semin. Oncol. 3(1), March 1976, pp 35-47.

This article discusses special demographic situations which affect the distribution and patterns of cancers in various areas of the world. General demographic characteristics such as age of onset of various types of cancer and time trends in various populations with different types of cancer, are noted. Variation of international cancer risks is noted, and the Caspian variations in esophageal cancer incidence are highlighted. The studies by Kmet and Mahboubi are described, including the preliminary results which show the diet of the high incidence area as predominantly wheat, as opposed to the low incidence area's diet of rice. Low vitamin A, C and riboflavin intakes with few vegetables and fruits are described in the high incidence area. The relationship between aflatoxin load of peanuts in Kenya and the incidence of primary liver cancer is also discussed.

40. Nahapetian, A., and Bassiri, A. "Variations in concentrations and interrelationships of phytate, phosphorus, magnesium, calcium, zinc and iron in wheat varieties during two years". J. Agric. Food Chem. 24(5), September-October 1976, pp 947-950.

Variations in concentrations and interrelationships of phytate, P, Mg, Ca, Zn and Fe were studied in grains of seven Iranian (Deihim, Derakhshan, Jolgeh, Koohrang, Navid, Ommid and Roshan) and five foreign (Akowa, Inia, Penjamo, Ciano and Tobari) varieties of wheat (Triticum aestiuum L.) in two successive years. Protein concentrations and yields of the grains were also determined. There were significant annual variations in yield and concentrations of phytate, P, Mg, Ca and Zn. The effect of year was not significant for concentrations of protein and Fe. Significant varietal differences were also found for most of the variables. There was a highly significant relationship between total P and phytate P ($r = 0.93$). Estimation of phytate P from total P data and possibility of changing concentrations of the variables with emphasis on phytic acid in the wheat grain by agricultural practices are discussed. (Authors' abstract)

41. Reinhold, J. G. "Rickets in Asian immigrants." (letter) Lancet 2(7995), November 20, 1976, pp 1132-1133.

The relation of rickets incidence in Asian children and the consumption of chupatties, tanok, and bazari, which are all breads which have a high phytate content was discussed. All the breads are high in fiber content, which may cause a predisposition to rickets. The phytate, starch, protein, and fiber are all capable of binding strongly with calcium, iron, and zinc. Metals bound by starch or protein have been shown to be released in the intestine by the action of pancreatic amylase or tryptase, but the fiber-bound metal remained bound in studies simulating small gut conditions. The rickets of Indian and Iranian children was suggested to be connected with the binding of calcium and subsequent unavailability for absorption. The high fiber was thought to bind bile acids and possibly bind Vitamin D with the complex, thus wasting enough vitamin D to produce rickets.

42. Reinhold, J. G., Faradji, B., Abadi, P., and Ismail-Beigi, F. "Decreased absorption of calcium, magnesium, zinc and phosphorus by humans due to increased fiber and phosphorus consumption as wheat bread". J. Nutr. 106(4), April 1976, pp 493-503.

Two male Iranian volunteers, 24 and 35 years of age, were studied for metabolic behavior regarding zinc, calcium, magnesium, phosphorus, and nitrogen during low and high fiber consumption in two 20 day periods via high white bread and Bazari bread consumption, respectively. Bazari (Taftoon) bread is a leavened flat wholemeal wheat bread made from flour of 80 to 90% extraction used as a staple in Iranian cities. During the high fiber consumption period, only the men developed negative balances of all the studied minerals. This was caused by increased fecal excretion, which correlated with phosphorus excretion and fecal dry matter weight. The dry fecal matter weight correlated directly with the amount of fecal fiber excretion. Nitrogen balance was unaffected, remaining positive through both periods.

43. Russell, R. M., Isnail-Beigi, F., Alfrasiabi, K., Rahimifar, Pourkanal, D., and Ronaghy, H. "Folate levels among various populations in central Iran." Am. J. Clin. Nutr. 29(7), July 1976, pp 794-798.

Four hundred sixty-seven male and female adults in the city of Shiraz, the town of Marvdasht, and Marvdasht's surrounding villages, from various socioeconomic classes, were assessed for serum folate levels via Lactobacillus casei assay. 170 of the subjects were pregnant females in varying trimesters. Overall mean serum folate was within the normal range of 5.9 to 21.0 ng/ml for all groups, and it ranged from 7.5 to 11.1 ng/ml. Two subjects were found to be deficient with serum folic acid below 3.0 to 5.9 ng/ml. Red blood cell folate levels were significantly higher in anemic subjects, those with hematocrit less than 37%, than in nonanemic controls. Authors suggested that the locally common iron deficiency seen in central Iran might contribute to folate underutilization. The high folate content of local Iranian breads made from high extraction wheat flour was cited as contributing to the adequacy of serum folate observed.

44. Russell, R. M., Ismail-Beigi, F., Reinhold, J. G. "Folate content of Iranian breads and the effect of their fiber content on the intestinal absorption of folic acid". Am. J. Clin. Nutr. 29(7), July 1976, pp 799-802.

Local breads from bakeries in the city of Shiraz and outlying villages were analyzed for folic acid content. This was done to determine whether the staple breads' folic acid content was responsible for the rarity of folate deficiency in central Iran. Sangask and Bazari (Taftoon), leavened flat breads made from flours high extraction rates, had average "free" folate contents of 0.38 and 0.71 mUg/g, respectively. These breads are widely consumed in central Iranian towns and cities. Village wholemeal bread, called Tanok, had an average "free" folate content of 0.34 mUg/g. The white bread from refined flour and oatmeal bread had average 'free" folate of 0.13 and 0.09 mUg/g, respectively, much lower than that of the commonly consumed local breads. Sequential folate absorption tests using tritiated pteroylmonoglutamic acid performed in 4 subjects with meals of increasing fiber content and fasting established that the breads' high content of undigestible fiber did not interfere with folate absorption. In vitro studies also failed to show insoluble complex formations of folic acid and bread fiber. Thus the breads were seen as major contributors to local folate adequacy.

45. Sadre, M., and Ziai, M. "Urinary calculi in Iran: urolithiasis in childhood." Idiopathic urinary bladder stone disease. Van Reen, R., ed. NIH, DHEW No.77-1063, 1977, Bethesda W3 F049 No. 37, 1976, pp 199-207.

This is a report based on composite data accumulated in Iran on urinary calculi and bladder stone disease in Iranian children. Data on hospital experience from 1968 to 1971 from different regions, data from 1971 to 1975 on hospital experience, and findings in two hospitals of 60 cases of childhood bladder stone disease were analyzed. Total number of lower urinary calculi cases in Abadan was only 1/4 that of Masjed-i-Soleiman. Tabriz and Esfahan showed a higher relative incidence of bladder stones, but not upper urinary calculi, when compared with that from Teheran. The Caspian seashore area near Ramsir showed a very low incidence of bladder stones. The male/female ratio for upper urinary calculi and bladder stones is high. Incidence was very high in children less than 6 years old for bladder stones, and the male/female ratio was also high. Ammonium urate and calcium oxalate were the main constituents in 85.8% of the stones analyzed.

46. Schoenborn, C. A. "Breastfeeding as a contraceptive method among a low income group of Tehrani women." J. Trop. Pediatr. 22(6), December 1976, pp 274-276. (Environ. Child Health)

A random sample of 95 married Tehrani women, who were 40 years old or younger and who had had at least one child, were studied when they sought medical care at a health center in Tehran. The mean length of breastfeeding was 10 1/2 months, and 67% of breastfeeding mothers relied on it exclusively. The women were questioned as to their beliefs on the contraceptive efficacy of breastfeeding, and only 41% believed that it acted as a contraceptive. 12% professed a strong belief in its contraceptive effectiveness. 45% of the sample utilized technological birth control, and 26% utilized biological methods. The women practiced demand feeding as opposed to scheduled feeding.

47. Amirshahi, P., Salimpoor, R., Kamali, P., Hedayat, S., Kohansedgh, S., and Roohani, G. "The amino-acid ratio, serum proteins and haematological studies on marasmic children." J. Trop. Pediatr. 21(6), December 1975, pp 321-324. (Environ. Child Health)

The subjects of this study were 87 marasmic children, ages 5 to 24 months, who were admitted to the pediatric service of a state hospital in Teheran during 1973, usually with diarrhea. They were tested for changes in amino-acid ratio, serum proteins, calcium, and haematological values. The weight deficit was also correlated with the other measures. Weight and arm circumference deficits were much more marked than deficits in length, sitting height, chest and head circumference. In group I, with lower weight deficit, mean amino-acid ratio was 1.66. Group II, with higher weight deficit, had a mean amino-acid ratio of 1.77. Mean serum gamma-globulin was higher in the higher weight deficit group, but mean serum total protein, albumin, alpha-1, alpha-2, and beta-globulin were lower for the higher weight deficit group. Mean serum calcium was higher in the lower weight deficit group.

48. Dutz, W., Rossipal, E., Ghavami, H., Kohout, E., and Vessal, K. "Geographic patterns of immunity and vascular disease." Pathol. Microbiol. (Basel) 43(2-0) 1975, pp 173-181. S. Karger AG, Basel.

Underlying epidemiological factors are compared from 25 years of biopsies at the Medical College of Virginia, 10 years of biopsies and autopsies at Saadi Hospital in Shiraz, Iran, and 9 years of medical records of a Shiraz orphanage. A discussion highlights the differences in vascular and immune-related disease in Iran and the U.S. Disseminated lupus erythematosis is absent in Shiraz and prominent in the U.S., while acute rheumatic disease is frequent in Iran and almost extinct in the U.S. These differences are explained in terms of environmental conditions, including nutrition, parasites, and viral disease influences. Early protein-energy malnutrition, as experienced in developing countries, can lead to reduced T-cell-mediated immunity with an active B-cell or humoral immune response. In high living standard environments with good hygiene, cell-mediated immunity develops undisturbed, but B-cell response is not stimulated.

49. Hormozdiara, H., Day, N. E., Aramesh, B., and Mahboubi, E. "Dietary factors and esophageal cancer in the Caspian Littoral of Iran." Cancer Res. 35(11 Pt. 2), November 1975, pp 3493-3498.

The dietary, social, and cultural features of 38 villages chosen at random in 14 regions in the Caspian Littoral of Iran were studied. These villages were well defined for esophageal cancer incidence and environmental characteristics. Six randomly selected households in each of the 38 villages were also studied for 5 days via measured dietary intake, clinical examinations of adults, and historical food consumption questionnaire. There were some major dietary differences between the regions with varying esophageal cancer rates. Low-incidence areas used rice as the chief staple food, whereas high-incidence areas used bread for this purpose. Low intake of riboflavin, animal protein, vitamins A and C, and fresh vegetables and fruit was seen in high-incidence areas, along with a higher consumption of goat and sheep's milk. Carcinogens in the food samples, polycyclic aromatic hydrocarbons, nitrosamines, and aflatoxins, were found in low concentrations in all areas. Alcohol and tobacco were not significant factors in Iran.

50. Kopito, L. E., and Shwachman, H. "Lead in human scalp hair: some factors affecting its variability." J. Invest. Dermatol. 64(5), May 1975, pp 342-348.

A study relating accumulation of lead in human scalp hair to environmental factors such as exogenous sources of contamination and dietary intake, age, sex, nutritional deficiencies, and place of residence, was conducted on samples from male and female adults and children subjects. Hair samples were collected from Iran, South Africa, Japan, Yugoslavia, and the United States. Sex and nutritional deficiencies were the least significant variables. The most significant correlates of lead concentration were place of residence, exposure to environmentally introduced lead, consumption of lead-containing substances, age, and the site from which the hair specimen was sampled relative to its distance from the scale.

51. Mahloudji, M., Reinhold, J. G., Haghshenass, M., Ronaghy, H. A., Fox, M. R., and Halsted, J. A. "Combined zinc and iron compared with iron supplementation of diets of 6- to 12-year-old village school children in southern Iran." Am. J. Clin. Nutr. 28(7), July 1975, pp 721-725.

Sixty-nine boys and 6 girls aged 6 to 12 years attending school in the village of Kherak near Shiraz in Iran were randomly assigned to one of three supplementation groups for 8 months. Group A received 20 mg each of elemental zinc and iron as carbonate and fumarate, respectively, along with supplements of vitamins, minerals, egg white, and corn oil. Group B received these supplements minus the zinc. Group C received lactose simulated-supplement placebo capsules. These supplements were given on a daily basis. Initially, 48 to 59 children, representing all groups, had low zinc concentrations (below 75 ug/100 ml). After 8 months of treatment, the zinc means dropped further and 38 of 40 had subnormal zinc values. Zinc supplementation at 20 mg/day failed to increase plasma zinc levels or stimulate growth or bone development, but iron supplementation alone was associated with accelerated height and weight accretion. High phytate and fiber content of local unleavened wholemeal village breads, which decreases biological availability of dietary zinc, may be the cause of the failure of 20 mg zinc/day to produce effects. Iron-zinc competition for absorption may also be a contributory factor in this lack of effect.

52. Nasseh, G. A., and Khadivi, B. "Epidemiological and clinical aspects of echinococcosis in East Iran." J. Trop. Med. Hyg. 78(6), June 1975, pp 120-122.

Three hundred and fifty-two cases of hydatid disease were diagnosed in a three year study in East Iran, where the disease is found frequently in rural areas. Camel meat is consumed in this region and the offal given to domestic carnivorous animals, for example sheep dogs. In these circumstances camels could contribute to the cyclozoonotic spread of the disease. Clinical symptoms are briefly mentioned. (Author's abstract)

53. Reinhold, J. G. "Phytate destruction by yeast fermentation in whole wheat meals. Study of high-extraction rate meals." J. Am. Diet Assoc. 66(1), January 1975, pp 38-41.

Destruction of phytate by yeast fermentation is compared in sponges prepared from Iranian whole wheat meals of different extraction rates. Phytate was destroyed rapidly in whole meals of 75 to 85 and 85 to 90 percent extraction, but destruction was retarded in those of 95 to 100 percent extraction. Production of acid-soluble phosphorus kept pace with phytate destruction in the two whole meals of lower extraction rates, but was delayed with less-than-expected yield in those of 95 to 100 percent rate. Unleavened whole meal bread contains little acid-soluble phosphorus. Leavened breads made from whole meals of slightly lower extraction rate average five times as much. Since phytate phosphorus appears to remain unavailable in the small intestine in many circumstances, dependence on unleavened whole meal bread may result in critically low intakes of available phosphorus when other sources are lacking in the diet. It is concluded that replacement of the whole meals of 95 to 100 percent extraction rate, presently the main staple of the diet of rural Iran, by those of somewhat lower rate is an important preliminary to the introduction of leavening and fermentation into village bread-making methods. (Authors' abstract)

54. Ronaghy, H. A., and Halsted, J. A. "Zinc deficiency occurring in females. Report of two cases." Am. J. Clin. Nutr. 28(8), August 1975, pp 831-836.

Two young females, 19 and 20 years of age, were admitted to Saadi Hospital, Shiraz, Iran in 1971-72 complaining of extreme chronic weakness. They were observed over a period of 14 months. They exhibited the syndrome of dwarfism, hypogonadism, iron deficiency anemia, and geophagia on admittance which had previously been seen in severely zinc-deficient males. Their anemia was treated with and responded to 100 mg of iron as ferrous fumarate daily. 2500 kcal/day diets were given. Then a supplement of 120 mg zinc sulfate containing 27 mg elemental zinc/day was instituted. Growth and sexual development after zinc supplementation was much more rapid than prior to it. Human zinc deficiency in females was confirmed with the rapid response to large amounts of zinc supplementation.

55. Sabbaghian, H. "Fresh white cheese as a source of Brucella infection." Public Health 89(4), May 1975, pp 165-169.

Human and animal brucellosis is a disease of public health and economic significance in Iran. The consumption of unpasteurized dairy products is one of the important sources of human brucellosis. Fresh white cheese, which is produced locally and sometimes privately in country houses from raw goat and sheep milk, is probably the most important way of transmission.

Out of 1220 fresh white cheese specimens, 86(7%) were found infected with Brucella melitensis biotype I. These specimens were collected from retail shops in three highly infected villages over a period of 12 months. The average number of organisms per gram of infected cheese was 2120 after collection, which decreased until the ninth week when no Brucella could be isolated. About 40% of infected cheese became free of Brucella one week after collection and in weekly culture 50% of the specimens continued to be infected up to the third week. At the eighth week, only 1.1% of the 86 infected cheeses showed infection with B. melitensis. The cheese collected from retail shops had a low pH and during weekly culture in the laboratory, B. melitensis was isolated from the specimens within a wide range of pH (5.0-7.6).

The seasonal fluctuation of infected cheese corresponds to human brucellosis in which most cases are seen from April through August with the maximum rate in May and June. (Author's abstract)

56. Salimpour, R. "Rickets in Tehran. Study of 200 cases." Arch. Dis. Child. 50(1), January 1975, pp 63-66.

Radiologically diagnosed rickets was found to be common in children of the poorer classes in Tehran. It was frequently associated with gastroenteritis or bronchopneumonia, and a large proportion of the children were severely underweight for their age. In children below the age of 1 year, malnutrition tended to mask the signs of rickets. Convulsions were much less frequent in the malnourished children; the concentration of calcium in the serum was higher and that of alkaline phosphatase was lower than in those who were well nourished. Biochemistry is of little value in the diagnosis of rickets in the presence of malnutrition. (Authors' abstract)

57. Amirhakimi, G. H. "Growth from birth to two years of rich urban and poor rural Iranian children compared with Western norms." Ann. Hum. Biol. 1(4), October 1974, pp 427-441.

1. Length, weight and head circumference were measured from birth to age 2 years in 63 boys and 68 girls of a high-income Iranian group living in Shiraz in economic and cultural conditions similar to high income groups in Western Europe and North America. The 10th, 50th and 90th percentiles of the measurements were very similar to the London and Boston standards.

2. The high-income Iranian group was compared with racially similar village and poor urban groups in Shiraz and the nearby countryside. The 50th percentiles of these groups for length and weight were at or below the 3rd percentile of the high-income group from 3 to 24 months; head circumference 50th percentile was at the 3rd to 10th percentile.

3. It is concluded that the growth potential of Iranian children is no less than that of West Europeans, though the majority of the population grow along a very much lower curve. (Author's abstract)

58. Ghassemi, H., Massoudi, M., and Azordegan, F. "State of nutrition in preschool children in Tehran. I. Calorie and protein intake." Am. J. Clin. Nutr. 27(10), October 1974, pp 1088-1094.

Calorie and protein intake of 286 preschool age children in low income families in Tehran was evaluated by the use of the direct weighing method for 3 consecutive days. It was shown that 37% of the children received adequate calories and protein. Of the remaining children, 62% were deficient in calories and only 15% were deficient in protein. Protein deficiency was strongly associated with deficiency of calories (r=0.67 and P less than 0.01).

Variation in dietary quantity and quality was substantial and sulfur amino acids were most limiting in most of the diets of the children. (Authors' Abstract).

59. Mohammadiha, H. "Resistance to ketonuria and ketosis in obese subjects". Am. J. Clin. Nutr. 27(11), November 1974, pp 1212-1213.

Eighteen obese subjects and 25 nonobese controls have been under observation during 20 days in Ramadan (fasting time). Urine and blood were examined for ketone bodies (diacetic acid, beta-hydroxybutyric acid and acetone). It was found that the normal controls developed ketosis after 3-6 days and beta-hydroxybutyric and diacetic acids were found in their urine, whereas the obese group did not show ketosis even after 20 days. Eating habit, kind of diet and energy expenditures were similar in both groups. (Author's abstract)

60. Prasad, A. S., and Oberleas, D. "Letter: Zinc deficiency in man." Lancet 1(855), March 16, 1974, pp 463-464.

The letter was a response to Dr. Caughey's contention (Lancet, May 1974) that zinc deficiency was not an important factor in adolescent malnutrition as seen in Iran and Egypt. The authors measured serum-albumin in Middle Eastern patients with zinc deficiency, and found the levels to be inconsistent with protein deficiency. They took exception to the equation of low serum-albumin with protein malnutrition without consideration of other biochemical and clinical factors, since the serum-albumin is affected in several other disorders. They also noted that investigators have found that zinc deficiency results in lower serum-albumin levels. The concentration of phytate in native unleavened Middle Eastern breads has been recognized to lower the bioavailability of zinc in the diet. Reversal of growth and gonadal effects support their view that zinc deficiency does indeed exist in man as a clinical entity.

61. Ronaghy, H. A., Reinhold, J. G., Mahloudji, M., Ghavami, P., Spivey Fox, M. R., and Halsted, J. A. "Zinc supplementation of malnourished schoolboys in Iran: increased growth and other effects." Am. J. Clin. Nutr. 27(2), February 1974, pp 112-121.

Effects of zinc, 40 mg daily given as zinc carbonate, in combination with a supplement of egg-white protein (10 g daily), corn oil, minerals, and vitamins were evaluated in 13-year-old prepubertal village schoolboys in southern Iran for 18 months. Thirty-five of the 49 boys had subnormal plasma zinc concentrations. The boys continued their usual diets in which unleavened, wholemeal wheat bread rich in phytate was the main staple. A similar group serving as controls received the same supplements without zinc.

Significantly increased heights, weights, and bone ages occurred in those receiving supplementary zinc, despite plasma zinc concentrations that remained subnormal throughout the study. Serum total protein and albumin concentrations were moderately decreased initially in approximately 75% of the boys, but became normal during the first 3 months of treatment.

The results demonstrate a stimulus to growth brought about by supplementation with zinc when adequate amounts are given. Contrary to findings in a previous study, no statistically significant stimulation of gonadal development was detected in the zinc-supplemented group compared with the controls. However, a tendency toward accelerated sexual development in the zinc-supplemented boys was evident. (Adapted from authors' abstract).

62. Sabbaghian, H., and Nadim, A. "Epidemiology of human brucellosis in Isfahan, Iran." J. Hyg. (Camb.) 73(2), October 1974, pp 221-228.

Studies on brucellosis were carried out to elucidate epidemiology in Isfahan province, where Brucella melitensis is highly prevalent in animals and man. A positive milk ring test of 32% and 23% was found in unvaccinated goats and sheep respectively. Card and tube agglutination tests showed an infection rate of about 12% in sheep and goats and 42% in cattle. B. melitensis was isolated from 8% of 677 samples of fresh cheese examined.

Of 1526 clinically suspected human cases, 476 showed laboratory evidence of brucellosis. Of these patients, 291 cases were from urban and 185 cases from rural areas. Cases from urban and rural areas were seen principally in younger age groups. Median age of infection was 19.7 in urban and 15.7 in rural patients respectively. Infection was encountered mainly from April to August. This correlates with animal parturition and the greatest amount of sheep and goat milk production, which is introduced to the local market as fresh cheese. Raw dairy product consumption is the most probable way of Brucella transmission in urban patients. In rural areas, both dairy product consumption and contact with animals are sources of infection. (Authors' abstract)

63. Tabibi, M., and Salehian, A. A. "Food poisoning in bread caused by Aspergillus flavatoxin: winter of 1967, Tehran" Acta Med. Iran 17(1-2), August 1974, pp 63-69.

Mycotoxins and their significance in food poisoning are the subject of this communication.

All four toxins attributed to Aspergillus could cause the toxic reactions such as the recent occurrence of food poisoning among a limited number of Teheran inhabitants 1967.

This brief communication signifies the importance of mycotoxins in food poisoning. (Adapted from authors' English abstract.)

64. Ter-Sarkissian, N., Azar, M., Ghavifekr, H., Ferguson, T., and Hedayat, H. "High phytic acid in Iranian breads." J. Am. Diet. Assoc. 65(6), December 1974, pp 651-653.

The phytic acid content of two native Iranian breads, Sangak and Taftoon, are compared with that of European-type breads made locally. Sangak, Taftoon, and village breads have short fermentation times, whereas commercial urban-baked breads have a longer fermentation time.

Mean phytate contents in the breads were: 525 mg for village breads, 329 mg for Sangak, and 209 mg for Taftoon. Fermentation was important for reducing phytate in the breads. Sangak, with a 2 hour fermentation, showed a mean reduction of 43.9%. Taftoon showed a mean decrease of 28.6% in 1 hour. Village bread, not fermented or fermented very little, showed a mean decrease of 18.2%. European-type white breads and their white flours showed almost no phytate. Authors suggested increasing fermentation time of breads where possible.

65. Vaghefi, S. B., Ghassemi, H., and Kaighobadi, K. "Availability of iron in an enrichment mixture added to bread." J. Am. Diet. Assoc. 64(3), March 1974, pp 275-280.

A simple to use vitamin mineral mixture developed and tested to enrich Iranian bread is described. The formula would provide the recommended allowances for iron, riboflavin, and calcium for adults if 400 to 500 grams of daily bread were consumed. Variations were negligible among the 100 samples analyzed for iron, calcium, and riboflavin and recovery was 101, 95, and 93% respectively. The mean change in serum iron two hours after ingestion of the enriched bread was 21 mcg per 100 ml. Because of the widespread anemia in Iran, the use of the enrichment mixture was recommended.

66. Amidi, S., Dutz, W., Kohout, E., and Ronaghy, H. A. "Anthrax in Iran." Z. Tropenmed. Parasitol. 24(2), June 1973, pp 250-255.

The charts of 329 human anthrax cases seen between 1961 and 1971 in hospitals affiliated with Pahlavi University in Shiraz were examined for probable source of infection. 25 additional cases seen in the early 1970s were studied for caloric intake and food quality. The main prevalence occured in summer, and was inversely related to the amount of rainfall. Persons coming into direct contact with livestock or their products, such as wool, were most affected. The exposed body regions coming into frequent contact with infected material or subject to frequent minor abrasions usually showed skin lesions. Human and animal malnutrition increased the incidence. This was most likely due to reduction of leukocyte mobilization in both, and in the case of livestock, also due to increased mouth abrasions from poor, thorny pasteurage during the dry season. Village diets were poor in protein, 19 of 25 patients eating animal protein less than once per week. Rice and bread constituted the dietary staples.

67. Amirhakimi, G. H. "Rickets in a developing country. Observations of general interest from Southern Iran." Clin. Pediatr. (Phila) 12(2), February 1973, pp 88-92.

This is a report of 25 children with vitamin-D deficiency rickets who were admitted to Nemazee Hospital, Shiraz, Iran between January 1958 and December 1967. The immediate cause of admission was most commonly respiratory and gastrointestinal problems and diagnosis of rickets was incidental to hospitalization. All children were from poor socioeconomic status families and all had been breast fed with no vitamin supplementation. All but three patients had low serum calcium of 9.0 mg/100 ml or less. Alkaline phosphatase was elevated in most of the children. Seven patients died in the hospital, with the usual immediate cause of death being malnutrition, bronchopneumonia, or gastroenteritis.

The author noted that breast milk is a poor source of vitamin D, and that swaddling is practiced up to 12 to 14 months of age, with avoidance of sunlight for the children. The high phytate content of the unleavened bread, common in the diet, may play a contributing role; phytate can chelate minerals such as iron, zinc, and calcium and make them unavailable for absorption. Treatment with several small doses and with a single large dose of vitamin D were described. Preventive measures such as general socioeconomic improvement, education and use of fortified dried milks and better diet were mentioned.

68. Anonymous "Editorial: Oesophageal cancer on the Caspian littoral." Lancet 2(842), December 15, 1973, pp 1365-1367.

The incidence of esophageal cancer on the Caspian littoral of Iran is reviewed. The three principle areas of the littoral, the East with high incidence, the middle area with intermediate incidence, and the West with low incidence, were studied for etiologic factors. The high incidence area was found to have a dry climate, with the main crop being wheat. The interlocking features of crops, soil, and diet were explored. Trace metals deficiencies such as iron were studied. The high risk area was seen to have diets which were very deficient in animal protein, vitamin A, vitamin C, and riboflavin.

69. Caughey, J. E. "Zinc deficiency in man." Lancet 2(825), August 1973, pp 376-377.

This letter was Dr. Caughey's response to replies, published in Lancet in June and July refuting Dr. Caughey's contention in a May article that zinc deficiency in man was not a clinical entity. He again stated that the serum albumin levels in the 19 patients with severe or marginal protein-deficiency were very low, and that the hypoalbuminemia was responsible for the low serum zinc levels. He cited results of South African studies which showed a correlation between the two, and reiterated that in his opinion, the significance of zinc deficiency as a cause of adolescent malnutrition in Iran and Egypt had been over emphasized.

70. Caughey, J. E. "Zinc deficiency in man." A letter. Lancet May 5, 1973, p 993.

This letter was written in response to a letter concerning the Shiraz, Iran studies of zinc metabolism published in the Feb. 10, 1973 Lancet. The author contends that protein-energy malnutrition, stemming initially from diets of less than 2000 calories per day in 70% of Iranian families and then from secondary malnutrition from infections and absorption defects, was the underlying cause of adolescent malnutrition seen in Shiraz and other areas of Iran. He cited studies in which zinc supplementation did not show greater growth than protein supplementation to support his contention.

71. Caughey, J. E. "Aetiological factors in adolescent malnutrition in Iran." NZ Med. J. 77(489), February 1973, pp. 90-95.

Severe malnutrition was observed in six adolescents in Iran, 5 boys and a girl aged 15 to 18 years. A description of the appearance and some biochemical observations of each case were given. All the subjects were severely malnourished, with dehydration or edema, history of poor growth and appetite, lack of sexual maturation, repeated diarrheal episodes, geophagia, and lack of pubic, axillary or facial hair. Plasma zinc was determined in five subjects, and was low in all of them, as was serum albumin. The author concluded that protein-calorie malnutrition was the main deficiency, and that the low zinc observed was due to the hypoalbuminemia, since albumin is a major zinc blood ligand and transporter. He suggested that the significance of zinc deficiency as a cause of adolescent malnutrition has been overemphasized.

72. Daneche Pajouh, M., Montazami, K., Hedayat, Ch., Kamali, P., and Pirouzmande, B. "Natural history of coronary atherosclerosis in Iranian workers." Arch. Mal Coeur. 66(9), September 1973, pp 1201-1210.

Precipitating or risk factors for coronary artery atherosclerosis were analyzed in two groups of workers, control and patients. The summarized results are:

-The age of patients was within the same range as that of patients from other countries.

-The various blood lipids were studied, and a definite increase of these was found for every age group in the patients when compared with the controls.

-Arterial hypertension, obesity, and diabetes were more common in patients than in controls.

-Smoking was clearly a risk factor.

-Among patients there was a high percentage of opium-addicts by comparison with normal controls.

-Physical activity and hard work were less commonly found in patients than in controls.

-Anxiety and stress resulting from work had a clear predisposing effect, shown by a percentage of anxious people of 41% in the patients and 12.5% in controls. (Adapted from authors' abstract.)

73. Djamei, P. "Ca, P, and Mg content in Iranian "YASDI" alfalfa during various flowering stages." Z. Tierphysiol. 32(3), November 1973, pp 172-176.

Iran alfalfa "Yasdi" was used in three crops and evaluated at 6 different stages of growth to determine mineral content depending upon crops and stage of growth.

There was no influence on the content of Ca and Mg except a decrease in Ca at the end of flowering stage and an increase for Mg at the same time. The P-concentration decreased continuously during the whole investigation period depending upon stage of growth. (Adapted from author's abstract)

74. Halsted, J. A. "Zinc deficiency in man." Lancet 1(817), June 1973, pp 1447-1448.

This letter was written in reply to an article by Dr. Caughey in May 5 Lancet, p 993 in which Dr. Coughey doubted that zinc deficiency in man was a clinical entity. The author cited data gathered by workers in Egypt and Iran in various studies, as well as in Denver, Colorado to refute this claim. He noted that sexual maturation occurred rapidly in response to zinc supplementation, but not in response to protein supplementation. He did not disparage the importance of protein malnutrition, but noted that the Iranian villagers subsist chiefly on an unleavened flat bread diet heavily laden with phytate. The resultant mineral complexes which make dietary minerals unavailable was cited as a factor in widespread zinc deficiency in these populations.

75. Hedayat, S. H., Faghih, M. A., Montazamy, K., Khorvash, P., Amirshahy, P., and Kamali, P. "Urinary urea-creatinine and plasma amino acid ratios and patterns of growth in school children in Iran." J. Trop. Pediatr. 19(1), September 1973, pp 19-27.

Anthropometric data from 2,936 Iranian primary school children were analyzed; first, to assess the growth and health of Iranian school children living in rural areas; second, to investigate further the inter-relationships between these measurements. Significant correlations were found between weight and height, arm circumference and weight, and head circumference and weight. The same result was noticed when the arm circumference with height and head circumference with height were correlated.

The relationships between physical characteristics and the ratios of plasma amino acid and urea nitrogen to creatinine nitrogen were demonstrated. The correlation between both weight and height deficits and the two above-mentioned ratios, although significant, was low. (Authors' abstract).

76. Hedayat, H., Shahbazi, H., Payan, R., Azar, M., Bavendi, M., and Donoso, G. "The effect of lysine fortification of Iranian bread on

the nutritional status of school children." Acta Paediatr. Scand. 62(3), May 1973, pp 297-303.

The effect of enrichment of bread with lysine was studied on a group of Iranian village children receiving free school lunch over a period of 210 days. Two groups received typical dishes, which were purposely modified to make them limited by lysine, one with enriched and the other with non-enriched bread. The third group did not receive lunch and served as control to assess the changes in the nutritional status of the former groups. The food intake at the homes was not controlled.

Markedly greater increases in weight and mid-arm circumference were observed in groups which received the school lunch (with or without lysine) than in the control group. Lysine enrichment showed no significant effect in improving the nutritional status, except that children who received the amino acid supplementation exhibited significantly higher increments in mid-arm circumferences. An increment in height and weight was observed in children of non-lysine group over those who received lysine which was significant with respect to height. The latter group also showed a small but significant decrease in serum albumin. (Authors' abstract)

77. Mobedi, I., Arfaa, F., Madadi, H., and Movafagh, K. "Sylvatic focus of trichiniasis in the Caspian region, Northern Iran". Am. J. Trop. Med. Hyg. 22(6), November 1, 1973, pp 720-722.

Trichinella spiralis larvae were found in 5 of 21,143 wild boars and 1 of 16 brown bears examined in the 5-year period from 1967 to 1971 and in 38 of 63 golden jackals (Canis aureus), 2 of 3 jungle cats (Felis chaus) and none of 3 other carnivores, 30 rodents, and 20 shrews examined in 1972. Infection has not been reported in more than 500,000 domestic pigs examined for Trichinella in the Teheran abattoir, although most of the pigs were raised in the Caspian region. Human infection from eating undercooked infected wild boar or brown bear probably occurs; one suspected case has been reported. (Authors' abstract)

78. Reinhold, J. G., Nasr, K., Lahimgarzadeh, A., and Hedayati, H. "Effects of purified phytate and phytate-rich bread upon metabolism of zinc, calcium, phosphorus, and nitrogen in man." Lancet 1 (798), February 10, 1973, pp 283-288.

Three young men were given 2.5 g. of phytic acid daily, first as purified sodium phytate together with leavened flat wheat bread for 28 days, then for 32 days as tanok, the phytate-rich unleavened wholemeal flat wheat bread that is the staple food of many Iranian villagers. Purified phytate administration was accompanied by increased losses of zinc in faeces which varied in degree when compared with outputs during a control period preceeding the high phytate intakes. Phytate in the form of tanok led to negative zinc balances and strongly negative calcium balances in all. Negative calcium balances persisted after 60 days of phytate consumption. Urinary phosphate excretion decreased while tanok was the source of phytate, a change attributed to decreased phytate destruction in the gut probably due to an inhibitor present in the bread.

Plasma-zinc and serum-iron concentrations fell shortly after phytate consumption began, but later rose while phytate ingestion continued. However, plasma-calcium and serum-phosphorus fell and remained below normal. The results suggest that high-phytate intakes can cause the disturbances of zinc and calcium metabolism prevalent among Iranian villagers. They are applicable also to other populations who eat a lot of unleavened wholemeal bread. (Adapted from authors' abstract).

79. Reinhold, J. G., and Ronaghy, H. A. "Zinc deficiency in man." Lancet 2(819), July 1973, p 50.

This letter is in response to a May 5, Lancet article page 993 in which Dr. Caughey doubted that zinc deficiency in man was a clinical entity. The letter's authors found that a stimulus to growth did occur with zinc supplementation, provided sufficient zinc and time were allowed. They also noted that gonadal development was more advanced in zinc-supplemented boys compared to those not zinc-treated in their studies. They also noted that the diets of Egypt and Iran contained high unleavened bread components and the phytate content of the bread decreased the bioavailability of the zinc. They suggested that the low food intake of Iranian villagers was not due to lack of food available, but to the zinc deficient state itself, since zinc deficiency results in anorexia.

80. Sadre, M., Donoso, G., and Hedayat, H. "The fate of the hospitalized malnourished child in Iran." J. Trop. Pediatr. 19(1), September 1973, pp 28-31. (Environ. Child Health)

One hundred twenty-seven protein calorie malnutrition patients, newborn to 2 years of age, were followed from admission in the hospital to discharge, and visited six months after discharge (if they survived) to assess nutritional condition. 20% of the cases were less than six months old, and 41% were between six months and one year old. 77% of all cases were in the third degree of malnutrition according to the Gomez classification. 50% of malnourished patients stayed in the hospital for about one week. 36.2% of cases died during hospitalization, with 54% dying within one week of admission. 58% of all cases died by six months after discharge, and the children who survived six months following discharge showed minimal increase in weight. The authors called for better treatment and facilities for rehabilitation after hospitalization.

81. Sever, L. E. "Zinc deficiency in man." Lancet 1(808), April 1973, p 887.

This short letter noted that a relationship between maternal zinc deficiency and congenital malformations of the central nervous system may exist in man. The author based his hypothesis on finding high rates of CNS malformations in zinc-deficient pregnant rats and correlation of areas of high human CNS malformaton rates with high rates of zinc deficiency. He pointed out that zinc deficiency was more wide-spread than had been thought, and called for population studies to highlight the possible relationship between zinc deficiency and CNS malformations.

82. Wynder, E. L., and Mabuchi, K. "Cancer of the gastrointestinal tract. Etiological and environmental factors." JAMA 226(13), December 24, 1973, pp 1546-1548.

This review article presents information collected from several retrospective studies and prospective studies concerning the etiological and environmental factors associated with esophageal cancer. Demographic distribution is outlined, with emphasis on the high rates in France, in the Caspian littoral of Iran, and among South African Bantu. The mechanism of action of such factors as tobacco smoke, alcohol, and various nutritional deficiencies, such as iron and B vitamin complex constitutents, is discussed. Damage to mucosal epithelium is mentioned as one possible effect of some nutrient deficiencies.

83. Haghshenass, M. Mahlouidg, M., Reinhold, J. G., and Mohammadi, N. "Iron-deficiency anemia in an Iranian population associated with high intakes of iron." Am. J. Clin. Nutr. 25(11), November 1972, pp 1143-1146.

In five villages typical of those in southern Iran, 30% of the children, 24% females, and 7% of the males over 16, had hemoglobin concentrations of 12 g/100 ml or less. Packed red cell volumes were correspondingly low. Iron concentrations of representative village diets averaged 98.9 $\pm$ 10.1 (SE) ug/g dry diet. Iron intakes of 18 boys 13 to 14 years old in three villages averaged 44.4 $\pm$ 4.49 (SE) mg/day and exceeded 18 mg/day in 16.

Treatment of children and adults whose hemoglobin concentrations were below 10.5 g/100 ml or whose packed cell volume was less than 33% with 18 and 109 mg of iron (as ferrous sulfate) globin concentrations remained normal or nearly so 8 months after treatment was stopped. The occurrence of iron-deficiency anemia despite high content of iron in the diet is attributed to the substantial intakes of phytate present in the unleavened wholemeal wheat bread that is the main dietary staple of the villagers. (Authors' abstract)

84. Halsted, J. A., Ronaghy, H. A., Abadi, P., Haghshenass, M., and Amirhakemi, G. H. "Zinc defiency in man. The Shiraz experiment." Am. J. Med. 53(3), September 1972, pp 277-284.

A zinc supplementation study was undertaken for two women and fifteen Iranian army-rejected men who were malnourished. The subjects were 19 to 20 years old and were studied for 6 to 12 months. Three randomly selected groups were studied - a zinc-supplemented group, a placebo group, and a group which received no treatment for 6 months and then zinc supplementation. All groups were given adequate diets. The zinc supplementation brought about statistically significant enhancement of height increment and of onset of sexual functioning.

85. Kmet, J., and Mahboubi, E. "Esophageal cancer in the Caspian littoral of Iran: initial studies." Science 175(24), February 25, 1972, pp 846-853.

A report on the distribution of esophageal cancer incidence along the Caspian littoral of Iran is based on an ad hoc cancer registry in operation since 1968. The northeastern area, a semi-desert area, has the highest incidence in the world, with a higher incidence in women than in men: female--174.1/100,000 and male--108.8/100,000. The southeastern and central areas showed a lower incidence with a switch in the male/female ratio. Higher rainfall and nonsaline soils are in these areas. The western area has the highest rainfall, and the lowest incidence: males--17.2/100,000 and females--5.5/100,000. The worst food intake conditions were seen in two villages in the high incidence area. The diet was deficient in animal proteins, vitamin A, riboflavin, and vitamin C.

86. Sadre, M., Payan, R., Donoso, G., and Hedayat, H. "Protein food mixture for Iran. Acceptability and tolerance in infants and preschool children." J. Am Diet. Assoc. 60(2), February 1972, pp 131-134.

Acceptability and tolerance trials are reported for a low priced protein mixture for infants and preschool children compared with a regular diet. The "Protein Food Mixture" (PFM) was based on locally grown chick peas, split peas, and wheat. Forty-two children from 6 to 24 months old from a Teheran orphanage were divided into a control and a test group. All the children accepted the PFM formula quickly and without reservation. The weight increment in the PFM-consuming children was significantly higher than in the other children. However, they also received significantly higher calories and protein, being fed by spoon twice per day. The PFM-receiving children also showed an increase in the hematocrit, but not a significant increase over regularly fed children.

87. Borhanmanesh, F., Ghavami, A., Dutz, W., and Bagheri, S. "Cirrhosis of the liver in Iran. A prospective study on 66 cases." Reprinted by permission from J. Chronic Dis. 23(12), May 1971, pp 891-905. Pergamon Press, Ltd.

Sixty-six patients with cirrhosis of the liver were prospectively studied at Pahlavi University Medical Center, Shiraz, Iran. Of 51 in whom adequate tissue was available for pathological classification, 43 had post-necrotic cirrhosis (Gall's Type I) and 8 had post-hepatic cirrhosis (Gall's Type III), while none were found to have Laennec's cirrhosis. The posthepatic variety appeared to be in a better state in terms of the performed liver function studies. The main clinical features in our patients, who were approximately 20 years younger than their Western counterparts, included splenomegaly, massive ascites and a variety of herniations. Comparatively, there was a significantly decreased incidence of palmar erythema, clubbing of the fingers, parotid enlargement, and Dupuytren's contracture. Though the pathogenesis of these types of cirrhosis remains unclear, our observations suggest that malnutrition and viral hepatitis may be etiologically significant in the development of post-necrotic cirrhosis in Iran. (Authors' abstract)

88. Chapman, K. "Osteomalacia in Iran." J. Obstet. Gynaecol. Br. Commonw. 78(9), September 1971, pp 857-860.

Two osteomalacia cases are described in young multipara women in Iran who were carpet weavers from an early age until adulthood. The young women endured a life of long work hours, no medical care, no primary education and little exposure to sunlight. Both young women (23 and 26 years old) experienced difficulty in child-birth due to sacral deformities and outlet contraction secondary to osteomalacia, which had healed from the initial onset and left them deformed skeletally. One woman was delivered of her child with difficulty and the second woman was delivered by Casearean section. The author contends that the disease should be prevented by improvements in working conditions, compulsory yearly medical inspections, and free supply of cod liver oil and milk.

89. Hedayet, S., Koohestani, P. A., Ghassemi, H., and Kalami, P.

"Birthweight in relation to economic status and certain maternal factors, based on an Iranian sample." Trop. Geogr. Med. 23(4), December 1971, pp. 355-364.

This statistical survey is of 2123 single live births at three hospitals in Teheran, during the period October 1969 to August 1970. The patients admitted to the hospitals were from various socio-economic levels of the community. The results were as follows:

The male infants were found to be heavier than the females.

A significant direct positive correlation between economic status and birth weight was found.

There was a systematically increasing trend in the birth weight for the maternal age group up to 30 years. The correlation was significant.

The birth weight increased according to the order of birth up to the third with a significant correlation.

The mean birth weight according to level of education was significant when the illiterate was compared with secondary and the primary with university level of education.

A significant correlation between birth weight and the intake level of eggs and milk was found.

Maternal age at first delivery was significantly higher for those with a better economic status.

The occurrence of complications of pregnancy was higher in the lower income groups. (Authors' abstract)

90. Mahboubi, E. O. "Epidemiologic study of esophageal carcinoma in Iran." Int. Surg. 56(2), August 1971, pp 68-71.

The results of the first two years of an epidemiologic study of esophageal cancer in Mazandaran and one year's data from Gilan are reported. Three regions of the Caspian littoral are described - a high, an intermediate, and a low cancer incidence region. The dry region in the east had the highest incidence - 70 cases/100,000/year. The intermediate semi-dry region had an incidence of 17/100,000/year. The well watered western area had a low incidence of 6 cases/100,000/year. A retrospective case control interview study was also carried out to elucidate etiologic factors more clearly. Results indicated that in Iran alcohol, tobacco, opium, food and hot tea played no part in the etiology, but that certain foods eaten by pregnant women in the high incidence area might be a contributing factor.

91. McBean, L. D., Mahloudji, M., Reinhold, J. G., and Halsted, J. A. "Correlation of zinc concentrations in human plasma and hair." Amer. J. Clin. Nutr. 24(5), May 1971, pp 506-509.

Hair and plasma zinc concentrations were determined by atomic absorption spectrophotometry during October 1968 in 75 Iranian children aged 6 to 12 years. Plasma zinc was 72 $\pm$ 12 ug/100 ml (X $\pm$ SD). This was significantly lower than that found in 26 American children aged 3 to 13 years (P 0.001) (Halsted and Smith, 1970).

The mean hair zinc content (199 ± 22 ppm) reported is significantly greater than previously reported for Iranian village control males of similar ages. Paired plasma and hair samples zinc content correlation coefficient was 0.05 and was not statistically significant. Authors concluded that the data failed to show zinc hair content to be a reliable indicator of body stores in prepubescent children.

92. Motabar, M., Mofidi, C., Saebi, A., Ghiassedin, M., and Rouhani, F. "A medicated salt project in the Kazeroun area, Iran--1962-1967." <u>J. Trop. Med. Hyg.</u> 74(2), February 1971, pp 39-44.

A two-and-a-half years' experimental programme of chloroquinized and one-and-a-half years' of amodiaquinized salt distribution amongst villagers and nomads of Southern Iran has produced a considerable reduction in malaria prevalence of the order 400:1 in the stable, and 100:1 in the nomadic population-over-all. Parasite incidences have dropped to 0.05 percent and 0.12 percent, respectively. (Authors' abstract)

93. Reinhold, J. G. "High phytate content of rural Iranian bread: a possible caue of human zinc deficiency." <u>Amer. J. Clin. Nutr.</u> 24(10), October 1971, pp 1204-1206.

Phytic acid concentrations of three types of Iranian bread were determined. Tanok, an unleavened high extraction wheat bread, was sampled from 17 villages near Shiraz during November through March. Bazari and sangak, leavened breads baked in commercial bakeries in Shiraz, were sampled from September through March. Results showed that the village bread tanok contained more than twice as much phytate as bazari, and one and a half times as much as sangak. The author ascribed this to the effect of leavening and fermentation in destroying the phytate. He concluded that villagers consume far more phytate than urban dwellers, and that the phytate may be instrumental in producing deficiencies of iron, calcium, and zinc by complexing with them in the intestinal tract.

94. Tahernia, A. C., Moatamed, F., and Sharif, H. "Some clinical observations on rheumatic fever in childhood. Pattern of the disease as seen in Southern Iran." <u>Clin. Pediatr.</u> (Phila) 10(9), September 1971, pp 530-536.

One hundred children with rheumatic fever (RF) and rheumatic heart disease (RHD) were examined clinically, with emphasis on severity of infection and incidence of carditis and congestive heart failure (CHF). The children were between 5 and 14 years old, and were admitted to Nemazee Hospital in Shiraz between January 1, 1958 through December 31, 1969. May, June, November, and December were the peak months of admittance, and the age peak was 11 to 12 years. Fifty children were badly malnourished. Seventy-one children had significant fever in hospital. Twenty children were the products of consanguinous marriage. Carditis was seen in 83 children, pericarditis in 12, and cardiomegaly in 70. Treatment differed according to three different groups: 22 in group 1 received only steroid (prednisone), 18 in group 2 received prednisone and aspirin, and 32 in group 2 received only aspirin.

95. Caughey, J. E. "The spectrum of protein calorie malnutrition in adolescents." <u>Australas. Ann. Med.</u> 19(4), November 1970,

pp 341-349.

The physical and growth status of 452 boys in a high school in Marvdasht village and of a group of boys and a girl with moderate or severe malnutrition in a Saadi Hospital at Shiraz were measured. Heights, weights, serum protein levels, serum albumin, plasma zinc, degree of sexual maturation, haemoglobin levels, and size of liver were determined. Four phases of severity of malnutriton, dependent on age, state of sexual maturation, degree of malnutrition, and several other factors, were seen. Primary malnutritin due to low calorie and animal protein intake, and secondary malnutrition due to infections, geophagia, and parasitism were common. The first phase consisted of retarded body growth and development in otherwise healthy children. The second phase included susceptibility to infectious diseases and other illnesses, and further growth impairment and delay in sexual maturation. The third phase consisted of aggravated malnutrition with recurrent infections, diarrhoeal bouts, geophagia, and helminthiasis with low plasma zinc levels. Phase four consisted of acute diarrhoea, failure to grow and mature sexually, and flattened glucose tolerance curves and low pasma zinc. The author suggested that the clinical biochemical protein deficiency was the problem in the Iranian adolescents studied.

96. Creamer, B., Dutz, W., and Post, C. "Small-intestinal lesion of chronic diarrhoea and marasmus in Iran." Lancet 1(636), January 3, 1970, pp 18-20.

The small intestines of 11 infants who had died of chronic diarrhoea and marasmus in an orphanage in Shiraz, Iran, were examined at necropsy. Gross abnormalities were found throughout most of the small bowel in every case. The mucosa was severely flattened on the mucosal folds, and low ridges were present in between the folds. The findings are similar to those in tropical sprue and suggest that malabsorption is present in this syndrome. (Authors' abstract)

97. Rahmanian, M., Khouhestani, A., Ghavifekr, H., and Ter-Sarkissian, N. "High ascorbic acid content in some Iranian honeys. Chemical and biological assay." Nutr. Metab. 12(3), 1970, pp 131-135. S. Karger AG, Basel

A high content of Vitamin C (over 100 mg/100 g) in three samples of honey from a mountainous area (Damavand) in Iran is reported. The vitamin was determined by thin layer chromatography of its 2,4 dinitrophenyl osazone, as well as by the less specific 2,6 dichlorophenol indophenol method. The effect of one of these samples on the prevention and cure of scurvy in the guinea pig indicates that it contained compounds with vitamin C activity. (Authors' abstract).

98. Ronaghy, H. A., Kohout, E., Hadidi, N. "Body height and chronic malnutrition in school children in Iran." Amer. J. Clin. Nutr. 23(8), August 1970, pp 1080-1084.

To assess the extent and severity of malnutrition, 414 adolescent boys between 12 and 17 years of age from a town in southern Iran were measured anthropometrically; 100 of them were also clinically examined for nutritional deficiency; and 70 of them gave voluntary blood for laboratory tests. Almost 25% of the boys showed significant growth retardation, particularly those between the ages of 16 and 17 years. Average heights below the 3rd percentile, or 2 standard deviations of the Iowa Mean, correlated with increased incidence of lowered hemoglobin, serum protein, and serum albumin as well as with other signs and symptoms of retarded sexual maturation and vitamin deficiencies. Chronic malnutrition was indicated in the stunted boys, and stature was thus seen as a reliable indicator of malnutrition in adolescents.

99. Saadat-Noori, B., Nahani, J., Saedi, H., and Nikpour, K. "The incidence of vitamin E deficiency in poultry around Tehran." Poultry Sci. 49(3), May 1970, pp 675-678.

This study was conducted to compare blood plasma a-tocopherol content with biological indicator variation in poultry in the Tehran area. Spectrophotometric measurements of plasma a-tocopherol were done on 104 chicks slaughtered in various slaughter-houses to determine extent and range of deficiency levels. In addition, two groups of chicks were fed either an adequate or a Vitamin E deficient diet for 8 weeks and vitamin E in plasma was then measured. Brain changes in deficient chicks were also noted, and consisted of general disintegration of the cerebellum, hemorrhage, and edema, despite a lack of clinical signs. Plasma of ten other chicks diagnosed with encephalomalacia was analyzed for vitamin E. The authors' conclusions were two-fold: first, that clinical symptoms and depressed plasma a-tocopherol correlated directly; second, that vitamin E deficiency, as shown by low plasma vitamin E levels, was present with sub-clinical symptoms in poultry around Tehran.

Iraq

1. El-Radhi, A. S., Majeed, M., Mansor, N., and Ibrahim, M. "High incidence of rickets in children with wheezy bronchitis in a developing country". J. R. Soc. Med. 75(11), November 1982, pp 884-887.

   The incidence of rickets in 100 Iraqi infants with wheezy bronchitis (24%) exceeded by two and a half times that found in age-matched controls (9%) and by ten times the controls when only those with severe rickets were considered. The reason for this is not entirely clear, but could be related to the fact that the infants with wheezy bronchitis weighed more and therefore had grown faster than the control group. This itself could be related to the higher incidence of breastfeeding in the infants with wheezy bronchitis. We wish to stress the importance of screening for rickets, particularly in those with wheezy bronchitis. (Authors' abstract)

2. Shurri, N. A., and El-Abed, M. D. "Composition and some properties of the Janubi (Native Breed) cow's milk" Arab Gulf 13(1), 1981, pp 13-16.

   Milk of Janubi cows in Basrah, Iraq was studied from May, 1977 to May, 1978 at the local animal husbandry station. Composition studies showed Janubi cow's milk to be similar to Geurnsey and Jersey cow's milk. Studies on properties of the Janubi cow's milk showed it to be suitable for the production of butter and cream.

3. Al-Bahrani, Z. R., Al-Khateeb, A. K., Degayi, O., and Butrous, G. S. "Cancer of colon and rectum in Iraq." Am. J. Proctol. Gastroenterol. Colon Rectal Surg. 31(1) 1980, pp 20-22.

   This retrospective case study of colon and rectal cancer cases treated in hospital in Baghdad covers a period of 13 years, from 1965 to 1977 inclusive. For both sexes, the colon cancer incidence age averaged 49.84 years, and the rectal cancer incidence age averaged 43.42 years, with the ratio of males: females being 1.25:1, and 1.3:1, respectively. Pathology sites, gross appearance, microscopic examination, and staging are discussed. Resection was the principle treatment. 30.16% of colonic cancer patients were under 40 years old. The authors suggest that the high rate of intestinal infestation with amebiasis may play a role in the cancer pattern, and they noted the high prevalence of lymphoma in Iraq and other Middle East countries. They also noted that intestinal parasites such as amebiasis and bilharziasis may play a role in the relatively high percentage of squamous cell carcinoma of the rectum via irritation of the intestine.

4. Bakir, F., Rustam, H., Tikriti, S., Al-Damluji, S. F. and Shihristani, H. "Clinical and epidemiological aspects of methylmercury poisoning." Postgrad. Med. J. 56(651), January 1980, pp 1-10.

   The effects of methylmercury poisoning in humans was studied during the large outbreak in Iraq in 1971-2. In adults, poisoning resulted from home-made bread prepared from methylmercury-treated seed grain and there was a highly significant correlation between the amount of bread ingested and blood mercury levels. Poisonings in infants resulted either from prior exposure in utero or from suckling or both. Blood mercury levels were higher in infants and children than in adults. There was no increased incidence of congenital defects. Symptoms and signs of poisoning and histopathological changes were mainly confined to the CNS. Symptoms developed, on average, 1-2 months after exposure. In children there was mental retardation with delayed onset of speech and impaired motor, sensory and autonomic function. Severely affected children were blind and deaf. In adults, the clinical picture could be classified as 1-mild (mainly sensory symptoms), 2-moderate (sensory symptoms accompanied by cerebellar signs) and 3-severe (gross ataxia with marked visual and hearing loss which, sometimes progressed to akinetic mutism followed by coma). Improvement was observed among the mild and moderate group. Interference with transmission at the myoneural junction was found in 14% of patients studied. There was no evidence of peripheral nerve involvement per se and sensory symptoms may be of central origin. Clinical differences between Iraqi and Japanese outbreaks may be a result of the severe, prolonged and continuous exposure which occurred in the latter outbreak. Treatment with chelating agents, thiol resin, haemodialysis and exchange transfusion lowered blood mercury concentrations, but produced no convincing clinical benefits. (Adapted from authors' abstract)

5. Hegazi, F. Z., and Abo-Elnaga, I. G. "Characters of Lactobacillus coryniformis, isolated from an Iraqi cheese." Zentralbl. Bakterio. (Naturwiss) 135(3), 1980, pp 205-211.

Twenty-one strains of Lactobacillus coryniformis were isolated from Iraqi cheese and studied for biochemical, physiological, and cultural characteristics. L. coryniformis was found to differ from L. plantarum in the following ways: it did not contain DAP, it did not ferment ribose or trehalose, it failed to grow in 4% taurocholate, its morphology was different, and it did not decompose tartrate. None of the studied strains grew in 9% NaCL but did grow in 6.5% NaCL. 20 of the 21 strains produced CO_2 from gluconate. CO_2 was formed in the presence of glucose from the decomposition of CO_2 was formed in the presence of glucose from the decomposition of pyrivate, malate, and fumarate. After 41 days at 30 degrees C, 42.6 +/- 2.5 mumoles /ml average total lactate was produced, of which 42.3 +/- 1.7% was L(+) lactate. Milk coagulation occured within 3 to 60 days with a final pH of 4.05 and a final activity of 0.85 to 1.09%. Diacetyl plus acetoin production was also measured.

6. Jaddou, H., and Al-Hakim, M. "Gas-liquid chromatography of trimethylsilyl derivatives of sugars from Iraqi dates". J. Agric. Food Chem. 28(6), November-December 1980, pp 1208-1212.

A method for accurate measurement of sugars in dates was developed in which 95% ethanol was used for Soxhlet extraction of sugars from two varieties of Iraqi dates. Sugars were converted to their trimethylsilyl (Me_3Si) ether derivatives before application to GLC. Arabinose was used as an internal standard and the separation of the sugar derivatives was carried out on a 3% SE-30 column. Fructose, D-glucose, and sucrose were the major sugars present. Sorbitol and sorbose, which were not previously reported in the literature, were found in small quantities. The identification of sorbose and sorbitol was based on retention data using three different chromatographic columns. (Authors' abstract)

7. Marsh, D. O., Myers, G. J., Clarkson, T. W., Amin-Zaki, L., Tikritis, S., and Majeed, M. A. "Fetal methylmercury poisoning: clinical and toxicological data on 29 cases." Ann. Neurol. 7(4),

April 1980, pp 348-353. Little Brown and Co.

29 mother-infant pairs, exposed during pregnancy to varying amounts of methylmercury poisoning during the 1971-72 mercury poisoning outbreak in Iraq, were studied to discover minimal clinical psychomotor effects in infants and to relate such effects to maternal exposure to MeHg during pregnancy. Maternal hair mercury concentration was related to infants' neurological effects, which included delayed achievement of developmental milestones with or without neurological signs up to 4 1/2 to 5 years of age. Two groups of mothers with low to moderate hair mercury (0 to 11 and 12 to 85 ppm, respectively) had infants whose frequency of abnormal findings was significantly lower than those of the third group of mothers who had high hair mercury content at 99 to 384 ppm. Small subject numbers precluded the possibility of assigning a "threshold" point above which psychomotor effects could be expected. 80% of mothers in the high concentration group experienced transient parasthesias, while only 30% and 22% of mothers in the moderate and low concentration groups experience transient parasthesis. Some asymptomatic mothers produced children with neurologic abnormalities.

8. Shehata, A. A., and Thannoun, A. M. "Chemical and amino acid composition of Iraqi mung beans." Z. Lebensm. Unters. Forsch. 171(5), 1980, pp 360-362. Springer-Verlag Heidelberg.

Chemical composition and amino acid content studies were conducted on 5 samples of Iraqi mung beans collected from varying geographic areas in Iraq. Protein, carbohydrate, and mineral contents were good in all samples. The ranges observed were 0.86-0.96% crude fat, 64.15-66.32% carbohydrates, 24.95-28.04% protein, 3.37-4.05% ash, and 4.13-5.01% crude fiber. Lysine was particularly rich in all samples, at 5.85-8.24 gm/100 gm protein. Samples were also adequate in the other essential amino acids with the exception of methioine, at 0.96-1.48 gm/100 gm protein. On a dry weight basis, mineral contents were: phosphorus, 381-528; iron, 5.14-5.76; and calcium, 128-143 mg/100 gm of flour, respectively.

9. Al-hindawi, N., and Taha, R. R. "Salmonella species isolated from animal feed in Iraq." Appl. Environ. Microbiol. 37(4), April 1979, pp 676-679.

Of 700 animal feed samples, 32 (4.5%) harbored Salmonella. The highest percentage of contamination was found in sheep feed and local protein. A total of 17 Salmonella serotypes were identified. The most frequent serotypes were Salmonella melsagridis, S. bornum, S. montevideo and S. drypool. S. bornum was isolated for the first time in Iraq and from both local feed and its ingredients. The common somatic group found was that of Salmonella group C; than came groups E, G, B and D. Three serotypes (S. enteritidis, S. california and S. muanchan) seemed to form a link of infection among feed, food, patients and carriers. (Authors' abstract)

10. Nagi, N. A., and Al-Dubooni, H. M. "Severe protein-calorie malnutrition in Iraq, and its effect on immunity reactions." J. Trop. Med. Hyg. 80(4), April 1977, pp 78-82.

One hundred pre-school children hospitalized with protein calorie malnutrition (PCM) in Mosul, northern Iraq, were studied for physical features and influencing factors. Marasmus outnumbered marasmic kwashiorkor and kwashiorkor cases. Causative factors were early weaning, prolonged lactation, unsanitary dilution of bottle feeds, infection, poverty, and ignorance. Although infection was invariably the precipitating cause of hospitalization, patients did not always exhibit signs and symptoms of infection. For example, tuberculosis existed in some with a negative tuberculin skin test. Light developmental retardation was shown by the patients. Authors suggested urinanalysis and culture for each PCM patient.

11. Al-Damluji, S. F. "Organomercury poisoning in Iraq: history prior to the 1971-72 outbreak." Bull. WHO 53 suppl, 1976, pp 11-12.

Mercury has been used medically in the Middle East since time immemorial. Organomercury compounds were first used as seed dressings in Iraq in 1955. During the years 1955-59, 200 cases of poisoning occurred. A more clearly defined outbreak occurred in 1960, involving approximately 1000 hospital admissions. Twelve patients from two families affected in this outbreak were re-examined in 1973, and showed considerable improvement. (Author's abstract)

12. Al-Damluji, S. F. and the Clinical Committee on Mercury Poisoning "Intoxication due to alkylmercury-treated seed--1971-72 outbreak in Iraq: clinical aspects." Bull WHO 53 suppl, 1976, pp 65-81.

Sixty-six hospitalized patients between 4 and 70 years suffering from chronic methylmercury poisoning were examined in Baghdad during 1972. The poisoning was attributed to consumption of home-made bread prepared from seed wheat treated with mercurial fungicide.

Neurological symptoms and signs were predominant and included muscular weakness, numbness, unsteady gait, paraesthesia, dysarthria, mental disturbances and, in severe cases, blindness, partial deafness, stupor, coma, and death. Involvement of the cardiovascular, urinary, gastrointestinal and haemopoietic systems, which was commonly encountered in methylmercury poisoning in the 1960 outbreak in Iraq, was unusual. The severity of symptoms and signs was, broadly speaking, dose-dependent; high exposure led to severe clinical manifestations, but variations existed. The series included 2 asymptomatic cases, 20 mild, 20 moderate, 14 severe, and 10 very severe. In the latter group 5 patients died from failure of the central nervous system.

The severely poisoned patients died irrespective of the medical treatment received. After 2 years of observation, most patients graded as mild or moderate cases lost their symptoms completely. Severe cases improved slowly although ataxia, diminution of visual field and acuity, and paraesthesia were still present. Thus, the previously accepted view that neurological signs were irreversible has been disproved. (Adapted from authors' abstract).

13. Al-Falluji, N., Makkawi, T. A., Abou-el-azm, I. M., Sokkar, I. M., and Darraji, M. "Experimental studies on organomercury poisoning in chickens in Iraq." Bull. WHO 53 suppl, 1976, pp 119-127.

For 164 days, mature chickens received a daily diet containing 40 g of wheat treated with organomercurial fungicide and 80 g of untreated diet. A control group received 120 g of normal diet daily. The experimental group was then split - half receiving the same diet for a further 155 days, by which time all had been killed or had died, the other half being fed the same diet as the controls. No cases of mercurialism were seen in the experimental group, although 2 died after 143 and 319 days respectively. Egg production fluctuated between the groups. Mercury levels in egg albumin showed high peaks after 98 and 108 days. After the feeding of contaminated wheat had been discontinued, the albumin mercury level did not fall consistently below 0.5 mg/kg for 127 days. Levels in egg yolk always remained below the level in wheat and dropped to zero 49 days after feeding the dressed wheat had been discontinued. Mercury levels found in tissue were similar to those described by other authors. Levels in the edible parts of the single cock examined exceeded those in the hens. Implications of these findings for public health decisions on the use of chicken and eggs as food when the birds have had access to contaminated grain are discussed. (Authors' abstract)

14. Al-Saleem, T., and Clinical Committee on Mercury Poisoning "Levels of mercury and pathological changes in patients with organomercury poisoning." Bull. WHO 53 suppl, 1976, pp 99-104.

    Autopsies were carried out on 4 adults who died during the outbreak of mercury poisoning in Iraq and on 4 infants who were exposed to organomercury in utero. Mercury levels in tissues and in some body fluids were determined. The high levels of mercury in the central nervous system and the marked neuronal degeneration are noted. (Author's abstract)

15. Al-Shahristani, H., Shihab, K., and Al-Haddad, I. K. "Mercury in hair as an indicator of total body burden." Bull. WHO 53 suppl, 1976, pp 105-112.

    Hair concentrates mercury, and in general the concentration of mercury in hair is proportional to and many times higher than its concentration in blood. The variation of the mercury concentration in human head hair was used to follow the history of poisoning in people who ingested grain treated with methylmercury. Instrumental neutron activation analysis was used for mercury determination. The initial rising slope of mercury concentration along the hair was proportional to the daily intake of methylmercury per kg of body weight. The ratio of the concentration of methylmercury in human head hair to the average body concentration was about 137. By using this ratio and measuring mercury concentration in hair, the total body burden can be calculated. In patients studied, peak body burden ranged from 0.8 to 4.4 mg/kg in cases showing mild symptoms, from 1.5 to 6 mg/kg in cases with moderate symptoms, and from 3 to 12 mg/kg in cases with severe symptoms. The curve of variation in mercury concentrations along the hair was also used to calculate the biological half-life of methylmercury in man. Forty-eight cases were studied and it was found that the frequency curve (population distribution curve) was grouped into two distinct regions. In about 90% of the population the biological half-life of methylmercury was 35-100 days, and 10% showed high values of 110-120 days. (Authors' abstract)

16. Al-Mufti, A. W., Copplestone, J. F., Kazantzis, G., Mahmoud, R. M., and Majid, M. A. "Epidemiology of organomercury poisoning in Iraq. I. Incidence in a defined area and relationship to the eating of contaminated bread." Bull WHO 53 suppl, 1976, pp 23-36.

    A survey was carried out in rural Iraq where there had been

organomercury poisoning following consumption of bread contaminated by mercury. Results were compared with those of a similar rural area from which few cases were reported. A questionnaire determined the amount of contaminated bread eaten and frequency of symptoms; a simple clinical examination was performed and blood and hair samples were collected for estimation of total mercury concentration. Of 700 people over the age of 5 years in the high-exposure area, 66% admitted to eating contaminated bread; none of the 864 persons in the low exposure area had. The mean period during which contaminated bread was eaten was 32 days, but some had eaten it for 3 months. A mean of 121 loaves was eaten, the maximum being 480 loaves. For the mean number of loaves, methylmercury intake was likely between 80 mg and 250 mg, but people who consumed the largest amount may have ingested up to 1,000 mg of methylmercury over 3-months. Of those with signs of alkylmercury poisoning 80% ate more than 100 loaves, and 53 (71%) out of 75 persons who had more than 200 loaves showed evidence of poisoning. Incidence for poisoning was 271 per 1,000; these figures include mortality rate of 59 per 1,000, 32 per 1,000 cases with severe disability, 41 per 1,000 cases with mild or moderate disability, and 138 per 1,000 cases with only subjective evidence of poisoning. (Authors' abstract)

17. Al-Tikriti, K., and Al-Mufti, A. W. "An outbreak of organomercury poisoning among Iraqi farmers." Bull WHO 53 suppl, 1976, pp 15-21.

An outbreak of organomercury poisoning due to the consumption of treated grain by farmers and their families occurred in Iraq in 1971-72. A total of 6530 cases were admitted to hospital and of these 459 died. However, there were many more with minor symptoms of poisoning who consulted outpatient departments. This outbreak constituted the largest poisoning epidemic ever recorded. No age was exempt and no pronounced sex difference was apparent. The latent period of up to 60 days between dosage and the onset of symptoms was probably the major factor contributing to the size of the epidemic. Measures taken to limit the outbreak are outlined. (Authors' abstract)

18. Amin-Zaki, L., Elhassani, S., Majeed, M. A., Clarkson, T. W., Doherty, R. A., Greenwood, M. R., and Giovanoli-Jakubeczak, T. "Perinatal methylmercury poisoning in Iraq." Am. J. Dis. Child 130(10), October 1976, pp 1070-1076.

The signs and symptoms of methylmercury poisoning and the concentrations of mercury in samples of blood, hair, and milk are reported and compared in two infant-mother pairs exposed in the recent Iraq outbreak. In one pair, the infant was born prior to the exposure of the mother, and was exposed only from ingestion of methylmercury in mother's milk. In the other pair, the mother was exposed during pregnancy and did not breast feed the infant, who died 30 days after birth. Both mothers had some signs and symptoms of poisoning, but the infants did not. The infants had maximum estimated blood mercury levels between 500 and 1,000 ng/ml, well above the minimum toxic levels for adults. Hair and blood concentrations of mercury correlated closely, the average hair-blood ratio being about 250. Maternal milk averaged 8.6% of the simultaneous blood level, but the relationship was nonlinear at blood mercury levels below 50 ng/ml. Postnatal exposure by suckling led to substantial infant blood mercury concentration (over 600 ng/ml), and prenatal exposure resulted in blood mercury levels in the infant at birth higher than those in the mother, even after corrections for differences in hematocrit level. (Authors' abstract)

19. Bakir, F., Al-Khalidi, A., Clarkson, T. W., and Greenwood, R. "Clinical observations on treatment of alkylmercury poisoning in hospital patients." Bull. WHO 53 suppl, 1976, pp 87-92.

Twenty-six patients suffering from methylmercury poisoning were treated by different therapeutic regimes. Seven received penicillamine or N-acetyl-d-L-penicillamine, 10 were treated with dimercaprol sulfonate and 9, who could not be treated, were given a placebo and were used as controls. Penicillamine, N-acetyl-d-L-penicillamine, and dimercaprol sulfonate reduced the blood level of mercury and increased its urinary excretion. No appreciable clinical improvement was noticed among the severe or very severe cases, while mild or moderate cases improved clinically irrespective of the treatment given. (Authors' abstract)

20. Bakir, F., Al-Shahristani, H., Al-Rawi, N. Y., Khadouri, A., and Al-Mufti, A. W. "Indirect sources of mercury poisoning in the Iraq epidemic." Bull WHO 53 suppl, 1976, pp 129-132.

Secondary sources of intoxication with methylmercury poisoning other than homemade bread were explored. Mercury levels in various food items were below 0.05 mg/kg.

Over 30,000 specimens of meat and internal organs of sheep were analyzed because of the strong suspicion that the animals had been fed treated barley. It was found that 6-12% of the specimens analysed contained more than 0.5 mg/kg of mercury. Consumption of meat did not appear to constitute a danger of intoxication during the outbreak. (Authors' abstract)

21. Clarkson, R. W., Amin-Zaki, L., and Al-Tikriti, S. K. "An outbreak of methylmercury poisoning due to consumption of contaminated grain." Fed. Proc. 35(12), October 1976, pp 2395-2399.

An outbreak of methylmercury poisoning took place in the fall and winter of 1971-72 in Iraq. Six thousand five hundred thirty cases were admitted to hospitals throughout the country and 459 died in hospital. The outbreak was the result of eating homemade bread prepared from wheat treated with a methylmercury fungicide. The wheat was intended for planting purposes only. Signs and symptoms of poisonings in adults indicate that the major site of action of this form of mercury is the central nervous system. Severe brain damage also resulted from prenatal exposure when the mother ingested large amounts of the contaminated bread. The frequency of signs and symptoms in an exposed population was found to be related to the estimated maximum blood levels, i.e., the concentration in blood at the end of exposure. A small percentage of the population exhibited a significant increase in complaints of paresthesia at maximum blood levels in the range of 240 to 480 ng Hg/ml. At higher blood levels a greater proportion of the population complained of paresthesia and other signs and symptoms became apparent. (Authors' abstract)

22. Demarchi, M., Demian, H. G., Ali, M., and Azzawi, M. Nutritional status of preschool children in the area of Baghdad (Iraq)." Bull. Nutr. Inst. 6(1), 1976, pp 129-144.

The study revealed the following epidemiological factors associated with the prevalence of protein calorie malnutrition (PCM) among low socio-economic groups of children:

1. Malnutrition is most prevalent in the age group 7-24 months.

2. Girls are more affected than boys, probably due to better care given to boys.

3. Contrary to expectation, the number of children in the family does not affect the prevalence of malnutrition.

4. The prevalence of diarrhoea is higher among children affected with malnutrition.

5. Under one year of age the prevalence of diarrhea was less among breast fed children than bottle fed children. The latter group of infants are more subject to infection as a result of unsanitary and unhygenic handling of milk at home.

6. No difference in the prevalence of PCM was found among children in the age group 13-24 months, whether they were on the breast or on bottle feeding.

7. It appears that breast feeding favours the nutritional status of the child while it continues; once weaning has occurred there is little evidnce of a "carry over" effect in this population. (Authors' summary)

23. Jernelow, A. "Environmental contamination by mercury in Iraq." Bull. WHO 53 suppl, 1976, pp 115-118.

Following the outbreak of organomercury poisoning in Iraq, an investigation was carried out during spring and summer, 1972 to evaluate environmental contamination by organomercury. Analyses were performed on fish of several species (not typical predators) and on a few specimens of aquatic birds (not fish-eating). Most fish samples contained concentrations in muscle ranging from 0.01 to 0.15 mg/kg. These concentrations were within the range found in tropical rivers. Higher figures, 0.3-0.5 mg/kg, were found downstream from a caustic soda plant south of Baghdad. A few cases of very high mercury concentrations (25-30 mg/kg) were reported from an area where fish kills had occurred. Aquatic birds (ducks and waders) contained low concentrations of mercury (900-2750 ng/g). Tail feathers of seed-eating birds contained 13,500-21,000 ng/g of mercury, which is about 10 times higher than values reported from Ethiopia and within the range found in Sweden and Canada. Insect-eating birds contained 1850-5200 ng/g, which is slightly elevated. Extremely high concentrations of mercury were found in muscle tissue of dead seed-eating birds (15,000-40,000 ng/g), while feathers contained similar concentrations (9000-52,000 ng/g). These extremely high concentrations were found only in the vicinity of storehouses where treated seed was kept. No birds of prey could be caught and analyzed. (Author's abstract)

24. Kazantzis, G., Al-Mufti, A. W., Copplestone, J. F., Majid, M. A., and Mahmoud, R. M. "Epidemiology of organomercury poisoning in Iraq. III. Clinical features and their changes with time." Bull. WHO 53 suppl, 1976, pp 49-57.

Three categories of mercury poisoning were defined in the survey described by Al-Mufti et al. and the age-specific incidence rates given. Persons with physical signs consistent with a diagnosis of organomercury poisoning were allocated to categories of severe disability or mild/moderate disability. However, the largest category consisted of persons who had symptoms but no readily elicitable physical signs at the time of the survey. These symptoms followed a consistent pattern with paraesthesia involving the lips and/or circumoral region or trunk and difficulty with walking, described as weakness or unsteadiness of the legs, and in some cases repeated falls. Mean maximum hair mercury levels differentiated this group very clearly from the group with no symptoms of mercury poisoning. Very few people in the area of low exposure complained of such symptoms; where they did occur they were less well related to the time of the outbreak and showed little tendency to improve. It is not known whether those people with only symptoms at the time of the survey had had at an earlier stage mild signs which had cleared. It was thought unlikely that further substantial improvement would occur in those persons with disability at the time of the survey. (Adapted from authors' abstract)

25. Kazantzis, G., Al-Mufti, A. W., Al-Jawad, A., Al-Shahwani, Y., Majid, M. A., Mahmoud, R. M., Soufi, M., Tawfiq, K., Ibrahim, M. A., and Dabagh, H. "Epidemiology of organomercury poisoning in Iraq. II. Relationship of mercury levels in blood and hair to exposure and to clinical findings." Bull WHO 53 suppl, 1976, pp 37-48.

In the survey described by Al-Mufti et al blood and hair samples were analysed for total mercury by modified atomic absorption spectrophocometry. Hair samples were divided into 2.5cm segments and analysed consecutively. Mean blood levels were 34 ng/ml and 7 ng/ml, respectively in those who had and had not eaten contaminated bread. Corresponding mean maximum hair mercury values were 136 ug/g and 5 ug/g, respectively. Hair mercury values provided a better discrimination between categories of exposure than blood mercury values some months after the end of the outbreak. Those who had not eaten contaminated bread but who lived in the area of high exposure had hair mercury values between the values of those who had eaten and those who had not eaten contaminated bread and who lived in the area of low exposure. Sequential estimation of mercury in 2.5-cm segments of hair in women gave information on the period of accumulation of mercury more than 1 year before the time of collection of samples. It was possible to show an approximate relationship between the maximum hair mercury value and the amount of contaminated bread eaten. The match between the blood mercury level and the severity of poisoning was poor, owing to the length of time that had elapsed between the onset of poisoning and the sampling. With hair mercury, while the group results showed a good relation to severity of poisoning, in individual cases the match was less good, especially in those where insufficient length of hair was available for analysis. Biological variation in sensitivity to methylmercury was also an important factor. (Authors' abstract)

26. Magos, L., Bakir, F., Clarkson, T. W., Al-Jawad, A. M., and Al-Soffi, M. H. "Tissue levels of mercury in autopsy specimens of liver and kidney." Bull. WHO 53 suppl, 1976, pp 93-97.

Fifty-one autopsy specimens of liver were analysed for total mercury. Thirteen specimens contained less than 10 mg/kg of mercury, with a minimum value of 1.4 mg/kg, indicating that death was not always due to lethal exposure to methylmercury. The methylmercury concentration in 28 livers was 10-30 mg/kg. Limited additional estimations have shown that 71% of the liver mercury was organic and that the level of mercury in the liver of a 7-month-old fetus was only 25% of that in the liver of the mother. In a patient who died in hospital with a blood mercury level of 4.1 ug/ml, the liver contained 16.5 mg/kg of mercury.

Differences between these results and those found in the outbreak of methylmercury poisoning in Japan are discussed. Any extrapolation of tissue mercury levels in relation to the toxic effects of methylmercury must take account of the intensity and duration of exposure. (Authors' abstract)

27. Sabelaish, S., and Hilmi, G. "Ocular manifestations of mercury poisoning." Bull. WHO 53 suppl, 1976, pp 83-86.

One hundred patients suffering from organomercury poisoning who were hospitalized in the Medical City, University of Baghdad, were examined ophthalmologically in the period between March and December 1972, and were reviewed again about 10 months later.

The examination included clinical signs and symptoms, slit lamp examination of the anterior segment of the eyes, examination for visual field changes and, in the autopsied cases, analysis of the optic nerve and the occipital cortex. In addition, aqueous humour was aspirated in 10 patients and in 10 controls for the estimation of the mercury level. (Authors' abstract)

28. Skerfving, S. B., and Copplestone, J. F. "Poisoning caused by the consumption of organomercury-dressed seed in Iraq". Bull WHO 54(1), 1976, pp 101-112.

In 1971-72, a large outbreak of poisoning caused by the consumption of seed dressed with organomercury compounds occurred in Iraq. International assistance was requested by the Government of Iraq in investigating this outbreak. The results of the investigations to date were presented at the Conference on Intoxication due to Alkylmercury Treated Seed, held in Baghdad, Iraq on 9-13 November 1974. This paper summarizes the main findings and recommendations of the Conference. (Authors' abstract)

29. Smith, J. C., Farris, F. F., and Von Burg, R. "Chemical type of mercury in patients in the outbreak of organomercury poisoning in Iraq." Bull WHO 53 suppl, 1976, pp 61-63.

Gas chromatography was employed to identify the mercurial compound involved in the Iraq outbreak of organomercury poisoning. Only methylmercury was detected in human blood, hair, and tissues. The quantity of methylmercury present correlates well with the quantity of organic mercury determined by selective atomic absorption. (Authors' abstract)

30. Shakir, A. "Arm circumference in the surveillance of protein-calorie malnutrition in Baghdad." Am. J. Clin. Nutr. 28(6), June 1975, pp 661-665.

Seven hundred seventy-seven Baghdad children of known birthdates from 3 to 72 months of age and from varying socioeconomic groups and different nutritional status levels were measured for weight, height, and left mid-upper-arm circumference. The percentage of

Boston weight for age standards was compared with the percentages of mid-upper-arm for age standards and they were found to have a 0.92 correlation (P smaller than 0.001). Percentage arm for age standard predicted within plus or minus 16% the percentage weight for age standard. The author suggested use in the field of a constant midpoint arm circumference standard of 16.5 cm for children with imprecise age between 13 and 72 months of age on the basis of its age independence and its efficacy compared with age specific arm standards and weight for age standards for this age range.

31. Shakir, A. "The surveillance of protein-calorie malnutrition by simple and economical means" (a report to UNICEF) J. Trop. Pediatr. 21(2), April 1975, pp 69-85.

The methods used for diagnosing malnutrition in children in developing countries were summarized. The author discussed the tools used, their advantages and disadvantages, and the variations for differing field conditions. Criteria for practicality were given for the methods and the equipment needed. The various anthropometric measurements were listed with advantages and disadvantages. The arm/head ratio, advocated for both surveys and screening, was criticized because two difficult measurements were needed for it. The use of a single measurement such as the triceps skinfold thickness or the mid-upper arm circumference was advocated. A tri-colored arm string was suggested as a simple and accurate method of diagnosing malnutrtion in young children. Use of local anthropometric standards was recommended, and a simple child progress chart with the identification of edema was suggested. The appendix contained many tables of data based on a measurement survey of 777 Baghdad children from 7 to 32 months of age.

32. Amin-Zaki, L., Elhassani, S., Majeed, M. A., Clarkson, T. W., Doherty, R. A., and Greenwood, M. R. "Studies of infants postnatally exposed to methylmercury." J. Pediatr. 85(1), July 1974, pp 81-84.

The blood, hair, and milk of mother-infant pairs in Baghdad hospitals and from people in farms and villages within 100 kilometers of Baghdad were sampled and analyzed for total and inorganic mercury. The pairs were exposed postnatally from June 1972 to March 1973 to mercury poisoning. In first samples, mercury in infant blood was significantly lower than that in mothers' blood (50% of mothers'). In July, infant and mother levels were similar. After that, infant levels were higher than mothers. Milk levels were always lower than either mother's or infant's blood levels. Eight infants had blood mercury levels more than 200 p.p.b. presumably from ingesting mother's milk. No clinical signs of mercury poisoning were detected in infants.

33. Amin-Zaki, L., Elhassani, S., Majeed, M. A., Clarkson, T. W., Doherty, R. A., and Greenwood, M. "Intra-uterine methylmercury poisoning in Iraq." Pediatrics 54(5), November 1974, pp 587-595.

An epidemic of mercury poisoning occurred in rural Iraq in 1971-1972 as a result of ingestion of bread made from wheat and barley treated with methylmercury fungicide. The authors assessed 15 infant-mother pairs exposed to the mercury during gestation.

Mercury levels were obtained from blood samples of mothers and infants and from breast milk samples for seven months following the epidemic. The infants' blood mercury levels were higher than the mothers in 14 cases. The results suggest that the mercury is transmitted easily from mother to fetus and mercury is then ingested through breastfeeding.

Six infants and six mothers showed clinical signs of methylmercury poisoning. Five infants had gross impairment of mental and motor development. Only one pair had an affected infant and symptom-free mother.

34. Harland, P. S. "Letter: Measuring malnutrition." Lancet 1(863), May 11, 1974, p 925.

This very short letter lauds the three-color cord advocated by Drs. Shakir and Morley for measuring malnutrition in young children, but points out that in Iraq, where this method was studied, marasmus is the prevailing type of malnutrition. The author points out that in Kenya he used the cord on a small number of children, and that the only kwashiorkor case he observed measured well in the normal, green area of the cord. The author questions the usefulness of the cord in areas where kwashiorkor is the predominant form of malnutrition.

35. Nagi, N. A., and Yassin, A. K. "Organic mercury poisoning in children." J. Trop. Med. Hyg. 77(6), June 1974, pp 128-132.

An outbreak of organic mercury poisoning took place in Iraq in 1972. The paper describes the clinical picture encountered in 26 children admitted to a children's hospital over a one month period. Neurological manifestations included ataxia, decreased visual acuity, dysarthria, exaggerated tendon reflexes, tremor, and paresis in lower extremities. No evidence of toxic effect on the kidneys or cardiovascular and haemopoeitic effects were seen. Anaemia in patients was thought to be due to endemic iron deficiency. Treatment with BAL produced no satisfactory results, nor did EDTA treatment result in improvement. Prognosis for recovery from the mercury poisoning was poor.

36. Shakir, A. "The arm/head ratio in the assessment of protein-calorie malnutrition in Baghdad." J. Trop. Pediatr. 20(3), June 1974, pp 122-125. (Environ. Child Health)

A comparison is made between the Boston weight for age standard and the Arm/Head ratio of 777 Baghdad children aged 3 to 72 months. The coefficient of correlation between them was 0.88 (p less than 0.001). The Arm/Head ratio seems a suitable alternative and has many practical advantages, especially under field conditions, when the precise age is not known. A simple ruler is designed from which the ratio of the two measurements can be read directly and the nutritional status defined. (Author's abstract)

37. Shakir, A., and Morley, D. "Letter: Measuring malnutrition." Lancet 1(860), April 1974, pp 758-759.

A multi-colored arm band was designed for measuring simple arm-circumference in nutritional assessment of young children. Red, green, and yellow bands are used to denote normal, possible mild malnutrition, and malnutrition. The simplicity of the method as a quick and reliable method of identifying ill-nourished children was noted. A picture of the cord itself and of a child being measured with it were included, along with a chart relating cord color to arm circumference.

38. Amin, A., and Sternkopf, G. "The content of amino acids in beet molasses from Iraq." Nahrung 17(1), 1973, pp 87-89. (German)

The amino acid composition of two beet molasses, produced in 1970 and 1971 in Iraq is given. With regard to the determined content of non sugar compounds, a comparison is made with bibliographical data of German beet molasses. (Authors' abstract)

39. Bakir, F., Damluji, S. F., Amin-Zaki, L., Murtadaha, M., and Khalidi, A. "Methylmercury poisoning in Iraq." Science 181 (96), July 1973, pp. 230-241.

This is a comprehensive report of the methylmercury poisoning epidemic among Iraqi farmers and their families in 1971-72 as a result of their having ingested bread made from methylmercury-treated wheat and barley grain. The grains had been treated with a fungicide and imported to Iraq for planting purposes only. 90% of cases were admitted to hospital during January and February 1972, and of 6530 cases admitted, 459 hospital deaths occurred. Mercury in plasma, urine, milk and other body fluids was assessed. Symptoms were paresthesias, then ataxia, dysarthria, and hearing defects at increasing toxicity levels. Starting 2 to 3 months after cessation of ingestion, some functional recovery took place. Blood tests were the best indicators of methylmercury poisoning, and consecutive segments of hair samples were a good means of recapitulating the exposure history. Rate of clearance from blood and response to orally-administered mercury binders varied with individuals. Methylmercury was transferred into milk at 3% concentration of that of mother's blood. There was a high mortality (45%) of affected pregnant females admitted to hospital.

40. Magos, L., and Jawad, A. M. "Method for screening barley and wheat samples for mercury". J. Sci. Food Agric. 24(10), October 1973, pp 1305-1309.

A flameless atomic absorption method was used for screening large numbers of undigested crushed grain samples in Iraq in 1972 in an outbreak of methylmercury poisoning which occurred after the misuse of seed wheat treated with methyl-mercury fungicide. In the standard procedure 1 g of crushed grain was added to a reaction vessel with 1 ml of 1% cysteine, 20 ml of 1% saline and 10 ml of 16 N-H_2SO_4. Methylmercury and all the other forms of mercury were converted to atomic mercury by the combined $SnCl_2$-$CdCl_2$ reagent after the addition of 20 ml 45% NaOH. Atomic mercury was moved from the reaction vessel through the gas cell of a mercury vapour meter by an air pump. Deflection on the scale of the mercury vapour meter was recorded and by use of standard additions to the same sample mercury contents were calculated. It was found that from crushed grain approximately 60% of the mercury was released compared with estimations carried out on digests necessitating the use of a correction factor for quantitation. This screening technique, which does not need elaborate instruments or special skill and care, made it possible for two people to screen approximately 30 samples per hour and to overcome the emergency situation which had been presented by the large number of wheat stocks suspected of containing methylmercury. (Authors' abstract)

41. Damluji, S. F., and Tikriti, S. "Mercury poisoning from wheat." Br. Med. J. 1(803), March 24, 1972, p 804.

This short letter describes an outbreak of poisoning caused by the mercurial compound Granosan M in Iraq. The poisonng was caused by the ingestion of fungicide-dressed wheat grain by Iraqi farmers, with the number of deaths reaching 280 in two months' time, and a hospital case load of 5500. The author requested correspondence with any doctors who had experience in this field.

42. Nagi, N. A. "Vitamin D deficiency rickets in malnourished children." J. Trop. Med. Hyg. 75 (12), December 1972, pp 251-254.

The study of 50 children, in whom the male to female ratio was 3:2, with vitamin D deficiency rickets revealed that, contrary to current belief, rickets can take place in children suffering from malnourishment and growth failure. In such children the disease is not associated with elevated serum alkaline phosphatase, probably because of hypoproteinaemia. There was a reduction of inorganic phosphorus in the serum of most of the patients and this is considered a fairly sensitive index of the disease. However, serum calcium was not significantly altered. Breast feeding does not seem to provide protection against rickets. (Author's abstract)

43. Najuib, K., al-Sonaily, I. A., and al-Sultan, A. S. "A study on Iraqi date extract: "Dibis" as substrate for mycological fat production". J. Sci. Food Agric. 23(7), July 1972, pp 845-851.

A date extract known locally in Iraq as "dibis" was used as substrate for mycological fat formation by Penicillium lilacinum, P. soppii and Aspergillus nidulans. The three fungi were grown on dibis medium at three concentrations. Carbohydrates readily disappeared, but this was accompanied by poor fungal growth and low yields of fat.

Fungal growth on dibis media enriched with asparagine led to heavy mycelial yields together with higher fat contents. Both economic and fat coefficients rose considerably. It is concluded that nitrogen deficiency in dibis media is at least one of the major factors against good fungal growth and high fat formation. (Authors' abstract)

44. Najuib, K., al-Schaily, I. A., and al-Sultan, A. S. "On mycological fat production from Iraqi date extract: the dibis". Mycopathol. Mycol. 47(1), June 1972, pp 93-103.

Three strong fat-forming fungi, namely, Penicillin lilacinum, P. soppi and Aspergillus nidulans were grown on Iraqi date extract, "dibis" supplemented with an external source of nitrogen in the form of asparagine, ammonium carbonate or sodium nitrate.

P. lilacinum was the slowest in growth and fat formation, but later exceeded the two other fungi. Media supplemented with ammonium carbonate were the least conducive to growth and fat formation. Asparagine was most favorable for fat formation in case of P. lilacinum, sodium nitrate in case of A. nidulans; but in case of P. soppi, the two sources were equally good.

The use of different levels of nitrogen has shown that in the case of P. lilacinum, increase in nitrogen within the experimental limits was accompanied by an increase in fat yield. In the case of P. soppi and A. nidulans, the fat yield increased with decrease of nitrate nitrogen (increase in C:N ratio), but with asparagine, the medium concentration gave the heaviest yield.

The highest fat percentage or fat coefficients did not, however, coincide with the highest total fat yield nor with the complete exhaustion of the sugar content. It is concluded that addition of nitrogen at the proper concentration to dibis media can bring up growth and fat formation to a reasonable level. But dibis as substrate for fat formation seems to be yet inferior to synthetic media favourable for fat formation. (Authors' abstract)

45. Shakir, A. "The age at menarche in girls attending schools in Baghdad." Hum. Biol. 43(2), May 1971, pp 265-270.

4673 girls of Arab descent, belonging to one of three socioeconomic levels, were questioned in a school setting as to the age of onset of their menses. The girls all attended school in Baghdad, Iraq. The highest socioeconomic level, Group A, showed a mean age of onset of 13.59 years; the next level, Group A-, showed a mean age of onset of 13.39 years; and the lowest level, Group B, showed a mean age of onset of 13.96. The difference between Group A's and Group B's onset ages was significant, but the difference was not significant between Group A and Group A-. Dietary pattern analysis showed Group A girls consuming a higher proportion of fruits and eggs, and a lower proportion of legumes, than those in Groups A- and B.

46. Shakir, A., and Demarchi, M. "Dietary pattern of rural school children in the environment of Baghdad." Trop. Geogr. Med. 23 (3), September, 1971, pp 258-263.

Using the method of qualitative dietary survey, by questioning school children about food eaten during the previous 24 hours, it was shown that in the winter season school children in rural areas close to Baghdad have a better diet than children in rural areas further away. This is because of the more frequent consumption of meat, green vegetables and fruits. This method of study was sensitive enough to show the difference in the dietary pattern in children who were similar in every aspect, except the geographical situation from a major city.

The results of this study seem to correlate favourably with a detailed dietary study done previously in this area. (Authors' abstract)

Israel

1. Anderson, J. E., Becker, S., Guinena, A. H., and McCarthy, B. J. "Breastfeeding effects on birth interval components: a prospective child health study in Gaza. Stud. Fam. Plann. 17(3), May-June 1986, pp 153-60.

   Data that were collected prospectively from a child health study conducted in Gaza show a strong relationship between breastfeeding and two major components of birth intervals, the postpartum anovulatory period and the waiting time to conception. Having moderate durations of breastfeeding and short intervals between births, the Gaza population is similar to other populations in the Middle East. The strong positive association between breastfeeding and the length of postpartum amenorrhea is as expected from numerous other studies. Using hazard model analysis, the relationship between breastfeeding behavior and the waiting time to conception is examined. Women who are breastfeeding when menstration resumes and continue to do so are less likely to conceive than other women.

2. Kaufmann, N. A., Dennis, B. H., Heiss, G., Friedlander, Y., Kark, J. D., and Stein, Y. "Comparison of nutrient intakes of selected populations in the United States and Israel: the Lipid Research Clinics prevalence study." Am. J. Clin. Nutr. 43(4), April 1986, pp 604-620.

   The Lipid Research Clinics Program assessed nutrient intakes of 2,772 US and 2,680 Jerusalem participants by 24-hour dietary recall in men aged 15-19 and 40-59 year and women aged 15-19 and 35-59 year. Energy intake was higher in the US than in Jerusalem. The P:S ratio ranged between 0.80 and 1.01. The corresponding ranges for the US were 38.8-40.8% for fat, 14.3-15.9% for SFA, 5.9-6.8% for PFA, 38.9-46.2% for carbohydrates, 17.0-17.9% for starch, and 0.40-0.53 for the P:S ratio. In Jerusalem intake of total fat ranged between 32.2-33.7% of kcal, of saturated fatty acids (SFA) between 9.8-10.9%, of polyunsaturated fatty acids (PFA) between 7.9-8.6%, of carbohydrates between 50.5-53.9%, and of starch between 24.0-30.5%. Intake of cholesterol (mg/1000 kcal) was higher in Jerusalem than in the US. These data address the feasibility of reducing fat in diets of free-living, Western populations.

3. Kocturk, T. O. "Events leading to the decision to introduce complementary feeding to the breast among a group of mothers in Istanbul." Scand. J. Prim. Health Care 4(4), November 1986, pp 231-237.

   It was shown that the majority of infants began receiving regular complements or had been weaned before the age of three months in a cross-sectional study carried out among 269 mother-infant pairs in Istanbul. Beginning in the last month of pregnancy and continuing until the time of regular complementation, a prospective study carried out among 24 mothers demonstrated that the average duration of exclusive breastfeeding was 58 days. Within the early postnatal days the infants began receiving complements on a regular basis. Irregularly introduced complements often lead to gastro-intestinal reactions and weight loss. Mothers displayed sensitivity toward cues that suggested dissatisfaction in infants or other events that they conceived as threats to their milk yield in terms of quality and quantity. Mothers often discussed their decision to introduce complements with other people such as doctors and older female acquaintances who supported them toward complementation. Failure to gain sufficient weight with exclusive breastfeeding was seldom the cause of introducing complementary feeding.

4. Modan, M., Karasik, A., Halkin, H., Fuchs, Z., Lusky, A., Shitrit, A., and Modan, B. "Effect of past and concurrent body mass index on prevalence of glucose intolerance and type 2 (non-insulin-dependent) diabetes and on insulin response. The Israel study of glucose intolerance, obesity and hypertension. Diabetologia 29(2), February 1986, pp 82-89.

A representative sample (n=2140) of the Israeli Jewish population aged 40-70 (excluding known diabetic patients), whose body mass index had been measured 10 years earlier, underwent an oral glucose tolerance test and redetermination of body mass index. Irrespective of weight changes, high concurrent and high past body mass index values (greater than or equal to 27) were associated with similarly increased rates of glucose intolerance as compared with body mass index values less than 27 at both time-points (rate ratio 1.76, 90% confidence limits 1.56-1.99). Glucose intolerance here includes borderline and impaired tolerance as well as Type 2 diabetes. The rate of Type 2 diabetes increased only with increasing past body mass index, while concurrent body mass index had no effect [rate ratios: 2.36 (1.48-3.75) and 1.99 (1.48-2.68) respectively for the medium-(23-26.9) versus-low (less than 23) and high- (greater than or equal to 27) versus-medium past body-mass-index categories]. Weight reduction was associated with only slightly reduced rate of glucose intolerance and had no effect on the rate of diabetes. Mean sum insulin (summed 1 and 2 h levels, mU/l) increased significantly with increasing concurrent body mass index (123, 150 and 190 in the low, medium and high categories) with no effect of past body mass index. It also increased significantly (p less than 0.001) in all concurrent body mass index categories from normal tolerance through borderline to impaired tolerance, and decreased significantly (p less than 0.001) in diabetes relative to impaired tolerance, although it remained above normal.

5. Pascoe, J. M., and Berger, A. "Attitudes of high school girls in Israel and the United States toward breast feeding." J. Adolesc. Health Care 6(1), January 1985, pp 28-30.

Differences in the attitudes of the two countries might suggest interventions to increase breast feeding. Newborns are breast fed more frequently in Israel than in the United States (92% vs. 57%). The breast-feeding attitudes of high school girls in Israel and the United States using a 21-item questionnaire were examined. Israeli girls were significantly more positive about breast feeding than U.S. girls. Israeli girls answered 13 items positively more frequently than U.S. girls. Israeli girls were more likely to plan on breast feeding (68.2% vs. 42.4%). Interventions designed to improve the breast-feeding attitudes of young people may increase the prevalence of breast feeding.

6. Dagan, R., Sofer, S., Klish, W. J., Hundt, G., Saltz-Rennert, H., and Moses, S. W. "Infant feeding practices among Bedouins in transition from seminomadic to settlement conditions in the Negev area of Israel." Isr. J. Med. Sci. 20(11), November 1984, pp 1029-1034.

Infant feeding practices among 353 Bedouin families in the Negev area of Israel were compared with those of 302 Jewish families from the same area. Over 99% of the Bedouin infants were initially breast-fed, in contrast to 79% of the Jewish infants. By the end of the first year of life none of the Jewish infants continued to be breast-fed, while 63% of the Bedouins were. Fruits and vegetables were the first solids introduced to the Jewish infants while rice was the first for Bedouin infants. By 6 months, 93% of the Jewish infants were eating fruits and vegetables, 78% meat, 49% bread and 55% eggs, in contrast to 20, 13, 8 and 18% among the Bedouins, respectively. Introduction of meat lagged significantly among the Bedouin infants, taking place after the 8th month of life for greater than 50%. It is likely that with increasing modernization this pattern will gradually disappear and will be replaced by that prevalent among Western populations.

7. Kark, J. D., Troya, G., Friedlander, Y., Slater, P. E., and Stein, Y. "Validity of maternal reporting of breast feeding history and the association with blood lipids in 17 year olds in Jerusalem." J. Epidemiol. Community Health 38(3), September 1984, pp 218-225.

   The validity of 74 mothers' reporting of the breast feeding history more than 20 years later was studied in a Jerusalem population. Duration of breast feeding was well correlated with that recorded in mother and child health clinic charts. Concordance was of similar magnitude in subgroups of ethnicity, mother's education, family size, and sex of child. Duration of breast feeding in 101 youngsters was inversely associated with plasma cholesterol in 17 year old girls. The correlation was statistically significant on univariate analysis and of borderline significance on multivariable analysis. Among 17 year old boys, a statistically significant inverse association for plasma triglyceride was apparent on multivariable analysis. Reported breast feeding history may be a useful instrument for study of possible long term effects of breast feeding in their adolescent or adult progeny.

8. Mansbach, I. K., Palti, H., Pevsner, B., Pridan, H., and Palti, Z. "Advice from the obstetrician and other sources: do they affect women's breast feeding practices? A study among different Jewish groups in Jerusalem." Soc. Sci. Med. 19(2), 1984, pp 157-162.

   Breast feeding practices and the sources of advice that influenced them were studied in a sample of 276 women from North East Jerusalem for 4 1/2 months. It was found that 89.7% started breast feeding after parturition, 62.4% were breast feeding after 6 weeks, 40.3% were breast feeding after 3 months and 27.3% were still breast feeding at 4 1/2 months postpartum. Obstetrician's advice given at the 6 weeks postpartum examination was significantly associated with duration of breast feeding (P = 0.001). Analysis of variance indicated that women of higher social classes breast fed more and for a longer period of time. There was a strong relation between advice of the obstetrician and percentage of women breast feeding 4 1/2 months postpartum. Women of Western origin breast fed more and longer than women of Asian or North African origin. The differential relationship between advice of obstetrician and women belonging to different social classes is discussed and key elements in the relation between obstetrician's advice and women's breast feeding practices are considered.

9. Palti, H., Mansbach, I., Pridan, H., Adler, B., and Palti, Z. "Episodes of illness in breast-fed and bottle-fed infants in Jerusalem." Isr. J. Med. Sci. 20(5), May 1984, pp 395-399.

   274 middle-class Jewish women in Jerusalem were interviewed about their breast-feeding practices, symptoms and signs of disease, and episodes of illness and hospitalization of the infant. Infants exclusively breast-fed had significantly fewer symptoms of disease

than did those not breast-fed or partially breast-fed. The odds ratios for cough, respiratory difficulty, and diarrhea by breast-feeding practice were 3.66, 2.14 and 2.72 (P = 0.04). Significant differences in the number of illness episodes were found between breast-fed and bottle-fed infants at 20 weeks. A positive association was found between number of illness episodes and duration of breast-feeding. Infants who were breast-fed for 20 weeks had the least number of illness episodes; 52% of them had no episodes compared with only 15% who were not breast-fed. Comparison of the numbers of illness episodes among non-breast-fed infants of mothers with low and high education levels indicated that the infants of better educated mothers had a significantly lower percentage of illness episodes (P less than 0.05). Even infants of a middle-class and well-educated population benefit from the breast-feeding practice and its protective effect, more so if they are exclusively breast-fed and for a longer period.

10. Lazarus-Yafeh, H. "Some Halakhic differences between Judaism and Islam" Tarbiz 51(2), January 1983, pp 207-225.

An examination of the differences between Jewish and Islamic legal tradition (in spite of their striking similarity) in order to define their basic characteristics. A major distinction is the important agricultural aspect of Jewish law, almost absent from the mercantile Islamic civilization, which explains differences regarding inheritance laws. Other differences are in laws of purity and impurity and in dietary laws. The differences of the political aspects of both systems are also examined. (Author's abstract)

11. Palti, H., Taveedej, C. H., and Pevsner, B. "The effect of rises in food costs on food intake of three year olds in Jerusalem." Int. J. Epidemiol. 12(4), December 1983, pp 426-431.

The food intake of two samples of children born five years apart were determined in 1975 and 1980. The subjects were three years of age and lived in a low to middle class Jerusalem neighbourhood. No deficiency in caloric intake was noted in the 24-hour recall. The protein intake was twice the recommended dietary allowance (RDA). The mean daily iron intake was only 40% of the RDA. The main sources for protein were milk and milk products, poultry and eggs. Children from Asian origin had the lowest caloric and protein intake in 1975 and 1980 whereas those of European-American origin had the highest. The percentage expenditure on food was 25% of total income during both periods. The possible factors influencing the stability in dietary intake are governmental subsidy for the essential foods, correction of wages and increase in social security payments thus maintaining the buying power, as well as the educational effect of the preventive services--the Mother and Child Health Stations on feeding practices.

12. Abdel Qader, R. "Day care centre opens in Beit Hanina" Al-Fajr 3(115), July 16, 1982, p 13.

A report on a day care centre in Bayt Hanina near Jerusalem, established by the Women's Work Committee of Jerusalem in June, 1982. The centre supervises 35 children, who spend their time in reading, music and art sessions, and is equipped to handle up to seven infants. The centre also sponsors lectures for mothers on psychology, first aid and nutrition. (Author's abstract)

13. Blondheim, S. H., Horne, T., Abu-Rabia, Y., Lehmann, E. E., and

Heldenberg, D. "Polyunsaturation of subcutaneous fat and concentration of serum lipids of Israeli Bedouin Arabs." <u>Hum. Nutr. Clin. Nutr.</u> 36(6), 1982, pp 449-457.

In 55 Israeli Bedou~~in Arab~~s the ratio of polyunsaturated to saturated fatty acids in subcutaneous fat (which reflects the degree of unsaturation of dietary fat) and serum cholesterol and triglyceride concentrations were all significantly lower in men and women leading the typical seminomadic Bedouin life than in men doing western-type work and in housewives of a fixed Bedouin settlement. The values were 0.76, and 159 and 72 mg/dl, respectively, compared with 0.93, 187 and 108; p less than 0.001, less than 0.01 and less than 0.02, respectively. In the group as a whole, there was a paradoxically positive correlation between P/S ratio and cholesterol (r = 0.37, Pr = 0.025) and P/S ratio and triglycerides (r = 0.46, Pr less than 0.01). The expected cholesterol-lowering effect of the polyunsaturated Israeli diet (P/S ratio about 1.0) was apparently swamped by other factors, dietary and/or non-dietary, involved in acculturation to a western life style of Bedouin, among whom coronary heart disease has only recently begun to appear. (Authors' abstract)

14. Anonymous "No easy remedies for occupation" <u>Middle East</u> 84, October 1981, pp 47-48.

A description of the state of medical services for Palestinians in the West Bank in 1981. The number of state hospital beds diminished in the 1970s and the remaining nine institutions suffer from underfinancing and a severe shortage of trained medical personnel. Local inhabitants have turned to foreign aid agencies which provide clinics, baby-care centers and women's health education classes. Nutritional deficiencies caused by the shortage of fresh food are blamed on the Israel occupation. (Author's abstract)

15. Ilia, R., Weitzman, S., Le Roith, D., Horowitz, J., and Sobel, R. "Prevalence of goiter and thyroid nodules among the Bedouin." <u>Harefuah</u> 98(7), April 1980, pp 293-295.

897 Bedouins were studied for the prevalence of goiter and thyroid nodules. 201 members of a nearby kibbutz served as a control group. In 11 Bedouins iodine 24 hour urinary excretion was determined and iodine concentration in various sources of drinking water was measured. 39.3% of adolescent and 20.4% of adult females showed a mild diffuse enlargement of the thyroid gland. These findings were not correlated with iodine intake. In spite of the high prevalence of mild thyroid enlargement, the prevalance of large goiters or thyroid nodules was similar to control group and other populations. (Authors' abstract translated by Dr. Menachem Sadeh.)

16. Biale, Y., Shany, S., Levi, M., Shainkin-Kestenbaum, R., and Berlyne, G. M. "25 hydroxycholecalciferol levels in Bedouin women in labor and in cord blood of their infants." <u>Am. J. Clin. Nutr.</u> 32(12), December 1979, pp 2380-2382.

25 Hydroxycholecalciferol levels were measured in eight Bedouin mothers in labor and in the cord blood of their infants, and compared with values in 42 Sephardi Israeli women in labor and the cord blood of their offspring. Bedouin baby cord blood had a mean 25 hydroxycholecalciferol concentration of 3.78 ng/ml +/- 3.22 (SD) being about half of their mothers' level in labor. Values in Sephardi women and cord blood were 3 times higher. PTH levels were

lower and calcium concentrations were higher in cord blood (p less than 0.001) in both groups when compared to their mothers' blood. The relevance of these findings to the higher incidence of infantile rickets and hypocalcemia in Bedouin children is discussed. (Authors' abstract)

17. Pogrund, H. "Osteomalacia" (letter) Clin. Orthop. (144), October 1979, pp 337-338.

The author of the letter recalls that Dr. Bid, 1978, found a 26.1% prevalence of osteomalacia in 69 patients with fractured neck of the femur in Qatar. A survey of 570 Jewish patients with fractured femur in Jerusalem however did not uncover a single case of osteomalacia. The author notes that habits and mode of life of Oriental Jews have changed little from that of their countries of origin, and expresses surprise at the lack of osteomalacia in them. He also notes that 32% of the series had osteoporosis, with the Oriental group showing a 35.7% prevalence.

18. Zmora, E., Gorodischer, R., and Bar-Ziv, J. "Multiple nutritional deficiencies in infants from a strict vegetarian community." Am. J. Dis. Child 133(2), February 1979, pp 141-144.

Severe nutritional deficiencies developed in four infants from a new vegan religous community. They had received breast milk until the age of 3 months; thereafter, breast milk was supplemented with or replaced by extremely low caloric-density preparations. All of the infants had profound protein-calorie malnutrition, severe rickets, osteoporosis, and vitamin B12 and other deficiencies. One infant died, while the three others had an uneventful recovery. After discharge of the infants from the hospital, the community responded well to a modification of the infants' diet, which did not violate their vegetarian philosophy. However, they refused to give their infants B12 on a regular basis. (Authors' abstract)

19. Guinena, A. H. "Protein-calorie malnutrition in young refugee children in the Gaza strip." J. Trop. Pediatr. 23(1), February 1977, pp 38-57.

Two studies were carried out in 1965 and 1967 in the Gaza strip on Palestinian refugee children. The first, a longitudinal study on growth, development and nutritional status of 1151 infants born in Jabalia camp, included clinical, anthropometric, and ecological and maternal investigations. The second, a transverse study on 4007 children from 24 to 60 months of age from four refugee camps in the Gaza strip area, evaluated growth and etiological factors responsible for protein-calorie malnutrition (PCM) in children under two years of age.

Growth retardation was seen in weight starting with the 8th month for males and the 6th month for females, with the poorest weight growth performance from 9 to 13 months for males and 6 to 13 months for females. The smallest length deviation occurred in the first six months and then increased by age, with 0.9 cm for males and 1.3 cm for females in the first year. The decline in linear growth attained its highest level at 15 and 18 months of age. The infant mortality rate was 78/1000 live births, the neonatal mortality rate 19.5/1000 live births, and the post-neonatal mortality rate 58.5/1000 live births. Of these deaths 33.4% were attributed to malnutrition, 29.8% indirectly and 3.6% directly. Early weaning, often secondary to mother's illness or pregnancy, as well as diarrheal diseases, respiratory infections and measles were major factors in PCM prevalence and related mortality.

20. Palti, H., Heiman, R., Adler, B., and Reshef, A. "Food intake in children." Harefuah, 93(9), November 1977, pp 225-228.

In a longitudinal study food intake of two groups of children was investigated. Each group was studied at ages 18, 24, and 30 months. The first group of children were born between 12/71 and 4/72 and the second group between 5/73 and 9/73. The caloric intake was close to the recommended intake, but there was a mild decrease at age 30 months. In 60% of the children protein intake was higher than 200% of recommended intake. Ferrous intake was close to that recommended by WHO. There was no difference between groups in caloric, protein, or iron intake. There was no significant difference between children from various social conditions. (Authors' abstract translated by Dr. Menachem Sadeh.)

21. de Vries, A., and Weinberger, A. "Stone disease in Israel." Idiopathic urinary bladder stone disease. Van Reen, R., ed., DHEW (NIH) 77-1063, Bethesda W3 F049 No. 37, 1976, pp 241-247.

Urolithiasis in Israel is mostly of the upper tract with bladder stones relatively rare. The incidence of uric acid lithiasis has decreased in recent years, except in the southern area of Israel, where immigrants from North Africa reside. Clusters of cystine lithiasis in Jews of Libyan origin were found in 1974. Calcium oxalate stones in patients seen in 1969-73 showed an idiopathic hypercalciuria in 19.6% of patients. Five studies of childhood lithiasis in Israel were cited. The age range was from less than 1 year of age to 13 years. The peak incidence was from 2 to 4 years of age, with Israeli Arabs having 8.4/1,000 admissions, Asian-African Jews 2.6/1,000 admissions, and European-American Jews 0.5/1,000 admissions. A marked preponderance of male patients, one-third below 5 years of age, were operated on for removal of urinary tract calculi in 1960-64 in northern Israel.

22. Shany, S., Hirsh, J., and Barlyne, G. M. "25-Hydroxycholecalciferol levels in Bedouins in the Negev." Am. J. Clin. Nutr. 29(10), October 1976, pp 1104-1107.

25-Hydroxycholecalciferol (25-HCC) levels were measured in 31 Bedouin females and eight Bedouin male tribesmen and compared with the levels in Jewish males and females in Beersheba. In nonpregnant Bedouin women the mean 25-HCC level was 25.4 ng/ml +/- 9.78. In pregnant Bedouin women the mean was 23.4 ng/ml +/- 8.52. In Bedouin males the mean level was 25.7 ng/ml +/- 3.03. In Jewish females, both pregnant and nonpregnant, the levels were higher (32.7 ng/ml +/- 6.02 and 44.3 ng/ml +/- 9.24). Jewish males had levels of 32.8 +/- 6.29 ng/ml. No Bedouin had plasma levels below 10 ng/ml, and there was no evidence to suggest deficiency of vitamin D in Bedouin males or females. (Authors' abstract)

23. Richardson, B. D., and Walker, A. R. "Letter: Bowlegs, knock-knees and vitamin D status in schoolchildren." N. Engl. J. Med. 290(6), February 7, 1974, p 346.

This short letter discussed the relationship between leg abnormalities, bowlegs and knock-knee, and vitamin D status in schoolchildren seen in South African black, colored, Indian, and white populations, and in Israel schoolboys 10 years old and older of Jewish, Druse, and Arab background. Boys from widely different backgrounds showed no difference in prevalences of bowleg and knock-knee. The authors concluded that a primary vitamin D deficiency appeared unlikely to be related to the leg abnormalities, but that a secondary deficiency of vitamin D may share responsibility for the abnormalities. They also suggested that the normal range of leg physiology may include many of the leg abnormalities.

24. Winter, S., Mainzer, W., Friedman, A., Muogbo, D., and Benderly, A. "Patterns of disease in hospitalized infants: changes over a decade." Harefuah 86(5), March 1, 1974, pp 242-244.

From a defined group of 5243 infants born in Haifa, 767 infants were hospitalized during their first 2 years and the total number of hospitalizations was 1078. Data was compared to another group investigated 10 years ago. More than 81% of the admissions and more than 76% of the main clinical problems during the hospitalizations were related to environmental factors, including diarrhea, infections, deficiency states and accidents. Anemia was very common around the age of 1 year. Average weights were usually satisfactory. (Authors' abstract translated by Dr. Menachem Sadeh)

25. Berlyne, G. M., Ben-Ari, J., Nord, E., and Shainkin, R. "Bedouin osteomalacia due to calcium deprivation caused by high phytic acid content of unleavened bread." Am. J. Clin. Nutr. 26(9), September 1973, pp 910-911.

A case of osteomalacia in a 30-year-old Negev Bedouin mother of six children was observed and treated. She was unable to walk due to severe bone pain in the lower back, pelvis and legs, and had numerous fractures and pseudofractures on admission to hospital. Vitamin D serum levels were in the low normal range, 30 U/100 ml. Dietary history revealed a low calcium intake of 500 mg/day as well as a high phytate and phosphorous intake of .528 mg/day which was attributable to consumption of the unleavened bread raghif as the main source of calories. Authors suggested that Bedouin osteomalacia was similar to that seen in United Kingdom Indians who consume the bread chapati as a staple.

26. Groen, J. J. "Why bread in the diet lowers serum cholesterol." Proc. Nutr. Soc. 32(3), December 1973, pp 159-167.

Some of the relationships between diet and serum cholesterol level are discussed. Studies of Trappist monks in Holland, Yemenite Jews, and Arab Bedouin in Israel show that low serum cholesterol levels in these populations are accompanied by an intake of diets lower in fat and cholesterol and higher in carbohydrates than that of a Western diet. The author cites several studies in which Western volunteers ingested, first, a Western diet, than a Yemenite diet. A low serum cholesterol level occurred with ingestion of the yemenite diet, and therefore was not a genetic or life-style result, but a result of diet composition. The Yemenite diet was characterized by low total and saturated fat and a high intake of starch and vegetable protein, achieved mainly by a high intake of bread. Another series of studies showed contradictory results in that protein content of bread was seen in one to have an effect on lowering serum cholesterol, and in another not to have an effect. The author also noted that the role of fibre could not be ignored, but considered it to be less than that of either starch or gluten. In conclusion, he noted that the American Heart Association in 1961 recommended the public eat less saturated fat and increase vegetable oil intake, but omitted a recommendation to substitute saturated fat with bread.

27. Vaisrub, S. "Epidemiologic vagaries of renal osteodystrophy." JAMA 224(13), June 1973, pp 1755-1756.

Renal osteodystrophy is rare in Israel, and the possible causative factors of this dearth of cases may be related to diet. Low milk and other protein intake in Israel is described, and the resulting low phosphate intake and high calcium intake from the drinking water are noted. The high Ca/P ratio is thought to produce a protective effect and prevent renal osteodystrophy.

28. Kanaaneh, H. "The relationship of bottle feeding to malnutrition and gastroenteritis in a pre-industrial setting." J. Trop. Pediatr. 18(4), December 1972, pp 302-306.

Gastroenteritis hospital morbidity before 6 months of age was studied by comparing feeding practices and weights at age 6 months in 610 infants. The infants were from three pre-industrial Arab villages in Israel and were divided by feeding experience into three groups. Diarrhoeal disease constituted the major cause of morbidity in infants and the second major cause of death. The incidence of malnutrition was nil among the two exclusively breast-fed groups and rose gradually to about 30% of those who were exclusively bottle fed for the greater part of the 6 month period. The difference was highly significant in both sexes. Authors suggested that, in these and similar communities, breast feeding should be used for the first 6 months of life exclusively.

29. Smith, P. "Diet and attrition in the Natufians." Am. J. Phys. Anthropol. 37(2), September 1972, pp 233-238.

There is a high correlation between the rate of dental attrition and the physical consistency of the diet. Hypotheses concerning types of diet and methods of food preparation in prehistoric populations may therefore be tested by comparing attrition rates in the specimens under investigation with standards derived from groups of known dietary status. For such comparisons the age factor is of paramount importance, but difficult to assess accurately in fragmentary skeletal material. The use of attrition gradients rather than mean attrition scores provides an age independent method for comparison of attrition rates. When Natufian specimens from three different sites (Kebara, El Wad and Eynan) were compared by this method, significant differences in the gradient of attrition were found at one site, Kebara. The incidences of caries and periodontal disease were also lower at this site and, taken in conjunction with the low level of attrition, were considered to relate to differences in the vegetable content of the diet between the individuals recovered from Kebara and those recovered from El Wad and Eynan. (Author's abstract)

30. Cohen, A. M. "Lessons from diabetes in Yemenites." Isr. J. Med. Sci. 7(12), December 1971, pp 1554-1557.

A study of the prevalence of diabetes in Israel showed differences in ethnic background and length of time of immigrant groups in Israel, and therefore in length of time to accommodate to a western-type diet. The incidence of diabetes was lower in Sephardic Jews than in Ashkenazi Jews, and lower in new Kurdish and Yemenite Jewish immigrants than in old Kurdish and Yemenite Jewish immigrants. The main dietary change was an increased sugar intake by the old settlers. The average daily intake of sucrose was 63 g in Israel while it was almost nonexistent in Yemen. The author also reported a human volunteer study in which adults were fed a high sucrose diet of 231 g/day for 21 days. Results showed an impairment of glucose tolerance and increased blood cholesterol which were reversed with a low sucrose diet.

31. Gilat, T., Malachi, E. G., and Shochet, S. B. "Lactose tolerance in an Arab population." Amer. J. Dig. Dis. 16(3), March 1971, pp 203-206.

Sixty-seven Arab adults from the coastal villages of Tira and Taybeah were given lactose tolerance tests after an all-night fast. Results of the tests showed that 80.6% of the subjects had a low rise in glucose and most of these had symptoms during the test. Four of 13 subjects with normal glucose rise also had symptoms, including diarrhea, abdominal pain, or abdominal distention. Thus a high incidence of lactose intolerance was seen in the studied Arab population and was not related to age or sex. A similarly high incidence seen in other studies of Jews and Greek Cypriots was cited, and the authors suggested that Southern Europeans be studied in the future to determine whether this phenomenon was pan-Mediterranean or not.

32. Chaimoff, C., Dinstman, M., and Nathan, P. "The frequency of dumping syndrome after partial gastrectomy and anterior anastomosis." Harefuah 78(2), January 1970, pp 57-60.

The incidence of dumping syndrome was investigated in 124 patients who underwent partial gastrectomy and anterior anastomosis for various causes, with the exception of malignancy. The general incidence was 46.8%, but only 27.4% had a severe form.

Ethnic origin played no role, but living conditions and length of residence in Israel were factors that apparently aggravated the symptoms. An increase in the number of daily meals or a decrease in the amount of food eaten at each meal did not alleviate the symptoms. The condition often leads to a change in occupation or else in difficulty in readjusting to the previous occupation. (Authors' abstract)

33. Davies, A. M. "Geographic and ethnic differences in incidence of the pregnancy toxemias." Pathol. Microbiol. (Basel) 35(1), 1970, pp 210-214. S. Karger, AG, Basel.

The problems of definition, control, and statistical analysis in determining ethnic and geographic differences in incidence of the pregnancy toxemias worldwide are discussed. Use of data gathered as part of the Jerusalem perinatal study since 1964, use of the definition of the American Committee on Maternal Welfare, and use of multivariate statistical approach, showed a significant difference in incidence by parity, maternal age, maternal education, and maternal country of origin. Highest toxemia rates were seen in first pregnancies and seventh and subsequent ones, in mothers aged 40 or over, and in the illiterate. Jewish immigrants from Iraq and Moslem Arabs showed incidence rates double those seen in Jews born in Israel or North Africa. The need for carefully controlled prospective studies to accurately determine ethnic differences in toxemias of pregnancy incidence was noted.

Lebanon

1. Henley, D. "Medical care in a Palestinian refugee camp: surprising absence of exotic diseases. Disabled children a major but neglected problem." Laekartidningen 80(4), January 26, 1983, pp 232-235. (In Swedish)

   Between October 1977 and June 1982 there was a medical clinic in the Palestinian refugee camp Rashediye in southern Lebanon. The clinic was run in conjunction with the Palestinian groups in Sweden and the "Palestinian Red Halfmoon." David Henley, medical superintendant in the county of Uppsala, and medical doctor Lars Jerden in Falun, who both have been working at the clinic, report the conditions at the clinic and describe the overall situation. (Author's abstract translated into English by Elizabeth Gustavsson.)

2. Sadler, C. "Dealing with disaster." Nurs. Mirror 156(10), March 9, 1983, pp 22-23.

   This report by a Save the Children Fund nurse describes various aspects of emergency relief medical work in Lebanon and Uganda based on personal experiences and observations. While the Karamoja, Uganda refugees suffered as a result of a famine due to drought and socioeconomic isolation, the southern Lebanon refugees suffered from war-related causes. STC health workers under auspices of the U.N. Relief and Works Agency, re-established, or set up, new UNRWA clinics in the Tyre and Sidon area. A noticeable lack of men and abundance of disoriented, homeless, and demoralized women and children were evident. Priorities included establishment of sanitation, vaccination against infectious disease, and rehydration of diarrheal disease victims. Workers replaced broken pipes and sprayed open sewage pools with disinfectant. War-related health problems included amputees needing physiotherapy and prostheses, phosphorous burn patients with skin contractures, and anxiety cases. Chronic health problems such as chronic bronchitis, malnutrition, and bronchopneumonia were related to poverty and poor housing. Home visits were seen as an important way to reassure terrified women and children.

3. Acra, A., Namaan, S., and Raffoul, Z. "Total mercury levels in canned and frozen fish imported into Lebanon." Bull. Environ. Contam. Toxicol. 27(2), August 1981, pp 209-212.

   Total mercury levels were measured in 407 samples of canned tuna and mackerel, and 98 specimens of a variety of frozen fish randomly collected from imported shipments. Overall mean values in 1974-75 were: canned tuna - .30 mg/kg, canned mackerel - .12 mg/kg, frozen fish - .16 mg/kg. The mean in 1974 for canned tuna, .3 mg/kg, was significantly higher than that for 1975, .05 mg/kg. Mean values were comparable with those for market fish elsewhere in the world. None of the imported fish samples contained mercury levels greater than the accepted tolerance level of .5 mg/kg. Authors urged Lebanese consumers to prefer locally caught fresh fish because they are smaller, and small size has been shown to be correlated with less mercury contamination.

4. Roumani, B. M., Abdelnoor, A. M., and Hilan, C. "Salmonella agona isolated from fish meal and a Salmonella strain isolated from shrimps in Lebanon." Zentralbl. Bakteriol. (B) 172(4-5) January 1981, pp 411-414.

   Salmonella agona was isolated from an imported fish meal specimen and a Salmonella strain not listed in the Kauffmann-White Scheme was isolated from a shrimp specimen obtained from the Mediterrenean coast of Lebanon. The biochemical and serological properties of the S. agona fish meal strain was identical to a standard strain. The serotype of the shrimp strain was 013,22 Vi. With the exception of hydrogen sulfide production, the biochemical properties of the shrimp strain were similar to S. agona.

5. Zurayk, H. C., and Shedid, H. E. "The trend away from breast feeding in a developing country: a women's perspective." J. Trop. Pediatr. 27(5), October 1981, pp 237-244.

This is an analysis of information obtained from two surveys conducted in southern Lebanon which pertained to contraceptive and breast-feeding practices in the area. The data, presented in a series of tables with textual discussion, highlights the most important factors contributing to a decreasing practice of breast-feeding among women who have moved away from traditional cultural influence via urban residency or educational level. These factors were: women's perception of breast-feeding as a negative influence on their health; an inadequate milk supply leading to early weaning; a majority of educated and urban women attended at delivery by trained health personnel who do not urge breastfeeding; and early weaning due to pregnancy. Recommendations for education campaigns to support breast feeding, for improved maternal health care systems, for inclusion of the breast-feeding process in health curricula, and for further research focussing on the women's perceptions and changing needs in the developing society were given.

6. Abdelnoor, A. M., and Roumani, B. M. "Characterization of some Vibrio parahaemolyticus strains isolated from seafoods in Lebanon." Zentralbl. Bakteriol. (B) 170(5-6), 1980, pp 502-507.

One hundred seventy seafood specimens were investigated for the presence of Vibrio parahaemolyticus. V. parahaemolyticus was isolated from two fish and one crab specimen, and V. alginolyticus was isolated from seven fish, three shrimp, two sea-urchin and one crab specimen. The V. parhaemolyticus isolates had biochemical characteristics that were similar to two standard strains. Like the standard strains, two of the V. parahaemolyticus isolates were Kangawa phenomenon positive and were serologically similar to one of the standard strains. One isolate exhibited slight cross reactivity with V. alginolyticus but no cross reactivity with E. Coli. One of the V. alginolyticus isolates was Kanasawa-phenomenon positive. (Authors' abstract)

7. Shiber, J. G. "Heavy metals in Ras Beirut prawns and sea urchin eggs." Reprinted from J. Environ. Sci. Health 14(1), (B) 1979, pp 73-95. Courtesy of Marcel Dekker, Inc., N.Y.

Whole samples of Palaemon elegans Rathke, 1837 and eggs of Paracentrotus lividus Lamarck, 1816 were collected on the coast of Ras Beirut, Lebanon in the summer and fall of 1977 and the spring of 1978. All were analyzed for lead, cadmium, copper and other heavy metals. Lead concentrations in both the prawns and sea urchin eggs appeared to be highest in the summer and lowest in the spring, whereas cadmium was low in all seasons with only a few elevated readings. The strongest tendency towards seasonal variation was seen in the copper levels of the prawns, which were high in summer, much lower in fall, and then high again in spring. Results of the analyses for nickel, iron, zinc and chromium and the various possible sources of chromium are also discussed. Of the various possible sources of heavy metals in the Ras Beirut coastal area, untreated sewage, pesticide residues, and automobile exhaust are the most important. (Author's abstract)

8. Edwards, J. A., Barnhardt, B., and Schnatz, J. D. "Hyperlipidemia in a Lebanese community: difficulties in definition, diagnosis and decision on when to treat." J. Med. 9(2), 1978, pp 157-182.

One hundred thirty-one male and female adults belonging to a Lebanese community in western New York were studied for fasting serum cholesterol and triglyceride levels. Average cholesterol levels in males were 217 mg% and in females were 234mg%. These values were comparable to those in most other populations, but were higher than those seen in Lebanon. Five point seven percent of the adults were hyperlipidemic at a level above the 90th percentile. Thirteen of the hyperlipidemic subjects were diagnosed as having two types of hyperlipidemia on the basis of family studies and clinical studies. Twenty-three percent of them had primary non-monogenic, and 77% had monogenic hyperlipidemia. A minimum of 0.7% were estimated to have familial hypercholesterolemia. This high frequency was similar to that found in Lebanon.

9. Nabbut, N. H. "Salmonella serotypes encountered in animal feed additives in Lebanon." Am. J. Vet. Re. 39(5), May 1978, pp 893-895.

Animal feed-additive samples (n = 300) were examined for the presence of salmonellae, using the selenite-F broth-enrichment method followed by subculturing on Salmonella-Shigella and brilliant green agar with sulfadizing selective agar plates. Samples consisted of a variety of feed additives: 119 bone meal samples, 77 meat meal samples, 40 fish meal samples, and 64 miscellaneous meal samples. Results of examination found 49 (41.2%) of the bone meal samples, 6 (7.8%) of the meat meal samples and 2 (5%) of the fish meal samples contained salmonellae. Of 57 isolates representing 24 serotypes, 4 most frequently isolated serotypes were Salmonella meleagridis (25.1%). Salmonella tennessee (7%), Salmonella chester (5.2%), and Salmonella senftenberg (5.2%). This study shows a high Salmonella-contamination rate of bone meal compared with meat meal and fish meal samples. Of 12 known positive bone meal samples that were examined, 100% of 25-g samples, compared with 70% to 100% of 2.5 g samples and 30% to 90% of 0.25 g samples, were positive for salmonella. (Authors' abstract)

10. Asfour, R., Wahbeh, N., Waslien, C.I., Guindi, S., and Darby, W. J. "Folacin requirement of children. III. Normal infants." Am. J. Clin. Nutr. 30(7), July 1977, pp 1098-1105.

Twenty children aged 2 to 11 months, and in apparent good health, were observed on nutritionally balanced diets that supplied folacin at levels of 3.6, 4.3, 5.0, and 16 ug/kg body weight. Similar growth, hemopoiesis, and clinical health, and slightly increased serum and red blood cell folate concentrations were seen with folacin intakes of 4.3 to 5.0 ug/kg body weight compared to 3.6 ug/kg body weight. The 3.6 ug/kg body weight per day intake level, equivalent to 70% of the Food & Agricultural Organization/World Health Organization allowance and 70% of the RDA, resulted in folate in serum and red blood cells which was termed borderline. The 3.6 ug/kg body weight per day intake was maintained in five of the children for 6 to 9 months, and they maintained hemopoiesis, clinical health, and growth for these periods. The highest intake level, 16 ug/kg body weight per day of folacin, failed to increase (or lower) growth, hematologic, or clinical parameters. It did, however, increase serum and red blood cell folate levels over those of the 4.3 to 5.0 ug/kg body weight per day folate intake range. The conclusion that the RDA and the FAO/WHO folate intake standards are adequate was reached. Investigators observed that the FAO/WHO and the RDA standards for tocopherol failed to sustain blood serum concentrations consistently above 0.5 mg/100 ml of tocopherol in the children. They therefore recommended that these standards be reviewed and possibly revised.

11. Kanawati, A. A. "At-Risk Factors and Health of Young Children: Geographical Studies in Lebanon." At Risk Factors and the Health and Nutrition of Young Children. Publication of the International Conference held in Cairo, June 23-27, 1975, pp 121-127. Printed by Al-Shaab Printing House.

This presentation reported results of a study of low socioeconomic status "thriving" vs "failure to thrive" preschool children in Lebanon. Infection was seen as the most harmful event in childhood, but the complexity of causality in childhood failure to thrive encompassed cultural, socioeconomic, health and hygiene, and psychological factors. Three reasons were seen as responsible for primary and secondary malnutrition: poor food supply availability, ignorance of proper food selection, and lack of means to obtain food. Education was highly correlated with child health. Decline in purchasing power endangered adequacy of energy intake. Living conditions, environmental sanitation and hygiene, as well as family income and parent's education levels were interrelated with each other and childhood malnutrition. Urbanization was found not to be especially harmful. The growth and feeding pattern of Lebanese preschoolers was: good growth during breastfeeding period to 6 months, declining growth during breastfeeding period to 6 months, declining growth from 6 to 18 months during weaning period, and catch-up growth spurt from 18 months onward with self-sufficiency in feeding established.

12. Loiselet, J., and Jarjouhi, L. "Levels of sugars in milk products in Lebanon." J. Med. Liban 28(2), 1975, pp 319-334.

We have examined 2 techniques of dosage of sugars, focussing on mixtures only fermenting galactose and lactose. The first technique utilizes oxidation of sugars in a strongly alkaline environment, an energetic oxidation which equally affects lactose and monosaccharides, and the same reaction in a more moderate environment, which only acts on the monosaccharides. The second technique utilizes the automatic dosage by ferricyanate (Technicon) after hydrolysis of lactose. The action of rising during baking permits separation of the effects of glucose and galactose. The results are identical and reproducible by the 2 techniques.

The application of these techniques to Lebanese milk products showed that the lactose of the original milk is hydrolyzed in the course of fermentation of milk in Lebanon. The glucose is utilized by the micro-organisms, and the galactose remains in the product. In making white cheese, the process of separation of the whey takes out the galactose and most of the remaining lactose. The white cheese contains no more than 15 grams of lactose/kg.

The Lebanese preference for using yoghurt, and even more for the white cheese explains why lactase can be absent (as it is known to be) from the population of Lebanon. (Translated by Cheryl Ritenbaugh, Ph.D., M.P.H.)

13. McLaren, D. S., and Read, W. W. "Weight/length classification of nutritional status." Lancet 2(7927), August 2, 1975, pp 219-221.

Three groups of young children were measured for nutritional status using two classifications of weight and length; McLaren And Read's (1972) and Waterlow and Rutishauser's (1974). The first group was 539 children from 3 to 48 months of age from a low socioeconomic population in a Beirut suburb. The second group was 154 patients of the Clinical Nutrition Unit in Beirut from 2 to 48 months of age with primary diagnosis of acute malnutrition. The third group was 87 acutely malnourished children in Luzmila Hospital, Amman, Jordan. Waterlow and Rutishauser's method underestimated malnutrition greatly, applying a "priority" grading to less than half of severely malnourished cases, and regarding 6.8% of them as needing "no action." Disregard for the effect of age on expected weight for length in young children was suggested as one basis for incorrect classification. Height deficit was also thought to be an unreliable indicator of present state of malnutrition. The authors devised a simple chart for use in the field with the McLaren and Read classification system.

14. Semine, A. A., and Damon, A. "Costochondral ossification and aging in five populations." Hum. Biol. 47(1), February 1975, pp 101-116.

Age changes in extent of costochondral ossification of the first rib and of the lower ribs were evaluated separately from chest roentgenograms in five populations: European Americans, Lebanese, Solomon Islanders (the Lau and the Baegu) and a special veterans group. Increase in the ossification was closely associated with age in all groups. The shapes of the age curves were similar in all populations within each measure and within sexes. However, the Solomon Islanders showed less ossification than the Caucasians, and the Baegu showed less ossification than the Lau. These findings may be explained by the dietary differences in the populations. With respect to sex differences, for the first rib, males showed greater ossification than females regardless of age in each of the groups. For the lower ribs, males generally showed most changes before age 45 and females after age 45. The sex differences may be related to endocrine factors. Ossification in the first rib cartilage was related to chest circumference in all three male groups investigated (the veterans, the Lau and the Baegu) but not in the females (the Lau and the Baegu). Ossification in the lower rib cartilages was related to chest expansion in the male veterans, the only group where such data were available. These latter findings supported the hypothesis that biomechanical factors influence costochondral ossification. (Authors' abstract)

15. Kanawati, A. A., Darwish, O., and McLaren, D. S. "Failure to thrive in Lebanon. 3. Family income, expenditure and possessions." Acta Paediatr. Scand. 63(1), January 1974, pp 108-112.

Seventy Lebanese Arab Moslem families, 40 of which had a young "thriving" child and 30 of which had a young "failing to thrive" child, all of low socioeconomic class, were investigated for causitive factors. Parents were questioned about sources and amount of income and expenditures on housing, furniture, home appliances, luxury items, clothes, food and miscellaneous categories. Inventory of possessions also took place.

Monthly income was markedly different in the 2 groups, with "thriving" families almost in a state of economic balance, and "failing to thrive" families having a monthly financial deficit. The value of possessions of "thriving" families was three times greater, 10% more of them owned homes, and the mean values of their home comfort appliances were much higher than that of the "failing to thrive" families. A smaller proportion of food expenditures was spent on expensive but more nutritious animal food products in "failing to thrive" families and more on cheaper cereals and legumes. Toys were also lacking in all but one of the failing families, indicating stimulative impoverishment for the preschool child.

16. Kanawati, A. A., McLaren, D. S., and Darwish, O. "Failure to thrive in Lebanon. IV. Longitudinal health and growth data." Acta Paediatr. Scand. 63(6), November 1974, pp 849-854.

Pre-school age Arab children of low socio-economic standard living in urban and suburban areas of Lebanon were divided into Thriving and Failing to Thrive groups according to an Index of Thriving. They were matched for age and their young siblings were also studied. Various somatic measurements were made and health-related data collected on three occasions over a period of approximately three years. Notable among the findings were (1) the very low mortality rate, (2) evidence of considerable spontaneous catch-up growth in the Failing to Thrive group, (3) a high rate of obstetric experience in both groups, greater in the Failing to Thrive, and (4) frequent occurrence of infections with a tendency to delay vaccination, especially in the Failing to Thrive group, as a probably consequence. (Authors' abstract)

17. Karayen, S. J. "Height and weight of Armenian college students in Lebanon." J. Med. Liban 27(2), 1974, pp 209-218.

The heights and weights of American college and university students were compared with those of young Armenian adults with elementary or a few years of secondary education. All subjects resided in Lebanon. The college and university group consisted of 247 females and 412 males; the control group consisted of 85 females and 54 males. Control females weighed a mean of 58.45 kg compared to student females' mean of 54.86 kg. Control males averaged 63.87 kg compared to student males' average 66.92. Male students averaged 6.56 cms., greater height than the control males, but there was no significant difference between the two groups of females.

18. Matossian, R. M., Rebeiz, J., and Stephan, E. "Outbreak of trichinosis in Lebanon, 1970. A clinical and epidemiological study." J. Med. Liban 27(3), 1974, pp 267-273.

Trichinosis, which is responsible for several epidemics in the past 100 years in Lebanon, was suspected as the cause of an epidemic in the village of Deir-el-Kamar in Mount Lebanon early in the fall of 1970. About 50 people were affected, and 37 were treated by a physician who noted that all his patients presented with nausea, malaise, chills, fever, muscle pain, weakness, and eosinophilia. 88% of them also presented with facial and periorbital edema, and 56% showed either macular (12 cases) or maculopapular (9 cases) rash. Initially seen were slight to moderate leukocytosis, a marked increase in eosinophils, negative blood smears for larvae, negative blood cultures, and elevated serum creatinine phosphokinase levels. T. spiralis-specific antibodies were detected in 9 of 10 patients who gave serum samples for this purpose. Negative muscle biopsy results were obtained up to the 34th day, but T. spiralis larvae were detected in 4 muscle samples obtained on the 44th day. This confirmed the diagnosis of trichinosis. The villagers had consumed the national dish of "kubbeh nayyeh", which consists of ground par-boiled wheat, meat, salt, and spices, kneaded together and eaten raw. The local butcher admitted to adulterating the mutton with pork.

19. McLaren, D. S. "Letters: Why under-five's clinics?" Trans. R. Soc. Trop. Mod. Hyg. 68(3), 1974, pp 260-1.

The author points out the need for models for comprehensive child care in growing slums of developing countries. He bases his suggestion on the results of a 10 years' progress report of a study by Morley, 1973, which centered on the predominantly rural African scene. Using information gathered in the failure to thrive Lebanese study of 7 years' duration (Kanawati, McLaren, and Darwish, 1974a), the author notes that the main form of malnutrition in peri-urban slum environment is marasmus, and is confined to the 3 to 18 month age period. He also notes that high catch-up growth and very low young child mortality occurs without any health intervention. A poor urban community is very mobile due to unpaid chronic debts, and the people are pre-occupied with survival and incapable of conscientious regular clinic attendance.

20. Kanawati, A. A., and McLaren, D. S. "Failure to thrive, in Lebanon. II. An investigation of the causes." Acta Paediatr. Scand. 62(6), November 1973, pp 571-576.

This is the second of a series of publications based on a health study of 1231 3- to 48-month-old Arab Lebanese children in three different locations. An Index of Thriving based on four anthropometric measurements identified 107 children classified as "thriving" and 92 as "failing to thrive". Questionnaires were completed in the homes concerning socioeconomic status, household data, and nutritional beliefs and practices. Categories of data formed were: family data, socioeconomic, living conditions, health, and dietary. The multi-factorial nature of causation was implied by numerous statistically significant differences in all categories of data, with poorer status in failure to thrive families. Living conditions and maternal care were major factors. Dietary factors were inadequate caloric intake, bottle feeding, and early weaning. The child's medical history was significant, with infection severity and illness duration more important than type.

21. Khouri, F. P., and McLaren, D. S. "Cytogenetic studies in protein-calorie malnutrition." Am. J. Hum. Genet. 25(5), September 1973, pp 465-470.

A sample of 17 children with severe protein-calorie malnutrition was investigated cytogenetically. Although the incidence of structural chromosome abnormalities was significantly greater among the patients than in a healthy control group, about half of the patients had aberration frequencies within the normal range. Furthermore, no correlation was found between the degree of malnutrition and the incidence of chromosomal lesions. Consequently, from our findings it is not possible to conclude that malnutrition per se produces chromosome damage. (Authors' abstract)

22. Davies, D. G., and Harvey, R. W. "Anthrax infection in bone meal from various countries of origin." J. Hyg. (Camb.) 70(3), September 1972, pp 455-457.

Using animal inoculation, three out of six Lebanese, three out of nine Argentinian, and two out of two Pakistani separate commercial consignments of bone meal imported during 1970 were found to be infected with anthrax. (Authors' abstract)

23. McLaren, D. S., and Read, W. W. "Classification of nutritional status in early childhood." Lancet 2(769), July 1972, pp 146-148.

Nutritional status classification for young children, according to weight/height/age and using the Boston standards for calculation, result in the following categories. Overweight is obesity at 110% of standard; normal is a range of 90% of standard; mild protein-calorie malnutrition (PCM) is 90-85% of standard; moderate PCM is 85-75% of standard; and severe PCM is less than 75% of standard. Subclassification of severe PCM on the basis of presence of edema, which correlates highly significantly with low serum albumin, is done as follows: marasmus shows no edema and kwashiorkor shows edema. The late effects of PCM are recognized with a separate category for nutritional dwarfism when length/age is less than 90% of standard but weight/length/age is more than 90%. A nomogram for rapid calculation makes the classification appropriate for hospital, clinic, and field use. The 1975 revision of the International Classification of Diseases should consider use of this classification system.

24. Abou-Daoud, K. T., and Hyg, H. M. S. "Cancer of the breast and breast-feeding. Study of 279 parous women and matched controls". Cancer 28(3), September 1971, pp 781-784.

Patients with cancer of the breast who were referred to the two radiation therapy centers in Lebanon for cobalt radiotherapy during a 2-year period were interviewed. Information was sought on parity, duration of breastfeeding, age at first childbirth and on other relevant variables. Controls were selected from among patients presenting for treatment of cancer of sites other than breast. A second control group was selected from non-cancer hospitalized patients. Matching was done for age, parity, treatment class, nationality and religion. A total of 289 patients with cancer of the breast was seen; 209 (79.4%) of these were parous, and, of this group, 279 (90.3%) were interviewed. There were virtually no differences in reported duration of breast-feeding between the cases and other cancer controls or non-cancer hospital controls. There was also no difference in average duration of breast-feeding a child between Lebanese and Syrian or Christian and Moslem mothers. Age at first childbirth was earlier for the control group than for the cases. (Authors' abstract)

25. Asfour, R. Y. "A new vehicle for supplementing an inadequate diet in children: use in Lebanon." Bull. NY Acad. Med. 71(1), January 1971, pp 5-16.

The use of nutritious "food rods" such as used for astronauts, was tested in 110 infants and young children up to five years of age in an orphanage in Beirut. The normal diet was found to be inadequate in caloric intake and to have a protein content of relatively poor quality. Separate studies were performed, with subjects of the first study between one and 2 1/2 years of age and the second between 3 1/2 and 5 years old. Control and treatment groups were chosen for each study and supplemented and non-supplemented periods of time were observed.

Results showed the food rods to be acceptable to the children in chocolate-flavored form taken ad-libitum at a snack period daily. The supplemented children gained a significantly increased amount of weight and height over the control children. The children spontaneously increased their daily calorie intake by 20% and daily protein intake by 16%.

26. Atiyeh, M. N., Uthman, S. M., and Shammaa, M. H. "Cancer of the esophagus in the Near East." J. Med. Liban 24(3), 1971, pp 273-277.

Esophageal carcinoma cases seen at the American University Hospital in Beirut were reviewed for the previous 15 year period. A statistical analysis of the cases showed a particularly high incidence of the disease in Saudis. The male to female ratio was three to one. The most frequent histopathological diagnosis was that of squamous cell carcinoma, with 60 out of 93 cases afflicted. Fourteen cases of adenocarcinoma were found, and the remainder were neurofibrosarcoma, unclassified, or leiomyosarcoma.

50.5% of the cases were from Saudi Arabia, 20.4% from Lebanon, and 16% from Syria. The Saudi case load was very high in view of the fact that Saudi admissions never exceeded 2% of the total hospital admissions. Authors noted that racial or hereditary factors were unlikely to explain the distribution of cases and stressed the environmental factors involved, such as spiciness of the food in Saudi Arabia.

27. Bickers, W. "Adventures in Arabian gynecology." Va. Med. Mon. 98(5), May 1971, pp 262-270.

This article highlights some of the different medical realities the author encountered in the Middle East while working at the American University of Beirut School of Medicine. Middle Eastern practices such as female circumcision and salt packing of the puerperal vagina after delivery and pathology such as acquired pelvic abnormalities of grand multiparas due to osteomalacia required a flexible approach to gynecology. There is a very low incidence of cervical cancer, but corrective surgery for genital fistula is common. The author briefly notes the range of pathology seen at the University Hospital and considers differences in mores and morals in the Middle East.

28. Bitar, J. G., and Andonian, K. "Viral hepatitis in Lebanon. With a review of recent advances." J. Med. Liban 24(4), 1971, pp 329-337.

224 cases of acute viral hepatitis admitted to the American University of Beirut Hospital were reviewed for clinical presentation and laboratory findings. Maximum incidence occurred in the third decade of life with 36% of cases, and 13% of cases were below 14 years of age. 66% of cases were foreigners, and the authors suggested that this was due to the life-long exposure of native Lebanese to the virus and subsequent build-up of immunity against it. Children experienced more cases in the autumn and winter months, with 25% of admissions occurring in November. Liver function tests were markedly deranged, with a 94% elevation in

total bilirubin. 88% of patients showed the elevated serum transaminases, SGOT and SGPT. Early ambulation and liberal diet, together with gammaglobulin therapy, were urged by the authors in treatment.

29. Haddah, N. E., and Harfouche, J. K. "Serum protein in Lebanese infants." J. Trop. Pediatr. 17(3), September 1971, pp 91-97.

Total serum protein and the electrophoretic patterns of 316 Lebanese infants from birth to 18 months were studied in relation to age, sex, dietary pattern and nutritional status.

The mean values of total serum protein and its fractions show some variations with age, especially in the gamma globulin level. No sex difference is observed, except for the globulin fraction, which is higher for females (9-15 months), probaby due to a higher incidence of infection among the females in this population. Completely breast-fed infants have a significantly higher albumin level at 3 months than the artificially-fed, but no similar difference is observed at 6 months of age. The values of the grouped data for well nourished (non-affected) and malnourished infants (affected) fall within the accepted levels or better when compared with values of others of essentially the same age.

The total serum protein is not a good index for the detection of marasmic infants, but is a reliable criterion in the kwashiorkor variety. However, if total serum protein is normal in a population suspected of having protein-calorie malnutrition, a serum albumin is indicated. (Authors' abstract)

30. Kanawati, A. A., McLaren, D. S., and Abu-Jawdeh, I. "Failure to thrive in Lebanon. I. Experience with some simple somatic measurements." Acta Paediatr. Scand. 60(3), May 1971, pp 309-316.

1231 Lebanese Arab children between 3 and 48 months of age living in 3 locations were measured anthropometrically during a 12 month period. Comparisons with national standards for boys and girls were done, and patterns of deviation from them established for weight, height, head circumference, and mid-arm circumference. A decline in weight and mid-arm circumference to 85% of standard was noted for both sexes between 6 and 18 months of age. There ws some recovery later in the second year until 4 years of age. Height and head circumference showed less decline as percent of standard, but no later recovery. An Index of Thriving was developed using the four somatic measurements to study and contrast control and failure to thrive children.

31. Wright, P. A. "Birth interval and malnutrition." Nurs. Times 67(50), December 1971, pp 1578-1581.

One Palestinian family was observed by a nurse to determine whether frequent pregnancies with a short bitth inverval were a significant factor in infant malnutrition. The author notes that the region's social organization is based almost entirely on the family unit, and that male children are most prized due to the reliance on the grown son to support his elderly parents. The family's home condition and family history are described, along with their diet, which is supported by family income and registered refugees' ration entitlement. A female child who died from third-degree malnutrition was followed from October to her death on May 23. She was breast-fed exclusively until December, then was sometimes given some orange juice. After her death, the mother gave birth to a very healthy boy who showed normal growth and development over a two-month period of observation. The author concluded that the short birth interval in this family did not influence the infant malnutrition status per se.

32. McLaren, D. S. "Nutrition in the medical school." Amer. J. Clin. Nutr. 23(10), October 1970, pp 1264-1266.

The author described the development since 1961 of the research interest and capability in nutrition at the American University of Beirut. The Nutrition Research Program was formed to investigate nutrition problems in the Middle East and eventually became an integral part of the medical school in 1967. No academic department status was accorded the Program, but faculty members and other personnel shared the same rights and responsibilities as staff of other departments. The four times when an undergraduate medical student is exposed to nutrition are: in the first year-hemeostasis; second year-nutritional diseases; third year-bedside presentations of nutritional aspects of various medical conditions; and classes in preventive medicine and community nutrition. The author suggested formal recognition for nutrition in medical school by combining metabolism and nutrition as a division in the department of medicine.

Middle East: Arab World and Islamic World

1. Al-Amadi, M. "Nutritional Security and Arab Cooperation" Shu'un 'Arabiyyah 23, February 1983, pp 30-57.

   There has been a dramatic increase in the dependency of Arab states on imported food throughout the late 1970s despite their continued development. The keys to maximizing agricultural potential of villages are development of a balanced policy and an emphasis on village life and agricultural development in each Arab state. In addition, financial resources must be mobilized more effectively to alleviate food supply problems in the 1980s throughout the Arab world.

2. El Sunni, M. "Arab scientists talk" Sudanow 8(1) January 1983, 28 pages.

   A description in 1983 of the work of the Arab Scientific Research Councils Federation, founded in 1977. Based in Iraq, which provides 50 per cent of the total budget, the federation aims to encourage research cooperation through the unification of scientific vocabulary in Arabic and the creation of joint research projects in the fields of agriculture, nutrition, industry, natural resources, housing, and sociolgoy. A journal is to be published. The federation held its sixth meeting in Khartoum in December, 1982. (Author's abstract)

3. Tarbush, S. "Reaching out to the rural poor" Middle East 12 (100), February 1983, pp 38-40.

   A report on the International Fund for Agricultural Development (IFAD), a UN agency devoted to increasing food production, improving nutrition and fighting rural poverty. Projects underway in the YAR, Egypt and Sudan concentrate on local needs, such as production of certain indigenous food crops, and tailors work to those conditions. IFAD suffers from logistical and manpower deficiencies, however, and squabbling over solutions to those problems and over funds tends to undermine IFAD's efficiency. (Author's abstract)

4. Anonymous "Conference of the Arab Gulf States' Health Ministers" Saudi Arabia Newsletter 67, March 15, 1982, p 11.

   A report on the Arab Gulf states' health ministers' conference held in San'a, YAR in March, 1982. The ministers agreed to put controls on imported foodstuffs and to check compliance with standards and nutritional value. A nutrition committee was formed with representatives from Kuwait, the UAE, Qatar, Saudi Arabia, Bahrain, Oman, and the General Secretariat of the GCC. The Gulf region imports 90 per cent of its food. (Author's abstract)

5. Fedail, S. S., Murphy, D., Salih, S. Y., Bolton, C. H., and Harvey, R. F. "Changes in certain blood constituents during Ramadan." Am. J. Clin. Nutr. 36(2), August 1982, pp 350-353.

   Fasting serum cholesterol, triglycerides, thyroxine, triiodothyronine, uric acid, gastrin, and insulin were measured in 24 Muslims at the beginning and end of Ramadan--the Muslim month of fasting. There was a significant increase in the levels of total serum cholesterol, thyroxine, and uric acid and a significant fall in body weight. There was no significant change in the levels of total serum triglycerides, triiodothyronine, gastrin, insulin (fasting), or in the rise in gastrin or insulin 1/2 hr after food.

These changes, although unlikely to affect normal people, may be significant in patients. Physicians working in Muslim countries should be aware that Ramadan may affect some laboratory findings. (Authors' abstract)

6. Schoeninger, M. J. "Diet and the evolution of modern human form in the Middle East." Am. J. Phys. Anthropol. 58(1), May 1982, pp 37-52.

Fully, modern human form more gracile than the antecedent archaic modern form was evident 30,000 years ago. One hypothesis to explain this decrease in skeletal robustness is that change occurred in human diet associated with a decrease in activity levels in both individual and group behavior. Dietary change can be studied directly using trace element analysis of strontium levels in bone which reflects the amount of strontium in diet. Since plants contain higher levels of strontium than do animal soft tissues, the level of bone strontium will differ according to the proportion of plant and animal products in the diet. In this study the ratio of strontium:calcium in human bone to strontium:calcium in faunal bone is compared for samples of archaic modern humans (from Mugharet et Tabun, Mugharet es-Skhul, and Jebel Qafzeh) and fully modern humans (from Mugharet el-Kebara and Mugharet el-Wad) from Israel. A ratio controls for potentially unequal strontium levels in soils at different sites and for different diagenetic histories between sites. The results of the analysis are internally reliable, reflecting bone strontium levels rather than technique error. It appears that a change occurred in the amount of animal protein in the diet of humans but it occurred almost 20,000 years after the first appearance of skeletally modern humans. These results refute the hypothesis that the morphological transformation to modern human form occurred as a result of behavioral changes involved in obtaining new foods. If any decrease in human activity level occurred between archaic modern and fully modern humans, it probably was due to alterations in the means of procuring or processing the same kinds of foods that had been utilized earlier in time. (Adapted from author's abstract).

7. Anonymous "Task analysis and priorities in programes to improve infant feeding." J. Trop. Pediatr. 27, December 1981, pp ii-iv.

Task analysis can be an important tool in studying child feeding practices and improving child nutrition within the cultural context and realities of the mothers' limited time. The involvement of parents in nutrition education, and the practical aspects of weaning foods as well as their nutritional content are factors which are seen as important in adapting nutrition education to local reality. There are three advantages to task analysis, as practiced by cultural anthropologists, in observing womens' preparation from food collecting through storage, preparation, and serving. First, observations enable one to choose which of two approaches, the family meal approach or special young child food approach, is appropriate in each instance. Second, the focus on nutrition education can be made more specific and realistic. Third, various appropriate culinary technologies can be suggested.

8. Anonymous "Nouveau Plan d'Action pour les 5 Prochaines Annees" Syrie et Monde Arabe 27(334), November 1981, pp 20-25. (Article in French)

A report on the joint Arab economic strategy for 1981-85, adopted by the Arab League's economic and social council in 1980, which is intended to complement individual member countries' plans. Breakdowns are given of the distribution of investment and loans in 1980. One estimate of the plan's cost is 62 billion dollars, divided between nutritional needs, industry, transport, communications, and other areas. Tables are given of exact sectoral distribution. The least advanced countries will profit most from the investment plans. (Author's abstract)

9. Barber, S. G., Fairweather, S., Wright, A. D., Fitzgerald, M. G., and Malins, J. M. "Muslims, Ramadan, and diabetes mellitus." (letter) Br. Med. J. 2(6181) July 1979, pp 46-47.

This letter discussed the effect of the Muslim fast month of Ramadan on Muslim diabetics. Thirty unselected Muslims attending the diabetic clinic during the 1978 fast were interviewed to determine if the fasting presented a problem. Half claimed exemption on medical grounds. All who fasted professed to do so strictly with no lapses. Only three patients noticed any change in diabetic control. Authors noted that there appeared to be little radical change in the apparent control of the patients. They felt it appropriate to advise Muslim diabetics not to fast during Ramadan, unless their diabetes was controlled on diet alone.

10. Barber, S. G., and Wright, A. D. "Muslims, Ramadan, and diabetes mellitus." (letter) Br. Med. J. 2(6191), September 15, 1979, p 675.

This short letter was a reply to a commentary concerning Muslims, Ramadan, and diabetes mellitus. The authors contend that they have not shown that diabetics can safely fast during Ramadan. They mention that the control they observed in their interviewed patients was not initially satisfactory, and conclude by saying that extra caution is preferable to unnecessary risk.

11. Born, M., Elmadfa, I., and Schmahl, F. W. "Effects of periodical fluid and food withdrawal. An inquiry conducted during the lenten month Ramadan on foreign workers." (author's translation) MMW 121(47) November 1979, pp 1569-1572.

The effects of fasting during the Moslem holy month of Ramadan were studied in 12 volunteer foreign workers. The subjects continued limited work and domestic chores throughout the study period. They experienced dehydration, with average increases of 11%-hematocrit, 12%-creatinine, 5%-total serum protein, 4%-albumin, 30%-blood glucose, and 11%-urea. The total fluid and food withdrawal which Orthodox Moslems practice from sunup to sundown during Ramadan also changed their electrolyte balance and several enzyme levels. Body weight and general state of health were assessed along with hematologic and biochemical clinical parameters. The largest change in a single parameter was seen in 3-hydroxybutyrate, which increased an average of 114% during fasting. The authors recommended avoidance of heavy work during day-long fluid and food withdrawal because of the dehydration observed in these subjects with restricted physicial activity.

12. Davidson, J. C. "Muslims, Ramadan, and diabetes mellitus." (letter) Br. Med. J. 2(6203), December 8, 1979, pp 1511-1512.

This letter was in response to those of Dr. Barber and associates, July 7 page 46, and Dr. Ebbing, August 2, page 333 in the same journal on Muslims, Ramadan, and diabetes mellitus. The author mentions that most of the 800 Muslim diabetic patients in the clinic in Qatar do not attend the clinic during Ramadan, but that no patient was admitted to hospital during Ramadan or in the following month. He also notes that no patients were found to have lost weight during or after Ramadan, and attributes this to the extra amount of food consumed during the month of Ramadan. Pregnant diabetics are usually willing to exempt themselves from fasting, and in the author's experience, fasting in practice seldom seems to cause trouble for the patients.

13. Ebbing, R. N. "Muslims, Ramadan, and diabetes mellitus." (letter) Br. Med. J. 2(6185), August 4, 1979, pp 333-334.

This short letter was written in response to a Birmingham diabetic clinic's televised warning to Muslim diabetic patients to refrain from fasting during Ramadan. The author found it difficult to understand why a warning was given because a letter by Dr. Barber and associates of July 7, page 46 in the same journal, showed that Muslims with diabetes mellitus come to no harm by observing the Ramadan fast. The author felt that the patients should have been seen weekly during Ramadan and should have been taught to test for ketones. He also mentioned specific instructions for adjusting insulin schedules.

14. James, E. O. "Cultural and religious taboos related to food." Prog. Food Nutr. Sci. 3(3), 1979, pp 67-77.

The paper traces the major food taboos of many cultures, including Polynesian, Hebrew/Judaic, Hellenic, Roman, Hindu, Buddhist, Islamic, and Christian, through history, from their ancient origins to modern times.

15. Anonymous. "Muslim patients during the Islamic month of fasting." Tijdschr, Ziekenverpl. 31(15), July 1978, p 702. (Article in Dutch)

The needs of Muslim patients who may be encountered by health personnel in hospital during the Islamic month of fasting known as Ramadan are discussed. Muslims are excused from fasting in cases such as illness, menstruation or lactation. However, special therapeutics may be needed for patients who still voluntarily fast, such as ulcer patients. Fasting Muslims tend to overeat compensatorily at night during Ramadan. The need for avoiding misunderstandings with the fasting Muslim patient is stressed.

16. Gumas, K. A., Mustafe, K. Y., Mahmoud, N. A., and Gader, A. M. "The effects of fasting in Ramadan. 1. Serum uric acid and lipid concentrations." Br. J. Nutr. 40(3), November 1978, pp 573-581.

The changes in serum levels of uric acid and lipids during 1 month of starvation-refeeding were measured in sixteen male volunteers. Uric acid levels increased linearly with the duration of the experiment. The increase was positively correlated with the increase in serum triglycerides but not with cholesterol or phospholipids. Triglycerides increased at a faster rate than uric acid implying that the increase in uric acid was secondary to that of the lipid. It was concluded that the purine and lipid synthetic pathways are linked through a common small-molecular-weight effector rather than through the sharing of a common enzyme. (Authors' abstract)

17. Last, G. "Overpopulation and Islam." Ther. Ggw. 117(11), November 1978, pp 1683-1710. (Article in German, no English abstract)

The interrelationships between Islam and overpopulation in the Muslim world are examined, including historical developments and modern methods of dealing with recent population increases. Traditional Islamic beliefs concerning the family, and how they relate to family planning goals and methods, including coitus interruptus, are featured.

18. Barakat, M. R. "Current information on nutritional problems in the Middle East". Practical Approaches to Combat Malnutrition with Special Reference to Mothers and Children Cairo, Egypt. Publication of Proceeding of IUNS Conference held May 25-29, 1977, pp 49-74.

This presentation focussed on Middle Eastern characteristics related to malnutrition. These included poverty, illiteracy, high birth rates, low life expectancy, young-aged populations, and food production vs. demand shortages within countries. Cultural factors included early marriages of girls, late start of supplementary feeding of infants, religious taboos, and unequal care for males and females in infancy. Ecological factors included poor home sanitation and prevalence of parasitic diseases such as ascariasis, ancylostoma and schistosomiasis, the latter two particularly in Egypt, Sudan, and Iraq. The nature and magnitude of malnutrition in the area was explored. Protein energy malnutrition (PEM) was the most serious nutritional problem in children below 5 years of age, most commonly in those 2 or 3 years old. Nutritional anemias, vitamin A deficiency, rickets, osteomalacia, goiter, pellagra, scurvy, and ariboflavinosis prevalences in various countries were cited. Priority approaches for nutritional measures, to be modified according to each country's needs and resources, included targeting at-risk subpopulations, focussing on breastfeeding, conducting nutrition education campaigns, and training health personnel in nutrition pre-service and in-service.

19. Auckland, A. K., and Singh, K. B. "The exploitation of natural genetic variability for the improvement of chickpea (Cicer arietinum L.)." Basic Life Sci. 8, March 1-7, 1976, pp 83-95.

An ACRISAT breeding program was begun in 1973 with the aim of producing elite lines and segregating populations of chickpeas of the small-seeded desi type and of the large-seeded kabuli types adapted to Eastern and Western Asia, respectively. The ultimate goal of the program is to strengthen national and regional programs for the chickpea-growing countries of the world. A 1975 summer crop was grown in Lebanon and provided information concerning divergencies between kabuli and desi types. Adaptability of coadaptation appeared to be most important in chickpeas. The introgression of desi germ plasm into kabuli germ plasm for the improvement of the kabuli crop in western Asia was indicated.

20. Halstead, S. B. "Studies on the epidemiology of idiopathic bladder stone disease." Idiopathic Urinary Bladder Stone Disease. Van Reen, R., ed. DHEW (NIH) 77-1063, Bethesda W3F049 No. 37. 1976, pp 121-134.

This report focused on the problems of idiopathic bladder stone disease in various countries, including Thailand and 9th century Great Britain. The infant feeding practice of hand feeding starchy foods is connected to incidence of stone disease in young children. The formation of insoluble urinary salts in the first few weeks of life is the suspected mechanism, and may be affected by a low milk diet in young infants. Relevance of the discussion to the Middle East is connected to infant weaning practices there.

21. Nikkila, E. M., Constantinides, S. M., and Meade, T. L. "Supplementation of Arabic and Indian breads with fish protein concentrate". J. Agric. Food Chem. 24(6), November-December 1976, pp 1144-1147.

The utilization of different kinds of fish protein concentrates (FPC) in the supplementation of Arabic bread and Indian bread (puri) was studied. Taste panel tests showed that the supplemented breads were well accepted when 10% of bread flour was replaced by FPC. Such a supplementation with the best test FPC used elevated the protein efficiency ratio of the bread to equal that of casein. It was demonstrated that extremely high dry heat (650°C) required for the Arabic bread or cooking in oil (190°C) for puri did little to decrease the protein value of FPC when the heating time was about 1 min. Significant differences in nutritional value were observed between the different kinds of FPC used. (Authors' abstract)

22. Armstrong, B., and Doll, R. "Environmental factors and cancer incidence and mortality in different countries, with special reference to dietary practices." Int. J. Cancer 15(4), April 1975, pp 617-631.

The incidence and mortality rates of various cancers in several countries have been correlated with various dietary and other environmental variables. A review of 23 countries' incidence rates for 27 cancers, and of 32 countries' mortality rates for 14 cancers showed dietary variables to be strongly correlated with several cancer types. Meat consumption was strongly correlated with cancer of the colon. Fat consumption was similarly correlated with breast and uterine cancers. Modification of cancer development at a number of other sites was indicated as a role for other dietary factors. Use of epidemiologic data to determine correlations and point out possible etiologic agents is discussed.

23. Malhotra, K. "Children of foreign workers from the viewpoint of medical practice". Fortschr. Med. 93(27), September 25, 1975, pp 1241-1242.

A comparison of the type of medical problems encountered in children of foreign workers compared to those in German children was conducted via a questionnaire of medical practitioners in Duisberg, Vilbert, Wuppertal, and Dusseldorf. Although most of the physicians noted no differences in health problems between groups, those who did note a difference cited a higher incidence of catarrhal disease and malnutrition and a lower incidence of neurotic problems in the foreign workers' children. Parental education concerning appropriate nutrition and apparal for the German environment may help to reduce the foreign childrens' higher illness and malnutrition incidences.

24. Sakr, A. H. "Fasting in Islam." Am. J. Diet. Assoc. 67(1), July 1975, pp 17-21.

The significance of fasting in Islam, the rules and regulations of fasting, types of fasting, nullification of fasting, and food practices and habits of Muslims during the month of Ramadan are summarized. Some problems pertaining to fasting and their solutions, and adaptations of fasting in America are considered.

25. Stoll, L. "Epidemiologic investigations of serum of foreign workers from the Mediterranean region in exposed and non-exposed occupations concerning toxoplasmosis infection." Oeff Gesundheitswes 37(2), February 1975, pp 99-107. (Author's translation)

A serologic study was conducted on newly arrived foreign workers in non-exposed occupations (Moroccans and Turks, Italians and Greeks) and on workers resident in W. Germany for some time in exposed occupations (Moroccans and Turks, Italians and Yugoslavs) to determine the incidence of toxoplasmosis infection. 676 sera were examined. Results showed 10.1% of Moroccans and Turks and 14.3% of Italians and Greeks who were non-exposed had antibodies against toxoplasmosis with the Sabin-Feldman-test (SFT). For exposed occupations held for some time, 80.9% of Italians and Yugoslavs, and 68.0% of Moroccans and Turks showed SFT Antibodies. In German controls in exposed occupations, a higher percentage of toxoplasmosis antibodies, 78.5%, was seen than was seen in non-exposed Germans, who showed 43.2% having antibodies to toxoplasmosis. The author concluded that pork could be excluded as a source of infection, and that one must assume increased risks of toxoplasmosis in people working in the sewage works and the cleansing works. He suggested that the oocysts were most probably inhaled by man.

26. Higazi, M. I., and Read, W. W. C. "A Method for determination of vicine in plant material and in blood." J. Agr. Food Chem. 22(4), July-August 1974, pp 570-571.

A colorimetric method for the determination of small quantities of vicine (2,6-diamino-4,5-dehydroxypyrimidine 5-(-D-glucopyranoside)) in biological materials is described. Folin and Ciocalteu's phenol reagent is used as the chromatogen after removal of proteins, amino acids, and phenolic materials from extracts of plants and from blood plasma. The method makes possible the study of variations in vicine concentrations in fava beans, due to habitat and maturity. Its use will help elucidate the role of vicine as a causative factor in favism. (Authors' abstract)

27. Anonymous "Zinc deficiency in man." Lancet 1(798), February 10, 1973, pp 299-300.

The history of zinc deficiency studies to date and the knowledge gained from them was reviewed. The initial possible syndrome of human zinc deficiency was described by workers in Iran and Egypt who obtained results with supplementation studies. Investigators showed a dietary connection between high phytate content of unleavened Middle Eastern breads and zinc biounavailability, and uncovered the possible effects of clay-eating in this area. Some researchers have speculated on the possibility of widespread, marginal zinc deficiency and a range of deficiency. Zinc deficiency may be connected with some conditions such as liver disease, diabetes and some renal diseases. Its loss through hemorrhage and sweat and the need for its addition to parenteral nutrition regimens in patients was noted. The need for further studies on the bioavailability of zinc and dose-effectiveness of zinc sulphate for therapeutic purposes was delineated.

28. Peruzy, A. D., and De Santis, A. M. "Statistical aspects of cardiovascular pathology in some Mediterranean countries." Minerva Med. 64(66), September 1973, pp 3423-3435. (Article in Italian)

Seven of the Mediterranean countries (France, Greece, Israel, Italy, Malta, and Gozo, Spain and Yugoslavia) have furnished reports on mortality rates for cardiovascular pathology during the period 1965-67. Statistics are considered in terms of sex, age, geographic-economic factors, and, for each median age of death, trends regarding the particular cardiovascular disease, as well as the correlation between cardiovascular deaths and diet.

As compared to a similar but uncomprehensive study for the period of 1955-1957, the general tendencies in the present study show an increase not only in arteriosclerotic and degenerative heart disease, but also for all cardiovascular pathology of endogenous origin, especially in countries with a more marked increase in the consumption of fats. (Translated and abstracted by Linda Manganaro and Gabriella Albanese.)

29. Patwardhan, V. N., Darby, W. J., (some chapters by Carter, P & Sandstead, H. H.) The State of Nutrition in the Arab Middle East, Vanderbilt University Press, Nashville, U.S., 1972.

This is a review of the nutritional observations, research findings, developments, and needs in several countries of the Arab Middle East. It summarizes information pertaining to food supplies and dietary habits and treats extensively the nutritional disorders endemic in the region.

Chapters on such diseases as pellagra, kwashiorkor, and marasmus (protein-calorie malnutrition), zinc deficiency, zerophthalmia, anemia, and parasitic infestations give the historical background of these conditions in the Middle East and reveal the prevalence of dietary deficiency and the intensive development of nutritional understanding that has occurred in the Middle East. Much information resulting from the work of WHO, FAO, and other international agencies, as well as bilateral programs, such as the ICNND, has been critically summarized and documented.

The findings are illustrated through ample charts and tables and the book presents a broad picture of the subject of nutrition, including the effects of food habits, limited food resources, and lack of development. The effects of nutritional ignorance, poverty, and displacement are depicted. Much information of historical interest also is included. (Adapted from book jacket abstract.)

30. Sakr, A. H. "Dietary regulations and food habits of Muslims." J. Amer. Diet. Assoc. 58(2), February 1971, pp 123-126.

Some two million persons of the Islamic faith, all of whom are expected to follow certain dietary regulations in practicing their religion, live in the United States. This description by a Muslim, of these dietary injunctions and regulations will help dietitians dealing with Muslim patients to understand their problems and to help them in planning dietary regimens. (Author's abstract)

31. Ronaghy, H. A. "Symposium on food science and nutritional diseases in the Middle East." Amer. J. Clin. Nutr. 23(11), November 1970, pp 1418-1421.

A Food Science and Nutritional Diseases symposium, held between April 27 and 30, 1970 in Shiraz, Iran, was reported. Segments were held on Growth and Development, Socioeconomic and Environmental Factors in Malnutrition, Food Science, Trace Metals, Vitamins, and Malnutrition and Disease during the symposium. Highlights from these segments are featured in the report, including the introduction of a simplified midarm-to-head circumference ratio for simplifying nutrition assessment, the epidemiologic characterization of nutritionally related problems such as zinc, vitamin A, iron, iodine, and vitamin D deficiencies, and synergism between folate deficiency and bacterial overgrowth on steatorrhea and abnormal mucosa during intestinal stasis.

Saudi Arabia

1. Elidrissy, A. T. H., Sedrani, S. H., and Lawson, D. E. M. "Vitamin D deficiency in mothers of rachitic infants." Calcif. Tissue. Int. 35, 1984, pp 266-268.

   Confirmed radiologically among infants there is an existence of nutritional deficiency rickets. The majority of the rachitic infants were breast-fed, some received unsupplemented infant feeding formulae and all lived in an environment that is devoid of sunlight. At the time of onset the mean age was 10.5 months. 25-Hydroxyvitamin D (25OHD) levels were found to be low in mothers of the rachitic infants. This maternal deficiency as a factor in pathogenesis of rickets in the infants is discussed. Proposals are made to prevent the occurrence of rickets on this scale.

2. Fonseca, V., Tongia, R., el-Hazmi, M., and Abu-Aisha, H. "Exposure to sunlight and vitamin D deficiency in Saudi Arabian women." Postgrad. Med. J. 60(707), September 1984, pp 589-591.

   Plasma 25-hydroxy cholecalciferol (25-OH vitamin D) concentrations were measured in 31 adult Saudi Arabian women with acute minor illness. The median plasma 25-OH vitamin D concentration was 6 ng/ml (range: 2-18 ng/ml). Plasma 25-OH vitamin D concentrations were significantly lower in subjects living in apartments than in those living in villas or rural areas (P less than 0.02). Plasma 25-OH vitamin D concentrations were significantly lower in those subjects whose average exposure to sunlight was less than 30 minutes daily than those whose exposure was more than 30 minutes daily (P = 0.002). The importance of inadequate exposure to sunlight in the aetiology of vitamin D deficiency was confirmed. Social customs may contribute to this deficiency in spite of abundant sunshine.

3. Sedrani, S. H. "Low 25-Hydroxyvitamin D and Normal Serum Calcium Concentrations in Saudi Arabia: Riyadh Region." Annals of Nutrition and Metabolism 28, 1984, pp 181-185.

   One hundred and four Saudis, 44 Jordanians, 17 Egyptians and 10 other subjects aged between 18 and 23 years were measured for serum levels of the circulating form of vitamin D, 25-hydroxyvitamin D, and calcium. Male university students living in Riyadh for more than 2 years compiled the entire subject population. 25-Hydroxyvitamin D levels were (mean SD) 12.8, 6.3, 11.0, 5.8, 11.9, 6.9 and 11.9, 5.0 ng/ml for normal Saudis, Jordanians, Egyptians and others, respectively. The percentages of subjects with serum 25-hydroxyvitamin D levels below 10 ng/ml were 35, 45, 53 and 50%, respectively. All subjects had normal serum calcium concentrations. There was no correlation between 25-hydroxyvitamin D and serum calcium levels in the subjects investigated. This study indicates a tendency for a low vitamin D status among residents of Saudi Arabia, in spite of abundant sunlight all the year round.

4. Sedrani, S. H. "Vitamin D status of Saudi men." Trop. Geogr. Med. 36(2), June 1984, pp 181-187.

   65 Saudis, 45 white and 12 dark-skinned non-Saudis serum levels of 25-hydroxyvitamin D and 1,25-dihydroxyvitamin D have been determined. The subjects were healthy male blood donors who lived in Riyadh for more than one year. A high percentage of the studied population were found to have low serum levels and to be at risk of developing vitamin D deficiency. The serum level of

1,25-dihydroxyvitamin D, were normal. Probably the main factor contributing to vitamin D deficiency in Saudi Arabia is avoidance of sunshine. Exposure to sunlight and fortification of food are indispensable measures for improving the vitamin D status of the population of Saudi Arabia.

5. Taha, S. A., Dost, S. M., and Sedrani, S. H. "25-Hydroxyvitamin D and total calcium: extraordinarily low plasma concentrations in Saudi mothers and their neonates." Pediatr. Res. 18(8), August 1984, pp 739-741.

   Plasma levels of 25-hydroxyvitamin D (25-OHD) and total calcium were measured in venous blood obtained from 100 consecutive and unselected Saudi Arabian mothers and their neonates within 48 hours after delivery. Fifty-nine mothers and 70 neonates had subnormal (less than 10 ng/ml) 25-OHD levels. Plasma Calcium concentrations were low in 61% of the mothers and 59% of the newborns consisting of 10 preterm and 38 full term babies. There were significant correlation between the plasma levels of maternal and neonatal 25-OHD ($r = 0.54$; $P = 0.0001$), maternal 25-OHD and Ca ($r = -0.22$; $P = 0.03$), neonatal 25-OHD and Ca ($r = -0.28$; $P = 0.0009$), and maternal and neonatal calcium levels ($r = 0.46$; $P = 0.0001$). Nevertheless, maternal 25-OHD was not invariably higher than that in the infant. Normocalcemia was observed in 29 neonates and 26 mothers (20 mother/baby pairs) in the presence of subnormal maternal 25-OHD. Twenty babies and 16 mothers including nine mother/baby pairs had hypocalcemia in the presence of normal levels of 25-OHD, indicating that vitamin D plays a crucial, but not exclusive, role in calcium homeostasis during pregnancy. This study revealed that vitamin D deficiency is very prevalent during pregnancy in Saudi Arabia, and it also showed that asymptomatic hypocalcemia in full term babies is far more common than expected. It is considered that vitamin D deficiency is primarily due to the lack of exposure to sunlight.

6. Haque, K. N. "Feeding pattern of children under two years of age in Riyadh, Saudi Arabia." Ann. Trop. Paediatr. 3(3), September 1983, pp 129-132.

   Feeding practices were discussed with mothers or other close relatives of children who were in a Riyadh hospital. Sixty-four percent of mothers of newborn babies had attended antenatal clinics, with 10% receiving instructions on feeding. Of the hospitalized children 27% were receiving breast milk alone by one month of age. However, of the 28% of mothers who had some education, 84% were breast feeding at three months of age. By three months of age, the average baby had consumed six of the 36 varieties of artifical milk. Less than 14% of mothers intending to bottle feed could read the instructions, and of those who believed they knew how, only 18% made up the formula correctly. Educational opportunities need to be exploited and easy availability of artificial milk curbed.

7. Sedrani, S. H., Elidrissy, A. W., and El Arabi, K. M. "Sunlight and vitamin D status in normal Saudi subjects." Am. J. Clin. Nutr. 38(1), July 1983, pp 129-132.

   Serum levels of the circulating form of vitamin D3, 25-hydroxycholecalciferol (25-(OH)D3), were determined in 59 university students, 26 males and 33 females aged 18 to 26 years and in 24 elderly subjects, 13 males and 11 females with a mean age of 62 +/- 13 yr. The level of 25-(OH)D3 was significantly lower in the elderly persons (p less than 0.001) than in young students of both sexes, and was significantly higher in females than in males. Serum levels of 1, 25- and 24, 25-dihydroxycholecalciferol were measured in adult males and found to be within the normal range. A group of elderly patients were exposed to natural uv light, and the circulating levels of 25-(OH)D3, serum phosphorus, and alkaline phosphatase were determined both before and 1 day after the last exposure. The exposure to natural uv light resulted in a 2 1/2-fold increase in the level of 25-(OH)D3 and a significant decrease in the activity of alkaline phosphatase, but no significant change in serum phosphorus concentrations was observed. It is concluded that the low vitamin D3 status in Saudis is mainly due to avoidance of sunlight exposure and other factors discussed. (Authors' abstract)

8. Sedrani, S. H., Elidrissy, A. W., and El Arabi, K. M. "Sunlight and vitamin D status in normal Saudi subjects." Am. J. Clin. Nutr. 38, July 1983, pp 129-132.

Fifty nine university students, 26 males and 33 females aged 18 to 26 years and in 24 elderly subjects 13 males and 11 females, with a mean age of 62, 13 years were tested to determine serum levels of the circulating form of vitamin D3, 25-hydroxycholecalciferol. The level of 25-hydroxycholecalciferol was significantly lower in the elderly (p 0.001) than in the male and female students and was significantly higher in female students than in males. Serum levels of 1, 25- and 24, 25-dihydroxycholecalciferol were measured in adult males and found to be within the normal range. The circulating levels of 25-(OH)D3, serum phosphorus, and alkaline phosphatase were determined in a group of elderly patients both before and 1 day after the last exposure to natural uv light. The exposure to natural uv light resulted in a 2-fold increase in the level of 25-(OH)D3 and a significant decrease in the activity of alkaline phosphatase, but no significant change in serum phosphorus concentrations was observed. It is concluded that the low vitamin D3 status in Saudis is mainly due to avoidance of sunlight exposure and other factors discussed.

9. Barbour, E. K., and Nabbut, N. H. "Isolation of salmonella and some other potential pathogens from two chicken breeding farms in Saudi Arabia." Avian Dis. 26(2), April-June 1982, pp 234-244.

Different salmonella serotypes were recovered from various sources in meat (A) and layer (B) poultry-breeder farms of Saudi Arabia. On farm A, salmonella were recovered from intestines of poultry breeders (7.41%), shelled chicken embryos (2.67%), day-old chicks (19.23%), and mice (21.43%). Salmonellae in shell contents and on shell surfaces of hatching eggs contaminated the same percentage of eggs (1.24%), and litter and feed contaminations were 4.0% and 1.67%, respectively. On farm B, salmonella were recovered from intestines of poultry breeders (27.59%), mice intestines (15.0%), shells of hatching eggs (2.48%), hatching egg contents (0.35%), litter (33.33%), and feed (5.0%). No salmonella were recovered from intestines of in shelled chick embryos or day-old chicks on farm B. The total number of salmonella serotypes indicated from both farms was 14, and the serotypes common to both farms were Salmonella concord and S. livingstone. Salmonella contamination of shells of hatching eggs, pooled from both farms, was higher for dirty floor eggs than for clean eggs collected from floors and nests. The percentages of hatching penetrated by bacteria other than salmonella on farms A and B, respectively, were: dirty floor eggs (25.53%, 22.83%), clean floor eggs (2.67%, 2.06%) and clean nest eggs (0.00%, 1.08%). The bacterial flora isolated from egg contents were staphylococcus, coliforms, streptococcus, Bacillus, Salmonella, and Proteus. (Authors' abstract)

10. El-Hazmi, M. A., Al-Faleh, F. Z., Al-Mofleh, I. A., Warszy, A. S., and Al-Askah, A. K. "Establishment of normal 'reference' ranges for haematological parameters for healthy Saudi Arabs." Trop. Geogr. Med. 34(4), 1982, pp 333-339.

The normal 'reference' ranges of haematological parameters vary considerably under the influence of different factors, such as the age and sex, and various environmental factors. Furthermore, diurnal variations have also been observed. In this study the normal 'reference' ranges of haematological parameters established by analysing samples from 804 healthy Saudi students (578 males and 226 females), with ages ranging between 20 and 29 years, are presented. Comparison of the results from males and females shows that all values are higher for the Saudi males than for the females except values for white blood cell counts. Comparison of the mean values for Saudi with the values for the western population show that for the Saudi male the mean value for HbF is slightly higher while for all other parameters the values are lower. Among the Saudi females, mean values for Hb F, white blood cell counts and and mean cell volume are slightly higher than those reported for western females. Mean values for all other parameters are lower than corresponding mean values in westerners. (Authors' abstract)

11. El-Hazmi, M. A., Al-Faleh, F. Z., Al-Mofleh, I. A., Warsy, A. S., and Al-Askah, A. K. "Establishment of normal "reference" ranges for biochemical parameters for healthy Saudi Arabs." Trop. Geogr. Med. 34(4), 1982, pp 323-332.

Biochemical constituents in the blood of healthy individuals are subject to variations under the influence of several factors. Differences can be seen in the normal ranges established for populations living under different environmental and dietary conditions. Age and sex also affect the normal range values considerably. Normal "reference" ranges for 29 biochemical parameters, established by using blood samples from 578 male and 226 female students aged 20 to 29 years at various colleges at King Saud University, are presented. Marked differences are found in the values for Saudi males and females. Comparison of the results obtained for Saudis with those reported for western populations also show differences in the majority of the parameters. The comparison of Saudi mean values with western mean values is presented. (Authors' abstract)

12. Nabbut, N. H., Barbour, E. K., and Al-Nakhli, H. M. "Occurrence of salmonellae in animal feed ingredients in Saudi Arabia." Am. J. Vet. Res. 43(9), September 1982, pp 1703-1705.

Of 346 samples of animal feed ingredients (144 complete feed, 88 feed concentrate, 42 calcium carbonate, 30 meat meal, 29 fish meal, and 13 mixed meat and bone meal), 42 (12.13%) were contaminated with salmonellae. The rate of Salmonella contamination varied according to the nature of the feed sample. Seven (58.84%) of the mixed meat and bone meal, 14 (48.27%) of the fish meal, 12 (13.63%) of the feed concentrate, 7 (4.86%) of the complete feed, and 2 (4.76%) of the calcium carbonate samples contained salmonellae.

The 49 Salmonella isolates represented 18 serotypes; the 5 most frequent serotypes in decreasing order were S. lille, S. new-haw, S. livingstone, S. kentucky, and S. typhimurium. The 4 most common somatic serogroups encountered were C1, E2, B and C3. (Authors' abstract)

13. Pegram, R. G., Hoogstraal, H., and Wassef, H. Y. "Hyalomma (Hyalommina) arabica sp. n. parasitizing goats and sheep in the Yemen Arab Republic and Saudi Arabia." J. Parasitol. 68(1), February 1982, pp 150-156.

Hyalomma (Hyalommina) arabica sp. n. is described from 62 adult specimens (29 males, 33 females) taken throughout the year from 23 goats and cwo sheep, mostly at 200 m altitude in the southern tihama foothills of Ta'izz Province, Yemen Arab Republic. One female from a goat at 2,300 m altitude in this Province may have attached to the host elsewhere and a male from Mecca, Saudi Arabia, was on a goat imported from an unknown source for the traditional religious pilgrimage feast. We postulate that the original host of adults was the Nubian ibex, Capra ibex rubiana F. Cuvier (Artiodactyla: Caprinae). This parasite is most closely related to H. (H.) Kumari Sharif, which infests chiefly wild and domestic caprinae from India to northwestern Iran and Tadzhik, SSR. It also shows relationships to H. (H.) punt Hoogstraal, Kaiser and Pedersen, which parasitizes gazelles and domestic mammals in Somalia and Ethiopia, but differs more widely from the third African-Arabian member of this subgenus, H. (H.) rhipicephaloides Neumann, which feeds on the Nubian ibex and gazelles in the Red Sea and Dead Sea areas. The Hyalomma subgenus Hyalommina now contains seven species, four confined to the Indian subcontinent (including Nepal, Burma, India, Sri Lanka, Pakistan, and Afghanistan) and Southwest Asia, and three in eastern Africa north of the equator and Arabia. (Authors' abstract)

14. Younes, S. A., and El-Angbawi, M. F. "Dental caries prevalence in intermediate Saudi schoolchildren in Riyad." Community Dent. Oral, Epidemiol. 10(2), April 1982, pp 74-76.

1389 Saudi schoolchildren, aged 13, 14, and 15, were studied for dental caries prevalence. The study population was evenly divided between males and females. Clinical criteria were based on a modified DMFT subdivision. The mean value of D_2F, secondary decay on the margins of formerly filled teeth, was significantly higher for females than for males. The mean M, or missing, value showed significant difference by age. No other statistically significant differences were seen between males and females and at different ages in the DMFT. In general, low caries prevalence was seen compared to that seen in similar Western populations, but the need for dental care was high as evidenced by a 77.65% incidence of dental caries, evenly distributed among males and females. The use of meat and rice staples in the diet as opposed to highly refined carbohydrates, as well as the use of the Arak plant's branch called miswak for brushing teeth, were cited as possible contributory factors in the low caries prevalence seen among the Saudi children studied.

15. Abaheseen, M. A., Harrison, G. G., and Pearson, P. B. "Nutritional status of Saudi Arab preschool children in the Eastern Province". Ecology of Food and Nutrition 10, 1981, pp 163-168.

Simple indices of nutrition status (height, weight, head

circumference, mid-upper arm circumference, triceps skinfold and hematocrit) were studied in a cross-sectional group of 198 Saudi Arab children aged birth to five years attending the ARAMCO Hospital Clinic for well child care in Dhahran, Saudi Arabia. Severe protein-energy malnutrition was rare, but mild undernutrition was highly prevalent, afflicting 35.4 percent of the children, based on the Gomez Index. There were significant differences in nutritional status by age and sex, with female children over the age of 30 months being most at risk for low values of all anthropometric indices of nutritional status. Older children were more likely to have low hematocrit values than younger ones, but there was no difference in prevalence of anemia by sex. (Authors' abstract)

16. Karrar, Z. A., and Abdullah, M. A. "Gastroenteritis among children in Riyadh: A prospective analysis of 254 hospital admissions." Ann. Trop. Paediatr. 1(2), June 1981, pp 119-122.

A prospective study was undertaken of 254 infants and children admitted with gastroenteritis to the Children's Hospital, Riyadh, Saudi Arabia during the period 1 September 1980 to 1 February 1981. Analysis of data showed that 80% of the admissions were less than one year of age, with a peak incidence of 0-five months of age. 65.4% were on bottle feeding. The incidence of second- and third-degree malnutrition was 38.9% and in marasmus was the commonest type of severe malnutrition. Hypernatraemic dehydration occurred in 12.6% of the cases. The parasitic and bacterial isolation rate was 23.8% salmonellae and entero-pathogenic E. coli being the commonest organisms. the mortality rate was 9.1% and was higher among malnournished patients, those with hypernatraemia and in the younger age groups. (Adapted from authors' abstract)

17. Lawson, M. "Infant feeding habits in Riyadh". Abstract found in Nutrition Research, 2, 1982, p 632, under "Country report-Egypt and Middle East." Original article in Saudi Med. J. Riyadh 2, 1981, pp 26-29.

A small survey was done among mothers attending Riyad El-Kharj Hospital. Seventy-two percent of babies were found to be entirely breast-fed at the end of the first week. By 3 months only 42% were entirely breast-fed and this decreased further so that at one year 11% of babies were still receiving breast milk as the only source of milk. Few infants (12%) were entirely bottle fed at one week, but by six months 41% were fed in this way and by the age of one year 55% of babies had ceased to receive any breast milk. Only 50% of mothers gave a correct answer when asked how to prepare a milk powder bottle feed. The age at which solid food was introduced varied between 5 and 7 months. The majority of the mothers gave rice, bread or vegetable soup as the first foods. The survey indicated that in the urban hospital population studied, breast feeding was on the decline. (Adapted from abstract)

18. Serenius, F., and Fougerouse, D. "Health and Nutritional Status in Rural Saudi Arabia"-Abstract found in Nutrition Research, 2, 1982, p 632, under "Country report-Egypt and Middle East." Original article in Saudi Med. J. Riyadh, 2, 1981, pp 10-22.

A Saudi study dealt with the results of village surveys carried out in 3 different areas: a desert area, a mountainous area and a coastal area. 452 families were studied. Over 90% of the mothers were unable to read. Poor sanitary conditions were prevalent; piped water supply existed in 10% of the houses, while 67% of the houses had latrines. Extended families were the rule, often with three generations living together. The birth intervals seemed to be short and the mothers had an average of 5.5 children each. The age pyramid from the community revealed a wide base, with 25% of the population less than 6 years of age, indicating high fertility and high wastage of child life. Infant mortality rates varied between 117 and 144/1000 population. Perinatal mortality rates, which are likely underestimated, ranged between 41 and 61/1000 live births. Breast feeding for more than a year was the rule; 53 to 76% of all children were still breast-fed at 12 months of age. There was, however, a considerable interest in bottle feeding. Health facilities were frequently underutilized; 84% of births occurred at home; vaccination coverage varied between 0.4 to 4.0%. Anthropometric evaluation of 827 preschool children revealed a point prevalence of acute malnutrition of 6% and of chronic malnutrition of 24%. Clinical examination of 256 preschool children revealed 3 children with marasmus, 7 with general wasting, 2 with rickets and 2 with goiter. No children had signs of vitamin A deficiency or clinical kwashiorkor. (Authors' abstract)

19. Abd El-Karim, H. A., and Bamheer, A. M. "Vitamin C content of vegetables and fruits available in Saudi Arabia." Z. Ernaehrungswiss 18(3), September 1979, pp 213-216. Dr. Dietrich Steinkopff Verlag.

The vitamin C content was determined in 27 samples of various vegetables and fruits commonly used for human consumption in the Western zone (Jeddah) of Saudi Arabia. Vitamin C content was assessed by N-bromo succinamide method on vegetables and fruits obtained in the morning during March, April, May, and June.

Peppers (both sweet and hot) spinach, cabbage, peas, parsley, sweet potato, radish, and cauliflower were found to have good amounts of vitamin C, but the levels in many cases were lower than those previously reported. Adverse effects due to the hot climate, and various effects by the sunlight which may speed synthesis of vitamin C in the growing plants but hasten its destruction in the cut plant, were suggested as possible reasons for the lower levels.

20. Hussein, M. A. "The effect of diet and mouth hygiene on the teeth health state of students at some schools of Saudi Arabia." J. Egypt Public Health Assoc. 54(1-2), 1979, pp 35-40.

Ninety girl assistant nurse students in Riyadh, 184 primary school boys and 156 primary school girls in Arka town Riyadh have been examined for the health of their teeth. Their diet was also investigated. The incidence of the tooth problems in the form of caries or DMF was high. The survey also revealed that the incidence was higher among girls 12 years and over than boys. The soft diet and low content of vitamin A, C, calcium, and iron may act as predisposing factors as well as the incomplete mouth hygiene. (Adapted from author's abstract)

21. Hussein, M. A "Nutrition activities in Saudi Arabia." J. Egypt Public Health Assoc. 52(4), 1977, pp 301-304.

This paper was a description of the nutrition activities in several ministries in Saudi Arabia. The Ministry of Agriculture stressed increase of cultivable land productivity and improved strains of crops and breeds of animals. The Ministry of Education supplied students with dry meal (50% of primary school students by 1971-72). The Municipal Department enforced subsidized bread, imported meat and sugar prices and inspected public restaurants. The Saudi Organization for Standards and Measures reviewed food laws and legislation and developed new laws.

The Ministry of Health carried out food analyses for cases needing hospital diets. The author evaluated the Ministry's nutrition activities at their request. He set up the Nutrition Division in 1973 to undertake research (nutriture surveys), nutrition training and education, and services such as the Nutrition Clinic and setting up National food tables. A High Committee of Nutrition was proposed to raise the Nutrition Division's functions to the planning level.

22. Wirths, W., Hamdan, M., Hayati, M., and Rajhi, H. "Nutritional status, food consumption and food consumption and food supply of studies in Saudi Arabia. I. Anthropometric data." Z. Ernaehrungswiss 16(1), March 1977, pp 1-11. Dr. Dietrich Steinkopff Verlag.

A field study of the nutritional status was made in school classes with boys 6 to 19 years old in different regions of Saudi-Arabia. The study measured 341 pupils for weight, height, skinfold-thickness, circumferences and other body-size measurements. In comparison with anthropometric measurements of comparable surveys in other countries, the Saudi-Arabian school boys were found to be smaller and leaner than boys from the USA, Europe, other Arabian countries and well-to-do Indian boys. (Adapted from authors' abstract.)

23. Wirths, W., Hamdan, M., Hayati, M., and Rajhi, H. "Nutritional condition, food consumption and nutritional intake in students in Saudi Arabia. II. Food consumption and nutritional intake." Z. Ernaehrungswiss. 16(3), September 1977, pp 184-197. Dr. Dietrich Steinkopff Verlag.

In field surveys in 13 schools in different regions of Saudi-Arabia, energy expenditure, food consumption, and nutrient intake were studied. Cereal products, especially bread, formed the bulk of the diet. Food consumption was generally low, but lowest in remote villages. In some age groups, the energy intake was very inadequate; 70% did not reach recommended dietary allowances for animal protein, and none consumed an adequate fat level. Intake of carbohydrates was too high, while intake of linoleic acid, minerals and vitamins was too low for nearly all test persons. To secure regularly a sufficient intake of essential nutrients, a school lunch program for the Saudi-Arabian boys is recommended. (Adapted from authors' abstract)

24. Cook, G. C., al-Torki, M. T. "High intestinal lactase concentrations in adult Arabs in Saudi Arabia." Br. Med. J. 3(5976), July 19, 1975, pp 135-136.

The maximum rise in blood glucose after 50 g lactose by mouth was determined in 40 adult Arabs. Out of 30 Bedouin, urban Saudi, and Yemeni and 9 of mixed ancestry (usually partly African), 25 (83%) and 2 (22%) respectively showed an increase of over 1.1 mmol/l (20mg/100 ml). In common with most northern Europeans and Hamitic people of northern Africa, Arabs in Saudi Arabia usually have high intestinal lactase concentrations in adult life. This persistence of high levels probably originated in the Arabian peninsula. Its selective advantage may have been associated with the fluid and calorie content of camels' milk, which is important for survival in desert nomads. (Authors' abstract)

25. el-Molla, A., el-Ghoroury, A., Hussein, M., Badr-el-Din, M. K., Hassen, A. H., Aref, G. H., and el-Araby, I. "Antibody production in protein calorie malnutrition." J. Trop. Med. Hyg. 76(9), September 1973, pp 248-250.

The antibody response to cholera antigen was tested in 26 children one to two years of age. Three subcutaneous doses of antigen were administered weekly to 11 normal infants, 8 kwashiorkoric children and 7 marasonic children. Blood samples taken 1, 2, and 3 weeks after vaccination showed significant rise in vibriocidal antibody titre in all groups, and differences between them were not significant at the 5% level. No agglutinating antibody rise occurred in most of the marasmus and kwashiorkor cases. This was a significant diminishment of response compared to control children. The children showed a competent IgG production, but defective IgM response; authors surmised that agglutinating antibodies to cholera reside in the IgM classes.

26. Busch-Petersen, D. "Pediatric specialist in South Arabia." Kinderaerztl. Prax. 38(6), June 1970, pp 266-276. (Article in German)

This subjective report describes medical facilities, treatment of illnesses in general, and specific diseases and their incidence rates in South Arabia. Diseases and parasites specifically discussed include tuberculosis, meningitis, gastroenteritis, Giardia lamblia, malaria, Ancylostoma duodenale, Hymenolepsis infection, leprosy, schistosomiasis, chronic tonsillitis, vitamin B_2 deficiency, and vitamin D deficiency rickets. (Translated by Brigette Woolsey.)

Sudan

1. Coulter, J. B., Suliman, G. I., Lamplugh, S. M., Mukhtar, B. I., and Hendrickse, R. G. "Aflatoxins in liver biopsies from Sudanese children." Am. J. Trop. Med. Hyg. 35(2), March 1986, pp 360-365.

   27 children with protein-energy malnutrition and 13 children with miscellaneous liver disease in Sudan were analysized for aflatoxin by percutaneous needle liver biopsies. Five of the 16 biopsies detected B1, B2 and aflatoxicol from kwashiorkor but none of the 11 biopsies detected aflatoxins from marasmus or marasmic kwashiorkor. Aflatoxins G1, G2 and M2 were detected in 5 of 12 children with chronic liver disease. A very high concentration of aflatoxicol was found in a breast-fed infant with neonatal hepatitis of unknown etiology.

2. Fedail, S. S., Badi, S. E., and Musa, A. R. "The effects of sorghum and wheat bran on the colonic functions of healthy Sudanese subjects." Am. J. Clin. Nutr. 40(4), October 1984, pp 776-779.

   The effects of surghum and wheat bran were compared and contrasted in a group of 10 healthy Sudanese medical students. The group took their normal diet, a diet of 20 g/day of sorghum bran and a diet of 20 g/day of wheat bran, each for 3 weeks. The wet stool weight, gut transmit time, and frequency of bowel evacuation were estimated at the end of each diet. The mean stool weight on normal diet was 136.6 +/-43.1 g/day on sorghum bran 173.3 +/- 48.4 g/day, and on wheat bran 219.1 +/- 98.3 g/day. The increase produced by wheat bran was significant, p less than 0.001. Both brans produced a similar number of bowel evacuations. The results suggest that sorghum bran, which is both cheap and readily available in Sudan, produces a similar number of bowel evacuations to those of wheat bran without significantly affecting stool weight or transit time.

3. Woodruff, A. W., Adamson, E. A., el Suni, A., Maughan, T. S., Kaku, M., and Bundru, W. "Children in Juba, southern Sudan: the second and third years of life." Lancet 2(8507) September 13, 1986, pp 615-618.

   A prospective study of child health was conducted until the children were 36 months old. The mortality rate in the second year was 8.1%, the most common cause of death being chronic undernutrition. Out of the 79 children seventy-six suffered episodes of faltering weight gain; 47 lost 0.5 kg, and most did not reach their former weight for 5 months. Eighteen faltering episodes were complicated with Marasmus; three were fatal. None of the 45 children remaining in Juba to their 36th month had marasmus, and their health was improved. Fifteen of 53 children, showed developmental delay with a mean age 2.25 years. After 10 months 7 showed continued delay. Hepatitis B seemed to be transmitted to the children from both mothers and other sources. Day-care centers can help chronically undernourished children, and health education should be directed towards the parents' capabilities.

4. Hendrickse, R. G., Coulter, J. B., Lamplugh, S. M., MacFarlane, S. B., Williams, T. E., Omer, M. I., Suliman, G. I., El-Zorgani, G. A. "Aflatoxins and kwashiorkor. Epidemiology and clinical studies in Sudanese children and findings in autopsy liver samples from Nigeria and South Africa." Bull. Soc. Pathol. Exot. Filiales 76(5), November 1983, pp 559-566.

   Clinical and epidemiological studies are in progress in Sudan to determine whether aflatoxins play a role in the pathogenesis of kwashiorkor. Local foods are screened for their aflatoxin content. Children with kwashiorkor and age and sex matched children with marasmus and with normal nutrition are being investigated for aflatoxins in their blood and urine. Autopsy liver samples of children with kwashiorkor and other nutritional disorders in Nigeria and South Africa have been examined. Results to date on over 350 children studied show that aflatoxins occur more frequently and at higher concentrations in the sera of children with kwashiorkor than in children with marasmus or in normal children. Urinary excretion of aflatoxins in kwashiorkor appears to be less than in other groups. These findings seem to implicate aflatoxins in the pathogenesis of kwashiorkor. If this is confirmed it would have very wide implications for the management and prevention of kwashiorkor.

5. Hummert, J. R. "Cortical bone growth and dietary stress among subadults from Nubia's Batn El Hajar." Am. J. Phys. Anthropol. 62(2), October 1983, pp 167-176.

   Cortical bone growth is analyzed for 174 children from a Medieval Christian population at Kulubnarti in the Batn el Hajar of Sudanese Nubia (550-1450 AD). Total subperiosteal area, cortical area, medullary area, and percent cortical area at midshaft were calculated on the tibia as a representative long bone. While growth in total and cortical areas, as well as in length, appear to be fairly well maintained, percent cortical area reveals unusual growth patterns which reflect excessive endosteal resorption. Compared to the relative reduction in bone mass which has been observed in malnourished living children, as well as with previously reported evidence for stress in the Kulubnarti population. The present data support an interpretation of nutritionally related stress and of no major diachronic dietary change.

6. Idris, S., and El Seed, A. M. "Measles vaccination in severely malnourished Sudanese children." Ann. Trop. Paediatr. 3(2), June 1983, pp 63-67.

   The clinical and serological responses to attenuated measles virus vaccine were compared in 35 severely malnourished and 35 well-nourished children for 3 weeks. A third group of severely malnourished children, who received an injection of vitamin B12, served as controls. Paired sera were collected from each child before and after administration of the vaccine or vitamin B12 and measles antibody titres were estimated using HAI technique. The malnourished children who received the measles vaccine developed fever which was higher and of longer duration and had more lower respiratory tract disease than the other two groups but had fewer skin rashes than the well-nourished group. Sero-conversion rates were 96% had 92.6% in the malnourished and well-nourished vaccinated children, respectively. Antibody titres were lower in children who had marasmic/kwashiorkor than in the marasmic children.

7. Mousa, H. M., Ali, K. E., and Hume, I. D. "Effects of water deprivation on urea metabolism in camels, desert sheep, and desert goats fed dry desert grass." Reprinted with permission from Comp. Biochem. Physiol. (A) 74(3), 1983, pp 715-720. Pergamon Press, Ltd.

   Camels, desert sheep, and desert goats were studied in Sudan for the effects of complete water deprivation and of partial water restriction on their urea recycling and nitrogen retention. The animals were fed a diet of dry desert grass which had 3.2% crude protein content. Urea recycling in goats and sheep increased from 79% to 95% and from 75% to 94%, respectively, during water deprivation. Urea recycling in camels remained high throughout the study at 94 to 97%. Nitrogen balance in sheep and goats improved to positive values during water deprivation, but did not change in camels. Dry matter intake decreased with water deprivation in all the animals, and they increased apparent digestibility of dry matter and nitrogen. Water restriction produced effects which were less than those of water deprivation. Short periods of water deprivation may actually improve nitrogen metabolism rather than harm it in these animals.

8. Al-Mokhalalati, J. "Factors influencing Sudanese food habits in Britain." Proc. Nutr. Soc. 41(2), June 1982, pp 239-242.

A survey was conducted by questionnaire among Sudanese students and their resident wives in Britain. Out of 404 respondents, the majority (59%) had changed food habits since moving to Britain. 38% had not changed their food habits, and 3% did not know if they had. A short-stay (SS) group and a long-stay (LS) group were questioned, and within each group a single versus a married group was differentiated. Results showed that length of stay had no effect on changing food habits in any group that was statistically significant. However, a trend in the married LS group was seen in that the longer they stayed in Britain, the more they adhered to their ethnic food habits after the initial switch to British foods. Marital status seemed to make no difference in food habits in the SS group, but again a trend toward a lower percentage of changers among the married vs. the single individuals was seen. Marital status did have a significant effect on changing food habits in the LS group. This was thought to be a result of the centrality of food preparation for an Arabic woman in caring for her family, and the unimportance of time of preparation of food in the lifestyle of the family. Food price was found to have no effect on the respondents' food habits.

9. Ostrowski, Z. L. and Heidrecheid, N. "Some aspects of nutritional status in the south of the Sudan (Preliminary study)." J. Trop. Pediatr. 28(3), June 1982, pp 153-158.

The purpose of this nutritional preliminary study of small children and pregnant women was to test the methodology and initiate the implementation of a longitudinal study. During this preliminary study, a sample of 183 individuals from 9 grouped villages was studied.

The study revealed that the members of the population are unusually tall. Their food intake was poor, with a very low fat intake. On the other hand, the protein intake was high, and formed 13% of the total caloric intake. (Authors' abstract)

10. El-Sunni, M. "Cultivating friends" Sudanow 6(9), September 1981, 11 pages.

A report on attempts to increase Sudanese production of sorghum, the country's most important nutritional crop, in the early 1980s. In 1967 it was recommended that extra land in the Gezira area should be cultivated with sorghum, but in the early 1980s the scheme was terminated because of heavy irrigation needs. The

Agricultural Research Center in Wad Medani is experimenting with different sorghum hybrids, including one which may be suited to the Gezira area. Other land use programmes are also under way. Figures for sorghum production and exports are included. (Author's abstract)

11. Khaittab, A. G. "Thought for food" Sudanow 6(11), November 1981, 35 pages.

A late 1981 review of proposals for the development of a national food and nutrition strategy for the Sudan. To achieve the long-term objective of a food technology appropriate to Sudan's disparate geographical, economic and social conditions, planners must stress increased productivity, diet quality and nutrition-related programs to promote better health. A multidisciplinary approach integrating national and local policy is advocated. (Author's abstract)

12. Ogilvy, S. M. "Food habits of the Dinka in the Jonglei area of Sudan-a preliminary study." J. Hum. Nutr. 35(4), August 1981, pp 296-301.

A food survey was conducted to determine the food habits of the Dinka tribe of Southern Sudan. The survey was part of a study program by the Sudanese government to determine the probable effects of the Jonglei canal on these people, including nutritional effects.

A dry season cattle camp was visited and interviews were conducted regarding food habits, infant and child feeding, cooking methods, foods grown and purchased, and seasonal availability of foods. Milk yield of cows in two households were measured and available quantity per person estimated. The marginal caloric character of the diet, especially for children during and after bad seasons, was delineated. The need for health and nutrition programmes to enable the Dinka to adapt to the canal-produced changes within their present life was highlighted.

13. Osman, A. K. "Urinary free amino acids pattern in protein-energy malnourished Sudanese children." Res. Exp. Med. (Berl) 179(3), 1981, pp 205-213.

Sudanese children in protein-energy malnourished states were tested for free amino acid pattern via the morning urine sample prior to and during the first two weeks of treatment. Kwashiorkor patients showed an almost constant amino acid/total urinary N of 3.62. The marasmic patients showed a mean amino acid/total urinary N of 27. Kwashiorkoric children had a lower, and marasmic children had a higher level of leucine, valine, phenylaline, methylhistidine, lysine, hydroxylysine, and beta-amino-isobutyric acid than normal.

14. Osman, A. K.,and Fatah, A. A. "Factors other than iodine deficiency contributing to the endemicity of goitre in Darfur Province (Sudan)." J. Hum. Nutr. 35(4), August 1981, pp 302-309.

Goitre is endemic in certain parts of Darfur Province, Sudan. 1604 school children of both sexes in nine schools from five Darfur villages were given physical examinations for goitre, and dietary surveys were done to determine adequacy of their nutritional intake. Results showed girls from three villages to have higher incidence of goitre than boys from these villages, with 55, 13, and

75% of girls vs. 35, 10, and 46% of boys affected in Tawaila, Nyala, and Kas, respectively. Dietary surveys showed a correlation between incidence of goitre and percentage of energy obtained from millet, which was 66.7% in Tawaila, 37.1% in Nyala, and 73.6% in Kas. A goitrogenic agent in millet was postulated to be a factor in the inter-village incidence differences. Other contributory factors included low iodine and vitamin A intakes, poor overall nutritional status, and high levels of the competing minerals, Na, K, and Fe in the water.

15. Zumrawi, F., Vaughan, J. P., Waterlow, J. C., and Kirkwood, B. R. "Dried skimmed milk, breast-feeding and illness episodes--a controlled trial in young children in Khartoum Province, Sudan." Int. J. Epidemiol. 10(4), December 1981, pp 303-308.

In a controlled trial, mothers and children attending urban maternal and child health (MCH) clinics in Khartoum Province were given a fortnightly take home food supplement of 1 kilogram of dried skimmed milk (DSM) or an equivalent amount of local beans. There were approximately 300 children aged 6-26 months in each group and each child was followed for 3 to 6 months. A comparison of the two groups showed: a) that the DSM group mothers were more likely to continue breastfeeding; b) there was no evidence to associate DSM with an increased incidence of episodes of diarrhoea, fever or vomiting; c) the utilisation of health institutions was very similar in the two groups; and d) there was no significant difference in the mothers' assessment of the proportion of children with a 'poor' appetite in either group. This trial met with considerable methodological problems and the results should therefore be interpreted cautiously. There is a great need for more and better designed trials to assess the possible adverse effects of DSM. (Authors' abstract)

16. Zumrawi, F., Vaughan, J. P., and Simmonds, S. P. "Baby milk in Khartoum Province--how many tins does a pharmacy sell?" J. Trop. Pediatr. 27(4), August 1981, pp 224-225.

This survey of 43 pharmacies in the cities of Khartoum and Omdurman was done to estimate the volume of sales of artifical baby milk powders. Nutrition workers interviewed shopowners about the prices for each brand and sales volume per month. The workers also counted the display tins for each brand. The five most popular brands and their countries of manufacture were: SMA, S26, and Similac (USA), Mamex (Denmark), and Beblac (Holland). Investigators estimated at least 300,000 Sudanese pounds were spent on baby milk powders per year in the survey towns. At the time, one representative brand, SMA from Wyeth Laboratories, was selling for more than twice the London price at the exchange rate currently effective, and three times the charge of the local welfare clinic. The large volume of sales and expensive prices of powders may constitute a substantial drain on the family income.

17. Anonymous "Malnutrition in Sudanese children as a function of socioeconomic change." Nutr. Rev. 38(2) February 1980, pp 76-79.

An ethnographic study in 1951 and a subsequent resurvey in 1978 were done of villages in the Gezira plain of southeastern Sudan. The villages were located in an area which had been developed in 1925 by an irrigation scheme into intensive cotton cropping land. The 1951 report indicated that no frank deficiencies existed, but that energy intake fluctuated seasonally. Low calcium, riboflavin, and vitamin A and C intakes were observed at that time. The 1978 study, done by 24-hour recall in 494 households in 5 villages, showed that two villages had intakes above energy needs, one had intakes of 94% of needs as calculated, and two had intakes of 73 and 63% of calculated needs. The protein intakes were more than adequate. The 1978 study was done in one summer season, when supplies of local staples started to dwindle.

A clinical study in 1979 of 1291 children under four years of age was done. Findings indicated that 24% of the children were weaned in the first year of life, most commonly due to subsequent pregnancy. PCM cases had been weaned in the first year in 39% of cases. Animal milk and sorghum pap were used for bottle feeding infants, and only after six months of age were supplements given. Malnutrition of children of educated (four years primary school) mothers was significantly less. The shortened breastfeeding time, the disappearance of usual food supplements for postpartum women and bottle feeding usage were cited as causes of young childhood malnutrition.

18. Taha, S. E., and Suleiman, S. I. "Volvulus of the sigmoid colon in the Gezira." Br. J. Surg. 67(6), June 1980, pp 433-435.

Out of 34 consecutive patients presenting with volvulus of the sigmoid colon in the Gezira area of The Sudan, 20 were western Sudanese farmers (age range 25-52 years) who habitually ate a single daily meal of high residue foods. Their colons were long and hypertrophied. In contrast, the four nothern Sudanese (age range 60-92 years) ate a Western European type of diet and had a thin colon. This factor may have been responsible for the finding that the five patients presenting with gangrene of the sigmoid colon included all four nothern Sudanese patients. Shock was a reliable indicator of gangrene, but rebound tenderness was valueless. Deflation of the sigmoid volvulus via the sigmoidoscope succeeded in curing 19 of 25 patients in whom there was no suspicion of gangrene (four later recurrences). Laparotomy was performed in the other 15 patients with operative untwisting in the absence of gangrene in 10 (two later reoccurrences) and resections in the presence of gangrene in 5 (three died). (Authors' abstract)

19. Dahlin, K. "Maternal and child health care among refugees in Sudan." Laekartidningen 76(22), May 30, 1979, pp 2115-2118. (Swedish)

In the discussions about health care in the developing countries, interest has more and more been focused on preventive care. Women of fertile age and children under the age of fifteen constitute together the majority of the population and bear the main burden of morbidity and mortality. The author served in Tanzania in the sixties and in 1976. In this article he describes maternal and child health care among refugees in eastern Sudan as seen between January-March 1978. (Author's abstract translated by Elizabeth Gustavsson.)

20. El Tinay, A. H., Abdel Gadir, A. M., and El Hidai, M. "Sorghum fermented Kisra bread. I--Nutritive value of Kisra". J. Sci. Food Agric. 30(9), September 1979, pp 859-863.

Kisra is a fermented sorghum bread which constitutes the staple diet of the Sudanese population. Kisra fermentation for three popular sorghum varieties was investigated. The objective was to determine the nutrient content as well as the amino acid pattern during this fermentation. The results indicated that there was a slight increase in protein content as a result of Kisra fermentation and an appreciable drop in starch. Total and non-reducing sugars decreased markedly at the commencement of the fermentation process, while crude fibre content increased. Threonine and lysine remained practically unchanged during Kisra fermentation. Tyrosine and methionine were enriched as a result of fermentation for all three sorghum varieties. Dabar and Fetirita Kisras were enriched in threonine and valine, while in Mayo Kisra these amino acids decreased compared to the grain. Tyrosine content improved in Dabar Kisra, but diminished in Fetirita Kisra. (Authors' abstract)

21. Mukhtar, N. D. "Chemical control of nitrification under rice in the central rainlands of the Sudan." Zentralbl. Bakteriol. (Naturwiss) 134(2), 1979, pp 125-132.

2-amino-4-chloro-6-methyl pyrimidine "AM" was used as a selective inhibitor of nitrifying organisms to prevent denitrification losses. Zero, 6, and 12 kg/ha of the chemical, 43 and 86 kg/ha urea-N or their equivalents were used in vitro and in vivo experiments. In the in vitro experiment, clear and significant inhibition lasted for 6 weeks. In both the pot and field experiments, inhibition time was shorter and only insignificant increases in yield and yield components were attained. The value of this chemical for rice under the soil and climatic conditions of the Central Rainlands seems to be small, though it seems promising for lighter (leaching) soils. (Author's abstract)

22. Mukhtar, N. D., and Yousif, Y. H. "Response of irrigated groundnuts (Arachis hypogaea L.) to urea fertilization in the central rainlands of the Sudan." Zentralbl. Bakteriol. (Naturwiss) 134(1), 1979, pp 25-33.

The response of 3 varieties of groundnuts, i.e., Ashford (A), Barberton (B), and Corinte (C), to different doses of urea nitrogen under irrigation was studied for three years. As a result of extensive tissue analysis, the critical needs of Barberton and Corinte for nitrogen were found to be 1500 ppm H03-11 and 3.7% total-N. Variety Ashford, which outyielded both, did not respond to urea nitrogen. A linear correlation coefficient of $r = 0.85$ for pod and straw yields gave a pod to straw ratio of 0.72. Kernel protein and oil content were not affected by nitrogen. Larger nodule counts and their total-N indicated better yields. (Authors' abstract)

23. Sukkar, M. Y., Kemm, J. R., Makeen, A. M., and Khalid, M. H. "Anthropometric survey of children in rural Khartoum, Sudan," Ann. Hum. Biol. 6(2), March-April 1979 pp 147-158.

The results of a cross-sectional anthropometric survey of Sudanese children up to the age of thirteen years six months is reported. Children in whom a quick clinical examination revealed pathology were excluded, as were children who did not have a true birth certificate. Height, weight and mid-arm circumference were measured in all children, head and chest circumference were measured in children up to the age of 5 years 6 months. Skinfold thickness at biceps, triceps, subscapular and suprailiac sites were measured in children above the age of 30 months. The children were found to be shorter and lighter, to have less subcutaneous fat than British children. The findings are also compared with those from other African populations. Comparison with a survey performed in the same village seven years earlier reveals that the heights and weights of the children have hardly changed despite a considerable improvement in economic status. The children have a lower weight for height than British and other African populations. (Authors' abstract)

24. Taha, S. A. "The pattern of severe protein-calorie malnutrition in Sudanese children attending a large hospital in The Sudan." Am. J. Clin. Nutr. 32(2), February 1979, pp 446-451.

One hundred fifty severely malnourished patients admitted in one month to Was Medani Hospital's Pediatric wards in Sudan were classified by the Wellcome classification as to type of protein calorie malnutrition. Marasmus was the predominant type seen, occurred mainly in children in the second year of life, and was associated with stunting and therefore chronic malnutriton. Marasmic-kwashiorkor patients were older and even more stunted, and had significantly lower hemoglobin levels than the other patients. Kwashiorkor patients showed an acute disease with minimal growth retardation and they were generally children less than one year of age. Most of the patients showed megaloblastic anemia. Several simple ratios and measurements commonly used to measure nutritional status were assessed, and the head-chest ratio was not reliable for children more than one year of age. Weight for head circumference correlated poorly with deficits in other variables. The weight for age ratio and presence of edema were the most crucial physical indicators of the type of malnutrition present.

25. Wilson, R. T. "Studies on the livestock of Southern Darfur, Sudan, VIII. Production of poultry under simulated traditional conditions." Trop. Anim. Health Prod. 11(3), August 1979, pp 143-150.

Observations were made on egg production, egg hatchability and fertility, liveweight and growth characteristics of domestic fowls, Muscovy ducks and pigeons kept under simulated traditional conditions in Southern Darfur. Fowl and ducks produced about 50 eggs a year in 4 1/2 clutches spaced at 80 day intervals and pigeons 17 in 8 1/2 clutches at 43 day intervals. First eggs were laid at about 240 days by the fowls, 213 days by ducks and 132 days by pigeons. The annual weight of eggs produced was 2,013; 3,596; and 286 g for fowl, ducks, and pigeons respectively, being 1.53, 2.33 and 0.88 times the mean adult female body weight for each species. Fertility and hatchability of eggs were higher in fowls than ducks which were in turn higher than in pigeons. Early growth in pigeons was very rapid. Muscovies achieved mature body weights at about 20 weeks while mature weights in fowls were achieved much later in males than in females. (Author's abstract)

26. Abu-Sin, A. Y., and Ahmed, M. A. "Pernicious anaemia in Sudanese patients." East Afr. Med. J. 55(12), December 1978, pp 568-571.

The clinical manifestations and laboratory findings in three patients with pernicious anaemia are described. The three are Sudanese individuals of a mixture of Arab and Negroid extraction. Pernicious anaemia is uncommon among people of Arab and African origin, but probably not as rare as generally assumed. The possible factors that might have contributed to the occurrence of the disease in the three patients are discussed. (Authors' abstract)

27. Mustafa, K. Y., Mahmoud, N. A., Gumaa, K. A., and Gader, A. M. "The effects of fasting in Ramadan. 2. Fluid and electrolyte balance". Br. J. Nutr. 40(3), November 1978, pp 583-589.

Fluid intake, urine output and evaporative water loss were measured and fluid balance calculated in sixteen subjects for 1 d before Ramadan, during weeks 1-5 of fasting and on the 10th day after the end of Ramadan. Plasma osmolality at 06.00 hours, the beginning of the fast, at 18.00 hours, before breaking the fast and at 19.00 hours, 1 h after breaking the fast, and urine osmolality during the day and night were measured before, during and after Ramadan.

All subjects developed an initial negative fluid balance which was maximum at the beginning of week 3 of fasting and that deficit was compensated for during the later weeks. Compensation was brought about by an increase in urine concentration, a decrease in urine volume by day and salt retention. No significant changes were observed in plasma osmolality during the days of fasting and the 'setting' of plasma osmolality during Ramadan also was not changed.

It was concluded that healthy young adults maintain good control of fluid and electrolytes during Ramadan. (Authors' abstract)

28. Suliman, G. I. "Coeliac disease in Sudanese children." Gut 19(2), February 1978, pp 121-125.

Coeliac disease has not hitherto been documented in Sudanese children. This report describes seven Sudanese children with coeliac disease of whom two are siblings. They all had evidence of impaired intestinal absorption, severe histological changes of their jejunal mucosa with clinical and histological improvement on gluten free/sorghum free diet. Subsequently one patient had a clinical relapse when gluten was reintroduced; four had positive gluten challenge using serial one hour blood xylose estimation. They all belonged to the upper socioeconomic group of the society in the north of the Sudan. (Author's abstract)

29. Taha, S. A. "The comprehensive child health care centres in the Sudan." Trans. R. Soc. Trop. Med. Hyg. 72(4), 1978, pp 333-337.

In 1963, Morley initiated the concept of clinics for children under five years old. This paper describes our experience in applying that concept in Omdurman town (Sudan) where existing maternity and child health centres and hospitals in the area were involved in the scheme. It was found necessary to establish a main centre to develop methodology and to provide a specialized training of staff. The medical problems were similar to those described by Morley. The approach to their solution was essentially the same except that we used more professional staff and placed more emphasis on nutrition education than higherto advocated. It is concluded that, in theory, Morley's concept provides a system of comprehensive child health care which suits the needs of developing countries. But our adaptation of Morley's ideas to existing health structures, even on the small scale we achieved in Omdurman, was difficult because of the high initial and running costs and in view of the long established dichotomy between curative and preventive medicine. (Author's abstract)

30. Taha, S. A. "The prevalence and severity of protein-calorie malnutrition in Sudanese children." J. Trop. Pediatr. 24(5), October 1978, pp 203-206.

One thousand two hundred ninety-one Sudanese children aged six months to four years, living in the Gezira, a farming community considered to be prosperous relative to other parts of the Sudan, were examined. Clinical and anthropometric measurements were recorded. These showed a tendency to drop below Caucasian standards of weight, height, mid-arm circumference and triceps skinfold thickness, starting about the age of six months. Only 47% of the children were found to be well nourished; of the remainder 1% had severe, 17% moderate and 35% mild protein-calorie malnutrition. Together with the data collected from two other different areas, the findings of this study indicate that malnutrition is a grave paediatric problem in the Sudan. (Authors' abstract)

31. Elmasri, S. H., and Khalil, T. "Volvulus of the sigmoid in Khartoum, Sudan." Trop. Geogr. Med. 28(4), December 1976, pp 297-302.

Twenty-six cases of acute volvulus of the sigmoid in Khartoum Hospital are analysed. The condition accounts for 17.8 percent of all cases of acute intestinal obstructuion. The majority of patients were from the Southern tribes whose diet contains a large amount of fibre. Of the different methods of surgical management, simple operative detorsion and deflation gave the best results. The overall mortality rate was 23.1 percent. (Authors' abstract)

32. Sukkar, M. Y., Vokac, Z., Nagdi, S., and Khogali, A. "The nutritional status of the Fur people of Jabel Marra." Afr. J. Med. Sci. 5(4), December 1976, pp 245-254.

The nutritional status of the adult Fur people of Jabel Marra of Western Studies was assessed by means of physical anthropometry, haematologic and serum protein measurements. The results of the anthropometry survey show a high incidence of low weight for height in comparison with Caucasian standards. The muscle mass as indicated by the upper arm circumference is also smaller than expected by European standards. The upper arm muscle circumference, however, is only marginally lower than the above standards. Subcutaneous adipose tissue is found to fall within the lower range of normal in comparison to available standards. The results are discussed in the light of findings in other African countries with similar ecology and socio-economic conditions. The haematological and serum protein results reveal a high incidence of anaemia especially in women. As the R.B.C. count was not done in this work the type of the anaemia cannot be ascertained. The value of cross-sectional nutritional surveys for the establishment of baseline data for future assessment of development is indicated. (Authors' abstract)

33. Sukkar, M. Y., Kemm, J. R., Makeen, A., and Habeeb, M. "Anthropometry in a Sudanese village; changes after 7 years." (Proceedings) Proc. Nutr. Soc. 35(3), December 1976, p 146A.

A repeat anthropometric survey was performed at the end of 1975 in the village of El Kalakla. The original survey had been done in 1968, and an increased standard of living had been achieved in the village, with higher incomes, improved health care facilities, a clean water supply, electricity, and a hard-surface road provided. Results showed that very little change had taken place between the two surveys. A small increase in the heights and weights of pre-school children and a small decrease in the heights and weights of the older schoolchildren were seen. Authors concluded that genetic constitution or other environmental factors such as hygiene may be the main contributors to the height and weight differences seen between Sudanese and Caucasian children.

34. Wilson, R. T., and Clarke, S. E. "Studies on the livestock of Southern Darfur, Sudan. II. Production traits in cattle". Trop. Anim. Health Prod. 8(1), February 1976, pp 47-57.

The results of an intensive 12 month study of a number of herds in the migratory and sedentary sectors of the livestock economy of Southern Darfur are recorded. In almost every production parameter the performance of the former is superior to that of the latter but, overall, production appears to be static or declining. During 1973, the cattle population of the areas is estimated to have declined 7 per cent. Meat production per kilogramme of breeding female was calculated to be 0-057 kg in the migratory sector but only 0-023 kg in the sedentary sector. Calculated calving rates are significantly higher at 65 per cent in the migratory sector than the 40 percent of the sedentary sector. Deaths in the former sector were only 15 per cent compared with the 35 per cent of the latter. It is concluded that total settlement of the migratory sector is not the answer to the current problem of the livestock sector of Southern Darfur. (Authors' abstract)

35. Omer, H. O., Omer, M. I., and Khalifa, O. O. "Pattern of protein-energy malnutrition in Sudanese children and comparison with some other Middle East countries." J. Trop. Pediatr. 21 (6), December 1975, pp 329-333. (Environ. Child Health)

The Wellcome Trust Working Party method of classifying malnutrition was used in 119 patients over a 6 month period. The incidence of marasmus was higher in the Sudanese children in the second year of life. The lack of supplementary food use and the frequency of gastrointestinal infections was seen as contributory to the malnutrition incidence. The sex incidence showed a preponderance of males. Anemia was very common, as evidenced by megalocytic changes in 45% of cases. Malaria parasites were found in 7% of cases. Almost 90% of cases had diarrhea on admission and 35% required rehydration therapy. 55% had been abruptly weaned, at an average age of 11.8 months. Causes of weaning were illness in the baby in 29 cases, subsequent pregnancy in 19, and mother's illness in 8.

36. Ibrahim, A. E. "Isolation of salmonella from the bile of meat animals." Bull. Epizoot. Dis. Afr. 22(3), September 1974, pp 234-237.

One hundred seventy samples of bile of cattle and sheep purchased from butcheries as a customer would, i.e., wrapped in a small piece of intestine, were compared for bacterial content and type with 194 samples collected aseptically from the gall bladder from cattle slaughtered in the central abattoir in Omdurman. Gram negative bacilli were isolated from all 170 samples of bile purchased from the butcheries, whereas only 137 of the 194 samples obtained aseptically contained gram negative bacilli. Salmonella was present in 2.35% of the first category of samples, and no Salmonella were isolated from the second category of samples. The handling and encasing of bile may cause contamination with Salmonella and other enteric organisms.

37. Ibrahim, A. E. "Milk hygiene and bacteriology in the Sudan: isolation of Brucella abortus from cow's milk." Bull. Epizoot. Dis. Afr. 22(3), September 1974, pp 231-234.

Dairy herds in the Sudan were experiencing a high incidence of Brucellosis as evidenced by "Milk Ring Test" (MRT) positive reactors. A study was conducted on 8 individual cows from three herds to isolate Brucella abortus from their milk. Milk from three of these cows tested Brucella abortus positive.

38. Osman, A. A. "Epidemiological study of appendicitis in Khartoum." Int. Surg. 59(4), April 1974, pp 218-221.

Appendicitis frequency in Khartoum and the factors affecting differential incidence in population subgroups and at different historical times were reported. A 25 fold increase in appendicitis incidence was seen in Khartoum from 1928 to 1961. From 1958 to 1961 the incidence shifted toward the 10 to 20 year old group from an older age group. The achievement of independence by Sudan and increased standard of living with accompanying ingestion of more refined diet were cited as possible etiologic factors. Northern tribes showed the highest incidence of appendicits (42%). Urbanization was seen as a correlate of increasing incidence, and shifting to a Western diet was also implicated. Low frequency in populations eating a traditional diet was seen. Observations by the author suggested increasing incidence during the fasting month of Ramadan.

39. Omer, A., el-Shazali, H., el-Karim, O. A., and el-Hassan, A. M. "Studies on the anaemia of kwashiorkor and marasmus in the Sudan." J. Trop. Pediatr. 19(2), June 1973, pp 91-97. (Environ. Child Health)

The peripheral blood picture, serum folate and Vitamin B_{12} levels, erythrocyte folate values, bone marrow morphology and stained iron stores were studied and compared in 31 cases of kwashiorkor and 23 cases of marasmus. A low serum or erythrocyte folate level was found in 85% of the cases, while in 74% bone marrow examination revealed megaloblastic erythropoiesis. The pattern of megaloblastic erythropoiesis fell into three distinct morphological groups and was in each case attributable to folate deficiency. The peripheral blood picture emerging from one of the megaloblastic groups showed unusual erythrocyte abnormalities. Similar reports on the anaemia of childhood protein-calorie malnutrition from other African countries were reviewed and compared with the present findings.

In view of these findings we recommend that folic acid be given routinely to Sudanese children with cases of kwashiorkor and marasmus. (Authors' abstract)

40. Beynon, K. I., Bosio, P., and Wright, A. N. "Absence of residues from crops irrigated with water treated with trifenmorph for schistosomiasis control." Bull WHO 46(6), 1972, pp 761-764.

The fate of the molluscicide trifenmorph (N-tritylmorpholine) following its use in irrigation systems to control the intermediate hosts of schistosomes was studied by laboratory and field experiments. Laboratory studies with ^{14}C-trifenmorph indicated that bean plants did not take up detectable residues when the soil in which they were grown was irrigated with water containing trifenmorph in concentrations likely to occur in the field. These laboratory studies have been complemented by field irrigation studies of growing crops in southern Africa and the Sudan. Residues of trifenmorph and its breakdown product triphenylmethanol could not be detected in the crops and the limit of detectability was 0.01-0.02 ppm. These results indicate that residues are not likely to be present in irrigated crops following the treatment of the irrigation water systems with trifenmorph. (Authors' abstract)

41. Greig, W. R., Gray, H. W., McGirr, E. M., Kambal, A., and Rahaman, I. A. "Investigation of endemic goitre in Sudan". Br. J. Surg. 57(1), January 1970, pp 11-16.

The total prevalence of goitre in people from the Khartoum area is 12.6 percent and 0.6 percent have large goitres; the total prevalence in West Sudan (Darfur Province) is 57.5 percent and 18.5 percent have large goitres. The plasma inorganic iodide concentration (PII), the thyroid uptake (150 minutes) of radioactive iodine and the serum protein-bound radio-iodine (PB ^{131}I at 150 minutes and at 48 hours) have been measured in goitrous and non-goitrous subjects from the Khartoum area and Darfur Province. The PII's are low in both areas but lower in Darfur; the mean thyroid uptake is high in both areas but higher in Darfur. The mean PB ^{131}I is low in Khartoum but very high in Darfur.

These results indicate that the major cause of endemic goitre in Sudan is iodine deficiency, and in Darfur Province where large goitre is a public health and surgical problem the iodine deficiency appears to be very severe. It is concluded that the iodine deficiency is dietary and if corrected, the high prevalence of large goitre in Sudan should be decreased. (Authors' abstract)

Turkey

1. Kocturk, T. O., and Mj'ones, S. "Consumption pattern of infant foods by Turkish immigrants." Scand. J. Prim Health Care 4(1), February 1986, pp 13-18.

   Food consumption patterns were studied from fifty-nine Turkish infants in metropolitan Stockholm and two adjacent communities. Breastfeeding was maintained for shorter periods of time in comparison with both Turkey and Swedish norms. Illiterate mothers breastfed longer than those who had received some kind of education in which formula feeding was extensively used. At 4-6 months supplementary semisolid feeding was introduced, which is much earlier than in Turkey but later than usual in Swedish families. Some problems were noted with bottle feeding, most importantly with regard to hygienic practices. Unsatisfactory handling of bottle feeding was linked to the mother's educational level. Further interest in nutrition education for this and other immigrant groups is important.

2. Kocturk, T. O., and Zetterstr"om, R. "Breastfeeding among Turkish mothers living in suburbs of Istanbul and Stockholm--a comparison." Acta. Paediatr. Scand. 75(2), March 1986, pp 216-221.

   The infant feeding pattern among working class was determined among 96 Turkish mothers living in a suburb of Istanbul and 30 living in a suburb of Stockholm. The duration of breastfeeding among the Stockholm immigrant group was significantly reduced compared with the group outside of Istanbul which has a similar social background and living in a native urban area. Infant feeding patterns among the Turkish immigrant mothers was more similar to that of Swedish populations in Stockholm. Attitudes to breastfeeding among the immigrant group had changed. Early weaning, reliance on commercially available infant foods and bottle feeding characterized their infant feeding practices. The majority of the infants of this group showed a tendency to be overweight.

3. Aktan, H., Ozden, A., Kesim, E., and Smith, A. N. "Colonic function in rural and urban populations of Turkey." Dis. Colon. Rectum 27(8), August 1984, pp 538-541.

   One urban and one rural Turkish population were compared in regard to their colonic function. Rural subjects consume a diet with higher fiber than urban people in Turkey. The rural group had a greater daily fecal output, faster intestinal transit, and lower intraluminal pressure, with a greater output of calcium in the feces than those living in an urban area in Turkey. The effects are similar to those described when fiber is added to the diet. Urban dwellers in Turkey who lack these effects may have a rising incidence of fiber-related diseases of the colon, such as diverticular disease.

4. Ozalp, I., Erdem, G., Cicliv, G., Kloksal, G., Metcoff, J., Costiloe, P., and Dolgramaci, I. "The incidence of fetal malnutrition in Turkey." Turk. J. Pediatr. 23(2), April-June 1982, pp 75-84.

   525 newborn babies and their mothers were studied to assess magnitude of fetal malnutrition in Turkey by considering deviations from expected birthweight obtained after adjusting for maternal age, height, pre-pregnancy weight, parity, gestational age and sex. Babies whose adjusted birthweights were 1 and 2 SD below the mean of expected birthweight were classified as moderate and

severely intrauterine growth retarded, respectively. Such cases in total constituted 28.7% (151 babies) of the population studied. Sixty of cases were severely malnourished (11.4%). Many babies weighed more than 2500 gr, or above the 25th percentile by the Lubchenco criterion, yet their observed birthweights were 1 or 2 SD below their expected birthweights. It was concluded that unless the adjusting factors are taken into account, infants who are actually considerably smaller than they should be given their sex, gestational age, and characteristics of their mothers may not be recognized to be undergrown. (Authors' abstract)

5. Merdol, T. O. "Nutritional traditions in Turkey (with reference to educational needs)." J. Trop. Pediatr. 27(6), December 1981, pp 273-278.

Traditional patterns and emerging trends in foodways in the rural and urban areas of Turkey were analyzed. Effects of urbanization included production of a market economy dependence in urban families and its contribution to the inferior nutritional status of urban slum families. Decreased income of migrant families significantly influenced lactational ability of mothers and therefore nutrition in early childhood. In addition, improper use of commercial formulas contributed to increasing infant and child mortality rate. The destruction of subsistence farming by the agricultural economic policy of encouraging cash or export crop production caused deterioration of the nutritional traditions of self-reliance and subjected peasants to commerical forces. Development of adequate new patterns to replace old disrupted ones was hindered by food industry advertisements which emphasized profit-producing food products. Two possible approaches to nutrition education were seen; one would operate despite and outside of all the negative trends and factors, and the other would take planned integral changes in these factors into account with nutrition education.

6. Cavdar, A. O., Babacan, E., Arcasoy, A., and Ertem, U. "Effect of nutrition on serum zinc concentration during pregnancy in Turkish women." Am. J. Clin. Nutr. 33(3), March 1980, pp 542-544.

The serum zinc concentration in 101 pregnant women and 40 control subjects was determined by using an atomic absorption spectrophotometer. The zinc levels were significantly low in 30 poorly nourished pregnant women compared to controls (P less than 0.01), whereas there was no statistical difference between the normal mean zinc values and that of well-nourished prengnant women (P greater than 0.05). This study revealed that nutrition is an important factor during pregnancy among Turkish women. In view of severe teratogenic effects of maternal zinc depletion in experimental animals as well as epidemiological evidence that maternal zinc deficiency could be a cause of severe congenital malformations of the central nervous system in humans, more extensive studies are definitely needed in Turkey. (Authors' abstract)

7. Hedstrom, M. "Semper persists: artificial feeding in Turkey via baby bottle." Vardfacket 4(8), April 24, 1980, pp 60-61. (Article in Swedish)

Only two percent of all women in the world are not able to nurse their children. Nevertheless, Semper produces formula for approximately 18 percent of all Turkish children. Bottle feeding costs a Turkish family one fourth of its wages compared to three percent for a Swedish family. Unemployment is about 20 percent and the population growth is the highest in the world. Now WHO (The World Health Organization) is examining "Semper's" role in Turkey. (Author's abstract translated by Elizabeth Gustavsson.)

8. Buckley, M. F., and Erten, O. "The epidemiology of anencephaly and spina bifida in Izmir, Turkey, in the light of recent aetiological theories." Br. J. Prev. Soc. Med. 33(3), September 1979, pp 186-190.

   A study of twins and other siblings investigated the incidence of anencephaly and spina bifida in Izmir, Turkey. Findings suggested that true concordance of a particular neural tube anomaly occurs only in monozygotic (MZ) twins. The concordance of anencephaly and spina bifida in dizygotic twins (DZ) was comparable with that of non-twin siblings. The genetic factor was thought to be important in the Izmir incidence distribution. Environmental factors of water hardness and potato consumption were not seen to be significant etiologic agents in the incidences of anencephaly and spina bifida in this area.

9. Mjones, S. "Child health care among Turkish immigrants--an attempt to bridge cultural cleavages." Nord. Med. 93(5-6), June 1978, pp 126-128. (Swedish)

   Attempts with new types of child health care in the Stockholm suburb, Tensta, where approximately 40 percent of the population are immigrants, show that a "contact assistant" can be of great help. The medical, child clinic at St. Goran's Hospital in Tensta has initiated an experimental study where increased cooperation between district child medical officers, child care clinics, and school health care centers has been focused on problems for immigrants. Since there were many problems concerning contacts, especially between Turkish immigrants and the health care system, special care was taken to examine the problems within this area. A Turkish "contact assistant" was employed. The experiment has constantly been followed by a social anthropologist. In this article the background of the Turkish group is examined as well as medical and social anthropological experiences. (Author's abstract translated by Elizabeth Gustavsson.)

10. Sutter, M., Riedler, G., and T'onz, O. "Juvenile pernicious anemia with congenital intrinsic factor deficiency and intermediate intrinsic factor secretion in the parents". Hel. Paediatr. Acta 33(3), August 1978, pp 267-274.

    An 11-1/2 year-old girl of Turkish origin showed symptoms and signs of pernicious anaemia with low B_{12} level in blood but normal gastric acid secretion. There were no antibodies to mucosal cells or intrinsic factor. Quantitative determination of intrinsic factor in gastric juice, done by a PIA method, proved absence of the factor. Both parents had normal values for haemoglobin, normal B_{12}-absorption tests and slightly decreased B_{12} blood levels. The gastric acid secretion was normal in both, but intrisnic factor in the gastric juice was decreased markedly. (Authors' abstract)

11. Sanli, Y., Fouassin, A., and Noirfalise, A. "Total mercury and methlmercury in canned fish of Turkish origin." Arch. Belg. Med. Soc. 35(3), March 1977, pp 161-167. (Original in French.)

Canned fish of Turkish origin on sale in Western Europe has been analyzed in order to measure its total mercury and its organic mercury contents.

The mercury concentration varied from 0.03 to 0.82 ppm depending on the nature of the analyzed samples. Three quarters of the mercury present in tuna was found to be in the organic forms, whereas in the other species that were examined the organic forms accounted for only two thirds of the whole. (Authors' abstract in English.)

12. Denizel, T., Jarvis, B., and Rolfe, E. J. "A field survey of pistachio (Pistacia vera) nut production and storage in Turkey with particular reference to aflatoxin contamination". J. Sci. Food Agric. 27(11), November 1976, pp 1021-1026.

A field study of soils and pistachio nuts in three major pistachio-growing areas of Turkey has been undertaken. The predominant soil fungus isolated from all three areas was Aspergillus niger; isolates of Fusarium, Trichoderma, Mucor and Rhizopus species were also common. A. flavus and A. ochraceus and related organisms were isolated only from the plateau of Gaziantep. The dominant external mycoflora of the immature nuts from all sites consisted of A. niger, A. flavus and Penicillium spp. There was no evidence for fungal contamination of immature endosperms nor of freshly dehulled nuts, but stored dehulled nuts and dust samples taken from warehouses were extensively contaminated with A. flavus, A. niger and A. ochraceus. Of 43 A. flavus isolates tested, 20 produced aflatoxins on laboratory media or on rice; all 11 isolates of A. ochraceus tested produced ochratoxin A on laboratory media. The results obtained are discussed in relation to agricultural and marketing pratices for Turkish pistachio nuts. (Authors' abstract)

13. Denizel, T., Rolfe, E. J., and Jarvis, B. "Moisture-equilibrium relative humidity relationships in pistachio nuts with particular regard to control of aflatoxin formation". J. Sci. Food Agric. 27(11), November 1976, pp 1027-1034.

Adsorption and desorption isotherms have been determined both manometrically and by weight equilibration for Turkish pistachio nut kernel, shell and hull. Comparison of the calculated and experimentally determined adsorption isotherms for whole nuts showed good correlation. Nuts inoculated with Aspergillus flavus conidia were equilibrated to various ERH levels and stored in controlled environment cabinets at 28°C. Competitive growth of xerophilic strains of A. amstelodami prevented growth and aflatoxin production by the A. flavus at ERHs of 86% and below. At 88% ERH, marked aflatoxin production occurred but competition was observed between the A. flavus and A. niger. In sealed containers metabolic moisture from growth of A. amstelodami raised the ERH from the initial 85% and permitted toxin production by A. flavus. The results are discussed in relation to post-harvest handling and storage of pistachio nuts. (Authors' abstract)

14. G'urson, C. T., Y'uksel, T., and Saner, G. "The short-term prognosis of protein-calorie malnutrition in Marmara region of Turkey." J. Trop. Pediatr. 22(2), April 1976, pp 59-62.

Two hundred cases of protein calorie malnutrition (PCM) admitted to a children's hospital in Istanbul during a five-year period were evaluated to determine the relative effect of different factors on the prognosis of PCM. Two groups, a "survived" and a "deceased" group, were studied. Results indicated that the statistically significant factors in short-term prognosis were hemoglobin levels, plasma total protein levels, chronological age, weight deficit, height deficit, and hyponatremia. However, no significant effect on mortality and/or recovery was shown by hair changes, edema, skin changes, hepatomegaly, potassium, and bicarbonate levels, and degree of stature relative to normal height for age or degree of weight deficit relative to measured height.

15. K'oksal, O. "Effects of nutrition on infant and maternal mortality and other vulnerable groups in special developing areas." <u>Turk. J. Pediatr.</u> 18(3-4), July-October 1976, pp 72-79.

This is a report on the association between insufficient feeding and the high infant mortality rate of infants in a developing area of Turkey. The mortality from 0 to 4 years of age is 15 times higher in Turkey than it is in Sweden. PCM and rickets are nutritional problems in the young, with women in the child bearing age range suffering disproportionately from protein malnutrition, anemia, and obesity. 17.6% of Etimesgut infants who survived 1 year had growth retardation, and 33.3% of those who died showed growth retardation, with the peak in the 6 to 12 month bracket. Maternal mortality rates are affected by rickets-induced pelvic deformities; 11% of mothers delivering in Ankara hospitals needed intervention during a survey. Malnutrition and diseases which could be related to malnutrition, such as enteric-diarrhea and bronchopneumonia, accounted for a majority of the infant deaths in Etimesgut.

16. Bremer, K., and Raatikainen, M. "Cereal diseases transmitted or caused by aphids and leafhoppers in Turkey." <u>Ann. Acad. Sci. Fenn.</u> 203, 1975, pp 1-14.

The following cereal diseases were found to occur in fields in Turkey 1) barley yellow dwarf, transmitted by the aphids <u>Rhopalosiphum maidis (Fitch.)</u>, <u>R. padi (L.)</u> and <u>Sipha kurdjumovi (Mordv.)</u>, 2) maise mosaic, transmitted by the aphids <u>Myzus persicae (Sulz.)</u>, <u>R. maidis</u>, <u>R. padi</u> and <u>S. kurdjumovi</u>, 3) toxaemia, caused by an aphid, <u>Brachycolus Bckt. sp.</u> 4) a disease similar to European wheat striate mosaic, transmitted by a planthopper, 5) barley yellow stripe disease, transmitted by the leafhopper <u>Euscelis plebjus (Fn.)</u> 6) a disease like aster yellows, transmitted by <u>E. plebejus</u>, 7) a histoid enation disease, caused or transmitted by <u>E. plebejus</u> and 8) toxaemia, which was caused by the planthopper <u>Metadelphax propinqua (Fieb.)</u>.

The occurrence and significance of these diseases were estimated in western Turkey in 1969 and 1970. Cool winters and hot summers greatly restricted the abundance of the insect vectors.

The occurrence of the expected vectors was investigated by netting insects from cereal fields, meadows, and field edges in western Turkey in 1969-1970. Vector populations were largest in autumn before the sowing-time, or in late spring when the cereals were heading. Therefore the diseases and insects did not do much damage to cereals. (Authors' abstract)

17. G'urson, C. T., Saner, G., and Y'uksel, T. "Some etiological aspects of protein-calorie malnutrition in the Marmara region of Turkey." J. Trop. Pediatr. 21(6), December 1975, pp 311-314.

In an effort to determine the effect of various factors in relation to etiology, 200 protein calorie malnutrition (PCM) cases and 50 normal controls from the same background were studied.

The comparison of the PCM groups with the normal controls showed that socio-economic level, area of residence, season and type of supplementary food had an important role in the etiology of PCM. The multiple regression analysis performed in PCM cases revealed that the major factors contributing to the development of the disease were in order of importance: age, length of breast-feeding, socio-economic level, weight at birth and size of family.

When these results were compared with those from other regions it was concluded that regional differences exist with regard to the epidemiologic and etiologic factors of PCM. (Authors' abstract)

18. Duff, G. "Letter: Turkish children, immunization and ascorbic acid." Med. J. Aust. 1(18), May 4, 1974, p 722.

This short letter reports a case of an eleven-year-old Turkish male who was found to be suffering from scurvy via a urinary ascorbic acid test. He had been thought on the basis of clinical exam to be suffering from leukemia. Oral ascorbic acid, 200 mg four times daily, and injections of 200 mg daily produced almost complete resolution of petechial rash and bruises to arms, legs, and trunk within 5 days of treatment. Gum bleeding ceased within 24 hours of treatment initiation. The author suggested that doctors should not assume children had an ample supply of vitamin C, and that doctors immunizing children should check scorbutic status. This could be done with the Ames dipstick.

19. Endl, J., and Tatra, G. "Geburtshilfliche Aspekte bei Gastarbeiterinnen." ("Special aspects of obstetrics in foreign workers" authors' transl.) Wiener Klinische Wochenschrift 86(4), February 22, 1974, pp 102-105. (German)

547 Yugoslavian and Turkish foreign workers were delivered at the Second Department of Obstetrics and Gynaecology, University of Vienna, during the years 1970 to 1972, i.e. 11.3% of the total number of births. These foreign workers were compared with an equivalent group of Austrian women. The analysis comprised a survey of pregnancy, delivery and the perinatal mortality of the infants of both groups. The foreign workers showed a significantly lower rate of attendance at the antenatal clinic, and the incidence of anaemia in pregnancy, both moderate and severe, was significantly higher in this group. EPH gestosis, especially the monosymptomatic form, is seen more frequently in the group of pregnant Austrians. The number of cases of Rh-antibody formation was as expected in the group of foreign workers, but a significantly higher rate was found in the Austrian control group as a consequence of the clinic's position as special centre for such cases. There is no difference in the frequency of operative obstetrics. The increasing percentage of births to foreign workers raises the perinatal mortality rate, as a result of the higher stillbirth rate in these women and a lower survival rate of the premature and dysmature infants. (Authors' abstract)

20. LeBlanc, S. A., and Black, B. "A long term trend in tooth size in the Eastern Mediterranean." Am. J. Phys. Anthropol. 41(3), November 1974, pp 417-422.

Posterior occlusal tooth areas were measured for a sample of Greek and Turkish populations spanning an 8500 year period. Rates of reduction of 2% per 1000 years for maxillary teeth and 1% per 1000 years for the mandibulary teeth were found. These rates are shown to be greater than those for earlier populations from Western Europe. (Authors' abstract)

21. Hildebrandt, G., Yurtyeri, A., Inal, T., and Aktan, H. T. "Tissue composition of Turkish raw sausage and quantitative analysis of its nutritional ingredients." Berl. Munch. Tieraerztl. Wochenschr. 86(16), August 15, 1973, pp 309-312. Reprinted with permission of Verlag Paul Perey.

Turkish sausage "Sucuk", which is meant to be eaten warm, consists mostly of beef, sometimes with added sheep musculature and fat. After 7-10 days dry pickling, it comes on the market without being smoked and should not be kept longer than 4 weeks without refrigeration. Because this period is often overlooked, and the production conditions are unsatisfactory from a hygienic point of view, there are many complaints of insufficient curing and rotten sausages in Turkey. Unsafe colouring materials may also be used, products may contain starches or inferior parts of the animal, or there may be mistakes in the production processes. However, when the sausages are made according to Turkish regulations, there could be no objection to their sale in Germany. They are rich in protein with low fat and water content and high collagen. In order to ensure the typical "Sucuk" character, the sausages to be produced in West Germany should contain 40% fat, 40% water and 18% raw protein. In sausages of medium quality, 40% connective tissue would be allowed as compensation for more than average muscle protein content. (Authors' abstract)

22. Hildebrandt, G., Yurtyeri, A., Tolgay, Z., Ambarci, I., and Siems, H. "Occurrence and significance of micrococci and sulfite reducing anaerobes from food of animal source in Turkey." Berl. Munch. Tieraerztl. Wochenschr. 86(5), March 1973, pp 88-93.

841 food samples of meat, meat products, and milk products were analyzed for type and amount of bacteria in Ankara. Control samples from a meat center run by the State showed a bacteria count, but fewer anaerobes than in goods offered for sale in shops. A high colony count was often found in cooked or fermented sausage, cooked meat special dishes, and in bottled pasteurized milk. Foods which had no serious defects were goulasch or prepared stews, grilled meat balls, or minced meat pizza. Staphylococcus aureus was found in salted cream cheese (6 egg yolk positive strains found from 82 samples). Clostridium perifringens A was found in 5 minced meat, 1 raw sausage, and 2 kebab samples. Authors concluded that increased supervision was necessary in production and marketing of the food, and that personnel needed intensive training.

23. Bozkurt, M., G'oksoy, N., Karaali, and Ak, sehirli, M. "A study on aflatoxins in Turkish pistachio nuts." Turk. Hij. Tecr. Biyol. Derg. 32(3), 1972, pp 221-223.

Forty samples representing 200 tons of pistachio nut ready for export were examined. Six of the 40 samples had aflatoxins in them. The tests were repeated after roasting the contaminated nuts, and dark, non fluorescent spots at the same R_f distances corresponding to that of aflatoxins were found. The authors concluded that aflatoxins changed chemically when exposed to heat, but it was not known if the new structure was carcinogenic.

24. Ogutman, R. "Brucellosis in eastern Turkey." J. Clin. Pathol. 25(6), June 1972, p 552.

This is a report on a limited survey conducted in the city of Erzurman in eastern Turkey on the incidence of brucellosis. Raising cattle is the main occupation of the region. Groups selected for survey were: 1, those with close animal contact -1.5% positives; 11, those with no animal contact - 1.3% positives; 111, those with close contact with meat or meat products-18% positives; IV, those with no contact with animals or meat or meat products with brucellosis but high consumption of milk or milk products - 7.4% positives; V, slaughtered cattle - 11.7% positives; VI, slaughtered sheep - 39.9% positives. All human groups showed no evidence of brucellosis clinically. Asymptomatic brucellosis was shown to be present in the area, with handlers of meat and meat products having a higher seropositivity than other groups.

25. K'oksal, O. "Nutritional problems in Turkey during the weaning period and some solutions." Turk. J. Pediatr. 13(2), April 1971, pp 59-71.

Protein-calorie deficiency was mainly marasmic type, and incidence was 16% from 6 to 30 months of age in Etimesgut (Ankara) area. 25% of children 0 to 3 years of age in low socio-economic levels in Ankara had signs of anemia. Rickets was common, with a prevalence of 8 to 20% in many parts of Turkey. Breast feeding for 24 or more months was common, with urban and western region mothers starting to give supplementary foods earlier than rural and eastern mothers, perhaps because of a higher average level of education. Main supplementary foods for babies were starches, sugar and cereals, with very little meat, eggs and dairy foods. Insufficient amounts of food were given in terms of protein, calories, and other nutrient needs. The shortage of production of good quality foods in Turkey, ignorance, infectious diseases, parasites, and the pressures of population have all been possible contributory factors to malnutrition in young children. Solutions have centered on use of soy protein in breads and main dishes.

26. Akseh'irl'i, M., and Bozkurt, M. "Turkish legislation regarding monosodium glutamate addition to foodstuffs." Turk. Hig. Tecr. Biyol. Derg. 30(2), 1970, pp 138-146.

An amino acid separation method is usually necessary to check for use of monosodium glutamate as a food additive. However, a new method was developed and tried in a study of 30 ready-made soups, 5 macaroni and bulgur mixtures, 2 tomato sauces, and 3 tomato paste samples. Glutamate was found in 25, 2, and 2 samples of the ready-made soup, bulgur mixture, and tomato sauce samples, respectively.

Adding monosodium glutamate to food products is prohibited by Turkish legislation, but some firms are using it to improve taste regardless of legislation. Authors pointed out that it is advisable to add bouillon and meat-powder to these products to improve nutritive value as well as taste.

27. Berkel, I., Kiran, O., and Say, B. "Jejunal mucosa in infantile malnutrition." Acta. Paediatr. Scand. 59(1), January 1970, pp 58-64.

Twenty-six infants with malnutrition and seven controls were studied by routine haematological tests, serum protein levels, glucose tolerance and D-Xylose absorption tests, jejunal biopsies and intestinal disaccharide assays. In conclusion, it can be said that in malnutrition the jejunal mucosa shows some mild or non-specific histologic changes compatible with malabsorption, which may be reversible. No correlation could be shown between these changes and absorption tests. Malnutrition may also result in secondary intestinal disaccharidase deficiencies which improve with correction of the nutritional state. These secondary enzyme deficiencies may be responsible for some of the diarrhoeas seen in marasmic children. No direct correlation between anaemia, iron-deficiency, folic acid levels, protein deficiency and intestinal mucosal changes could be established in this study. (Authors' abstract)

28. Kehrer, A. "Copper deficiency diseases of sheep in Turkey." Berl. Munch. Tieraerztl. Wochenschr. 83(19), October 1, 1970, pp 371-378. Reprinted with permission of Verlag Paul Perey.

Copper deficiency in sheep in Samsun and Denizli/Civril, Turkey areas was studied via copper analyses of soil, plant, and blood samples. Most tested soils in Samsun contained high copper, 5.6 to 16.3 mg copper to 1 kg air-dry soil, but soils in Denizli/Civril contained a low amount of copper, 0.1 to 0.4 mg Cu available for plant use. An extremely high calcium content in the soils of Civril could be greatly restricting the copper availability for plant use.

Serum copper levels in mother sheep and lambs were low, with lambs showing symptoms of enzootic ataxy.

Also, during winter stall-feeding periods, the protein and energy supply for pregnant and nursing animals is insufficient. (Author's abstract)

All Other Countries

1. Cadotsch, A. F. "Does selective intervention affect other areas of primary health care? Evaluation of a vaccination program in Somali refugee camps." Soz. Praventivmed. 31(6), 1986, pp 302-7.

   The present study examines how far a selective strategy with one target problem influences other areas of primary health care. It is based on the experiences with a vaccination program in the Somalia refugee camps. The program produced a reliable census of the refugee population which produced smaller figures than had been reported previously. Data on the nutritional status of all children under 5 was collected at the vaccination places. These data provided a new basis for the general food distribution. At the same time the data served to evaluate the supplementary feeding program for vulnerable groups. It also demonstrated that general food distribution was more important for the reduction of malnutrition than other interventions, such as curative health care, community water supplies, sanitation, supplementary feeding programs and vaccination programs.

2. Portoian-Shuhaiber, S. "Infantile diarrhoea due to water complementation of breast and bottle feeding." Arch. Dis. Child. 61(12), December 1986, pp 1215-8.

   This study of 204 mothers of infants aged 1-12 months, who were admitted with acute diarrhoea to the Kuwait national hospitals investigated the prevalence of unusual infant feeding practices. To prepare a powdered milk formula, ninety percent of the mothers boiled their water, but only 15% boiled water for drinking. Thirty nine infants (19%) were admitted more than once. Although not significant better Socioeconomic class, maternal education, and breast feeding gave some protection against re-admission. It seems that the condition of drinking water is an important cause of diarrhoea and hence of re-admission. The number of readmissions was twice as high among infants drinking boiled or unboiled but filtered water. Breast feeding is protective if no extra water is given.

3. Rolls, E. T., and de Waal, A. W. "Long-term sensory-specific satiety: evidence from an Ethiopian refugee camp." Physiol. Behav. 34(6), June 1985, pp 1017-20.

   "Sensory-specific satiety," is the reduction in appetite which occurs during a meal being partly specific to the foods which have been eaten earlier in a meal. A long-term form of sensory-specific satiety has been demonstrated. Refugees in an Ethiopian refugee camp reported that the taste of 3 foods which they had been eating for approximately 6 months was less pleasant than that of 3 new foods. Eating the regular diet for only two days the refugees found its taste as pleasant as that of the different foods. When only a limited variety of food is available, long-term sensory-specific satiety may have nutritional implications. It will be useful to determine the extent to which long-term sensory-specific satiety can be prevented by provision of perhaps even a limited range of spices, flavorings or foods.

4. Beckerleg, S. "Socio-religious factors affecting the breast-feeding performance of women in the Yemen Arab Republic." Hum. Nutr. Appl. Nutr. 38(5), October 1984, pp 368-76.

   The existing socio-religious perspective of women in Yemen may be expressed in, and reinforced by, their attitudes to breast-feeding.

Yemeni women consider breastfeeding to be a powerful, but a potentially destructive force. The attitudes of contemporary Yemeni society are upheld by the Quran which defines the worth of both women and breast-feeding. The practices and beliefs associated with the reproductive and menstrual cycles, indicate that they are to be considered hedged with danger and ambiguity. Breast-feeding, which is connected to both cycles, is no exception. Traditional breast-feeding beliefs and practices are best understood within the wider context of the perceived place and ritual status of women in Yemeni society.

5. Fransson, G. B., Gebre-Medhin, M., and Hambraeus, L. "The human milk contents of iron, copper, zinc, calcium and magnesium in a population with a habitually high intake of iron." Acta. Paediatr. Scand. 73(4), July 1984, pp 471-6.

Human milk samples from 18 Ethiopian and 23 Swedish women were examined for iron, copper, zinc, calcium and magnesium contents. Both the non-privileged and privileged group of Ethiopian women had an excessively high dietary iron intake. In spite of this, the mean concentrations of iron in the milk, as well as zinc and magnesium, were similar in all three groups. The mean copper concentration, however, was significantly lower in the Ethiopian than in the Swedish milk samples. In contrast, a significantly higher mean calcium concentration was found in milk samples from the Ethiopian women than from the Swedish. It is suggested that an excessively high dietary iron intake does not increase the breast milk content of iron in mothers with a good iron status. The reasons for the differences in the content of copper between the Ethiopian and Swedish milk samples are unclear. The higher calcium content in milk from the Ethiopian mothers, despite a low dietary calcium intake may be a result of an increased endogenous cholecalciferol synthesis due to greater exposure to sunshine.

6. Musaiger, A. O. "Nutrition Status in the Arabian Gulf Countries." Human Nutrition: Better Nutrition Better Life. Proceeding of the Fourth Asian Congress on Nutrition held in Bangkok, Thailand on November 1-4, 1983. Edited by V. Tanphaichitr, W. Dahlan, V. Suphakarn, and A. Valyasevi. Aksornsmai Press, Bangkok, Thailand. 1984, pp 549-554.

The nutritional status in the Arabian Gulf countries; mainly Bahrain, Kuwait, Oman, Qatar and United Arab Emirates (UAE), is similar. These states enjoy good economic situation with the highest per capita income in the world and sufficient supply of food; however undernutition and overnutrition continue to exist. First degree malnutrition exists in this area, though second degree malnutrition is more frequent. Marasmus and anemia are the main undernutrition problems. Gastroenteritis, intestinal parasitism and food habits are believed to be responsible for the prevalence of underweight and anemia among the children. On the other hand obesity, diabetes, hypertension and heart diseases are the common public health problems of the adults. There is no specific nutrition program in any of these countries. A food and nutrition policy as a component of social and economic development plan, therefore is highly recommended, in order to improve the nutritional status of the people in the Gulf area. (Author's abstract)

7. Rao, G. M., and Morghom, L. O. "Relationship of obesity to diabetes." Horm. Metab. Res. 16(4), April 1984, pp 209-10.

Of 201 diabetic patients of Tripoli, Libya, 138 were obese the age group 41-50 years had the highest percent of diabetics and obesity. In all age groups, there was a parallel increase/decrease in obesity with diabetes. Regulation of body weight should be considered very important in control of diabetes.

8. Duncan, M. E., Samson, R. R., McGrath, J., and McClelland, D. B. "Humoral defence factors in the breast milk of Ethiopian women with leprosy and healthy controls." Am. J. Clin. Nutr. 38(6), December 1983, pp 921-8.

Secretory IgA, lactoferrin, albumin, and total protein were determined in colostrum and milk samples obtained from 215 Ethiopian mothers from 1 day to 2 years postpartum. IgG, IgM, C3, and C4 complement components were determined in 11 day 1 samples. The subjects were classified into three groups: lepromatous leprosy, borderline lepromatous leprosy, and a nonlepromatous group consisting of women with tuberculoid leprosy and healthy controls. Results obtained were compared with a group from Edinburgh. No major variation in levels of secretory IgA, lactoferrin, albumin, and total protein was found between the three groups of Ethiopian women. Results from the Edinburgh group were significantly higher, mainly in the level of total protein. When the individual proteins were expressed as a percentage of the total protein, there was no difference between the milk samples from the Ethiopian and Edinburgh mothers.

9. Hadidy, S., Fahdi, L., Tabbakh, H., and Deebo, M. "Serum lipids and glucose in obese Syrian people." Trop. Geogr. Med. 35(3), September 1983, pp 259-62.

Along with a control group, ninety three obese individuals were selected to study serum levels of total lipids, cholesterol and triglycerides together with glucose. The four estimated parameters showed statistically significant higher values in obese individuals. Serum level of triglycerides was higher in obese males than in females.

10. Henderson, P. L., and Biellik, R. J. "Comparative nutrition and health services for victims of drought and hostilities in the Ogaden: Somalia and Ethiopia, 1980-1981." Int. J. Health Serv. 13(2), 1983, pp 289-306.

The civil chaos created by a combination of drought and hostilities in the Ogaden region of southern Ethiopia during the past five years has caused the majority of the indigenous, principally nomadic population to flee the area and seek refuge either in Somali refugee camps or in Ethiopian shelters for displaced persons. This paper compares the provision of basic food rations, selective feeding programs, primary health care, and preventive health measures between the two groups.

During 1980-1981, Somalia received more international assistance per capita than Ethiopia. Large numbers of Western personnel provided health and nutrition services in Somali refugee camps, whereas no foreigners were involved in Ethiopian shelters. These disparities were largely due to inadequate publicity concerning the problems Ethiopia faces, partly resulting from real and perceived political limitations related to the Soviet presence in that country. Refugee needs in Somalia have been publicized far more adequately, partly due to that country's alignment with the West.

Ethiopians nevertheless demonstrated greater efficiency in assisting their disaster victims; camp services comparable to those in Somalia were available despite greater logistic difficulties and fewer donated resources. Effectiveness of relief operations in Somalia was reduced by political constraints on governmental agencies. (Authors' abstract)

11. Kassim, A. A., Auckland, J. N., and Hunt, C. "The policy of the Peoples Democratic Republic of South Yemen concerning the feeding of boarding school children." J. R. Soc. Health 103(1), February 1983, pp 33-34, 44.

This report details the diet of boarding school students in South Yemen. The students are between 14 and 18 years of age and are all males. Staple foods are white bread and rice, the bread made from unfortified flour imported from Canada and the UK. Fish and beans supply most of the animal and vegetable protein. Eggs and animal offal are occasionally eaten with chapatti or bread. Common vegetables and fruits in the diet are okra, onions, garlic, radish, tomatoes, coriander, eggplant, potatoes, bananas, and dates. Carrots are seldom eaten, and milk available is dried imported milk. Serious deficiencies in energy, vitamins A, D, B2 and zinc were estimated in the diet. Adding carrots to the mid-day curry was suggested as a method of increasing vitamin A intake. Increasing the dried milk allowance by 50 g/day would increase the B2 intake. Replacement of fish with lamb or chicken 2 days/week would increase zinc intake, with supplementation with liver, beef, and whole wheat or rye bread as another possibility.

12. Lombeck, I., Al-Zubaidy, I. M., Kasperek, K., Feinendegen, L. E., and Bremer, H. J. "Zinc status of Libyan children -- a pilot study." Z. Ernahrungswiss. 22(1), January 1983, pp 1-5.

Hair zinc was investigated in North and South Libyan children. The zinc content was 213 +/- 36 micrograms/g in newborns. There was no difference between North Libya and South Libyan newborns. The zinc values decreased during infancy. In toddlers and school-children the zinc content was 88 +/- 35 micrograms/g and 89 +/- 25 micrograms/g respectively. These values are similar to those reported in American children with low height percentiles or nearly as low as those found in dwarfs with poor zinc status from Egypt and Iran.

13. Singh, M., Qureshi, M. A., Aram, G. N., Hadi, F., Atif, S. Y., Adel, S. S., Arya, L. S., and Rao, J. S. "Morbidity and mortality in childhood in Afghanistan: a study of 40,492 consecutive admissions to the Institute of Child Health, Kabul", Ann. Trop. Pediatr. 3(1), March 1983, pp 25-30.

During a three-year period, 336,029 children were accorded ambulatory care and 40,492 children were admitted to the Institute of Child Health, Kabul, for inpatient treatment. Sixty-three percent were male. Three-quarters (75.3%) were under five years of age and provided 81.7% of the overall mortality. Children with acute gastroenteritis and respiratory infections together accounted for 49.9% of all admissions and 34.5% of all deaths. Malnutrition of varying degrees was a core problem and was seen in 67% of hospitalized children. The infectious diseases as a single group accounted for 70.7% of the morbidity and 71.9% of the mortality. Septicaemia and infections of the central nervous system were associated with the highest case fatality rates, especially among newborn babies. Six target diseases and accidents accoanted respectively for 10.4 and 9.7% of all deaths. Sixty-three percent of children died within 24 hours of admission and the majority of deaths occurred after regula hospital working hours. In order to safeguard the well being of children in Afghanistan, and to reduce their morbidity and mortality, it will be mandatory to ensure effective delivery of primary health care, improve nutritional standards, provide safe drinking water, immunize the vulnerable population, make free elementary education universal and improve the lot of women and future mothers. (Authors' abstract)

14. Taylor, W. R. "An evaluation of supplementary feeding in Somali refugee camps." Int. J. Epidemiol. 12(4), December 1983, pp 433-6.

In order to describe their process of operation and to measure their effect on the refugees' nutritional status, supplementary feeding programs (SFP) that were functioning in Somali refugee camps were evaluated in March 1981. While those children enrolled in SFPs gained weight, because the programme's overall effectiveness was reduced, many malnourished children in camp had not been identified. The rate of weight gain diminished rapidly each succeeding month of attendance. It is suggested that supplementary feeding is a short-term, remedial measure in disaster relief and should be quickly incorporated into a borader plan for relief assistance so that resources can be used most efficiently.

15. Barnabas, G. "Nutrition and child care amongst Ethiopian refugees in Eastern Sudan. Perspectives in primary care." J. Trop. Pediatr. 28(4), August 1982, pp 218-220.

A cross-sectional nutritional survey of a sample of 151 refugee children from the camp of Um Gulja, Eastern Sudan, was done in July and August, 1981. Most children (up to 64%) were stunted and 6% percent were undernourished. Age groups less than 24 months, children born in the camp, and children who suffered from diarrhea, were more malnourished than others. The rainy season was related to diarrheal episodes due to the higher malaria incidence and the scarcity of food. Increased use of infant bottle feeding in the camps and the practice of abrupt weaning with next pregnancy, together with absence of suitable weaning diets traditionally, combined to produce malnutrition in the young children. Wheat, barley, Teff, and rice water were used as weaning foods. Priorities for the refugee children in terms of care were listed as malnutrition and infection, followed by promotion of positive child care practices.

16. Cowan, N. "Freedom fighting in Eritrea." Nurs. Mirror 154(7), February 17, 1982, pp 16-18.

The author worked as a nurse for 18 months in a clinic at Wad el Hilewa Camp for 30,000 Eritrean refugees. She also visited Eritrean-controlled areas as well as Eritrean-run schools, underground workshops and women's organizations, and interviewed teachers and nurses belonging to the Eritrean People's Liberation Front (EPLF). She describes reprisals on civilians by Ethiopian authorities, including a massacre of 545 villagers in Hirgigio near the Red Sea port of Massawa, and the torture of prisoners such as electric shocks applied to the genitals.

The EPLF's barefoot doctor system consisted of three months' training with continuing weekly study and discussion sessions with participation by all health workers. War-related measures such as location of hospitals and clinics undergound or in camouflaged tents, nighttime scheduling of operations, and use of mobile medical teams to treat civilians behind Ethiopian lines are described. The need for food as well as medical facilities is stressed. Problems most often seen in refugee camps were malnutrition, TB, malaria, parasitic infections, and respiratory infections.

17. Parvez, S. Z. "Eye Camp for Afghan Refugees at Jaluzai and Azakhel, Peshawar District, N.W.F.P." J.P.M.A. 32(5), May 1982, pp 130.

The first eye camp was established for Afghan refugees in Jaluzai, Peshawar District by the government of Pakistan in February 1982, includings beds, an operation theatre, and outpatient facilities providing glasses and medicines. Trachoma was a major problem, with cataract cases less frequent. Surgery obtained had a high success rate, and a similar eye camp was held subsequently at Azakhel, another Peshawar site. Statistics on types and incidence of eye diseases encountered in both camps are provided.

18. Popkin, B. M., Bilsborrow, R. E., and Akin, J. S. "Breast-feeding patterns in low-income countries". Science, 218, December 10, 1982, pp 1088-1093.

This paper is a discussion on breast-feeding patterns in low-income countries as evidenced by nationally representative World Fertility Surveys (WFS) and secondary sources. Jordan was the only Middle Eastern country represented in the 17 country WFS data.

Based on limited data, regional breast-feeding pattern appeared to be intermediate between that of Asia and Latin America. Urban-rural differences in Africa-Near East region were smaller than in the other two regions. The median age at weaning was eleven months in Jordan and limited evidence on trends seemed to indicate a decline in the duration of breast-feeding. Concern regarding adverse implications for infant health and nutrition was expressed in connection with this decline.

19. Shawky, R. M., and El Din, S. S. "Iron deficiency anaemia in children in Um Al-Quwain, United Arab Emirates." J. Egypt Soc. Parasitol. 12(1), June 1982, pp 217-224.

500 Arab children of both sexes between 4 months and 6 years of age who attended the Pediatric Clinic at U.A.E. Hospital in Um Al-Quwain were assessed for iron deficiency anaemia via hemoglobin, hematocrit, blood smear and reticulocyte count, glucose-6-phosphate dehydrogenase, serum iron level (on 50 patients), blood smear for malaria parasites, serum proteins, occult blood in stools, and routine urine and stool examination. A diagnosis of iron deficiency anaemia was reached in 232 children, or 46.4%. They had hemoglobin concentrations below 11 gm/100 ml and hematocrit values less than 33%. Although a high standard of living is maintained, malnutrition was implicated because dietary history showed 22% of infants to be breast fed with no supplemental foods during their first year of life, and 45% of infants to be bottle fed either cow's milk or dried milk which was generally not fortified with iron. From 2 to 6 years years of age, children were fed a staple

diet of rice and bread with little animal protein or green vegetables. 65% of the tract infections, and parasite infestations were ruled out as direct causative agents in the anaemia. Malnutrition secondary to illness was seen in 17% of the iron deficient cases, and malnutrition attributable to dietary deficiency was seen in 46% of the iron deficient cases.

20. Watson, W. "Tuberculosis programme in a Somali refugee camp." Trop. Doctor 12, April 1982, pp 92-93.

Oxfam representatives responded in February 1980 to a Somali government request to assess the need for a medical team to work in Saba'ad camp for Ogaden refugees. Need was obvious and a medical team was sent. This report described a camp programme to combat tuberculosis (TB). A similar camp in the area showed active TB incidence to be 1.7% of the population, with many malnourished children, particularly those who had survived measles, being affected. After a clinically-based tentative diagnosis, treatment by oral or parenteral penicillin daily for a week was given. If no clinical improvement was seen, TB diagnosis was made. Prime initial clue with malnourished children was failure to gain weight regardless of intensive feeding and treatment of anemia and infection. The contagiousness of TB in the camp of 65,000 who lived 2 or 3 families per shelter with the risk factors of malnutrition, infectious disease, and psychological shock was great. The team treated TB cases with .40 mg/kg BWt. of streptomycin intramuscularly daily for 3 months, and TB1 daily for 1 year initially. Of 237 registered TB cases, most had pulmonary TB, 6 had bone involvement, and 6 had involved enlarged neck glands.

21. Anonymous "Follow-up on refugees--Somalia." MMWR 30(7), February 27, 1981, pp 85-88.

In September and October 1980, Center for Disease Control epidemiologists assisted the Somali Ministry of Health in conducting follow-up nutritional surveys in nearly all settled refugee camps in the Waqoozi Galbleed, Hiran, and Gedo regions. Findings were compared with those of previous surveys done in May and July of 1980. Nutritional status, TB control, health surveillance, and camp feeding programs were assessed. Nutritional status of camp inhabitants was also compared with that of selected non-refugee children from nomad, farming, and urban backgrounds. Based on weight-for-height criteria, 8.9% of refugees 5 years or under, and 3.9% of comparable non-refugee children were deemed moderately or severely malnourished. Overall prevalence of PEM had decreased in all regions and moderately so in the Gedo region. Food shortages, irregular food distribution, and the very recent institution of the supplementary feeding programs in Gedo region were causative factors in continuing high PEM rates there. In summer cough, fever, diarrhea, and anemia were most prevalent. By October, childhood PEM, lack of firewood cooking fuel and water supplies, and shortages of essential medicines, shelter covers, blankets, and clothing items were ongoing problems. Dependable delivery of food supplies and supplemental feeding programs were pinpointed as high priorities.

22. Gastpar, H., Wilmes, E., and Wolf, H. "Epidemiologic, etiologic and immunologic aspects of nasopharyngeal carcinoma (NPC)". J. Med. 12(4), 1981, pp 257-284.

Common genetic characteristics in populations with a high risk of NPC include high nasal index, possible HLA-antigen profiles, and certain blood group frequencies of low A, high B, and High O. External factors such as inhaled domestic carcinogens in Hong Kong boatdwellers and intranasal fungus infection in Sudan are mentioned in connection with epithelial mucosal changes. Adenovirus infections, and Epstein-Barr virus infections are seen as being related to NPC incidence. A genetic predisposition seen in Chinese populations is noted. An additional environmental factor in their case may be linked to their ancestral living habits. African tribal incidences in Kenya and Nilotic peoples are given. An elevated incidence level is mentioned for Morocco, Algeria, and Tunisia.

23. Hussein, M. A., and Eid, N. M. "Nutrient components of truffles." Nahrung 24(8), 1981, pp 811-812.

Known as "Kameh" and "Fagaa" in the Arabian Peninsula, the truffle composition was: for nitrogen, 6.3% and 2.7% from Kuwait and Saudi Arabia, respectively; for fat, 7.2% and 6.8% from Kuwait and Saudi Arabia, respectively; for carbohydrate, 37.1% and 40.9% from Kuwait and Saudi Arabia, respectively. Fiber and ash contents were also given. The amino acid pattern was compared to that of the FAO pattern. Thiamin, riboflavin, and vitamin C contents were given as 0.02, 0.19, and 24.2 mg/100 g fresh sample, respectively. Potassium was the most concentrated mineral, with 1456 mg/100 g dry sample, followed by calcium with 512 mg/100 g dry sample and magnesium with 904 mg/100 g dry sample.

24. Kimball, A. M., Hamadeh, R., Mahmood, R. A., Khalfan, S., Muhsin, A., Ghabrial, F., and Armenian, H. K. "Gynaecomastia among children in Bahrain" (letter) Lancet 1(8221), March 21, 1981, pp 671-672.

The Directorate of Public Health of Bahrain in conjunction with the American University of Beirut and the Center for Disease Control conducted an investigation in response to a cluster of cases of significant breast enlargement outside infancy but before puberty in one village in Bahrain. Eight cases were found in the village, with all the children belonging to one of five families in three households. Cases contained normal chorionic gonadoptrophin and estradiol levels. Six of the affected children normally drank milk from a cow which had been given estrinyl injections monthly for 6 months prior to the first case report. The cow's sera contained normal levels of chorionic gonadotrophin and estradiol. When the samples were taken from the children, the cow had been sold, the gynaecomastia was subsiding, and all cases resolved spontaneously. The authors suggested the need for further studies and recommended the restriction of milk from distribution when cows are on treatment with biologically active hormones.

25. Musaiger, A. O. "A study of nutritional habits in Bahrain", 1981, 62 pages by the Ministry of Public Health, Department of Nutrition published in Manama, Bahrain (Arabic).

A random sample of 310 households from 8 geographical regions was surveyed to determine dietary habits of Bahraini families on social occasions. Housewives were interviewed at home to determine socioeconomic level, meal patterns, foods for social occasions, food beliefs and food preparation methods.

The major difference between rural and urban areas was type of food served at supper; rural meals included tea with milk, bread, cheese and/or eggs while urban suppers consisted of meat or chicken stew, bread, and tea with milk. Most families (71.6%) ate together while 13.2% segregated the sexes. 95% of housewives used canned foods.

For special occasions, certain foods were consumed. Al-harees and Al-threed were major dishes for Famadan, Gadoo for wedding guests and rice with meat for pilgrimage. Tea or coffee with sweets were prepared for mourning. Milk, eggs or sweets were given to male children after circumcision in 39% of households. Twenty-five percent of housewives believed nuts increased male sexual potency.

26. Simmonds, S. "Feeding the hungry." Nurs. Times 77(2), January 8, 1981, pp 57-62.

More and more refugee camps worldwide have taken on a "temporarily permanent" character. In recognition of this reality, the author emphasizes a community health approach, with the long-term goal of helping the refugee community to help itself upon ultimate withdrawal of relief agencies. The provision of adequate food, water, sanitation, clothing, transport, education, and health services is seen to be as crucial as medical services. A flexible approach, ongoing discussions with the refugee community, and integration of efforts with the local and central governments' health plans are essential for success. Necessary decision-making steps include evaluation discussions to assess national, district, and camp-perceived needs, prioritization of problems, establishment of short and long-term objectives, timed planning of precise activities and tasks, implementation, and reassessments to identify operational problems on a day-to-day basis.

27. Strong, P. "The recruitment and training of volunteers for emergency relief work." Nurs. Times 77(2), January 8, 1981, pp 62-64.

This report discusses the method by which a Shropshire Medical Relief Team of volunteer nurses was recruited and trained for short-notice emergency relief work under the aegis of Oxfam. Relevant details were published through the nursing network, a selection panel interviewed applicants, and 15 team members were selected. Ward sisters, charge nurses, health visitors, and a midwife comprised the team. Criteria for selection stressed capacity for harmonious teamwork in stressful and uncomfortable conditions. Lists of necessary articles were prepared for the team by Oxfam. Speakers and materials used to train the team were scheduled in evening sessions at 2-month intervals. Last-minute arrangments such as anti-malarial therapy, cholera protection, and human gamma globulin injections, and passport checks, were covered. Background reading on the area, which in this case ultimately was Somalia, was urged prior to departure.

28. Cowan, N. "Nursing overseas: after the bullets...." Nurs. Mirror 151(25), December 1980, pp 30-31.

A nurse reports her experience of the beginnings of a resettlement plan for Eritrean refugees who fled to Sudan. The wandering life of the refugees and harsh conditions, such as sleeping outside in all weather while searching for casual agricultural work, are described. The overcrowding and poverty which result in high TB incidence and the malnutrition which results from their dependence on World Food Programme rations are highlighted. The WFP rations are described as paltry and erratic, consisting of powdered milk, oil, beans, and sorghum. Suki refugee camp exhibits a high incidence of anaemia, malaria, and protein deficiency, as well as gastrointestinal infections and parasites. The author states that medicine alone is not a solution, that the refugees can only have their problems solved when they can return to their own country to live and work in freedom.

29. Jain, R. C. "Serum cholesterol in Libyans." J. Trop. Med. Hyg. 83(6), December 1980, pp 247-250.

The average diet consumed by Libyans resembles that in developed Western countries in being high in calories and containing a substantial amount of animal protein and fat. Total serum cholesterol and betalipoprotein cholesterol were determined in a section of the population of Benghazi and the figures were compared with those from other countries. In spite of consuming a high calorie and high animal fat diet, the total serum cholesterol and betalipoprotein cholesterol in Libyans were found to be much lower than those reported in the American population. The mean systolic and diastolic blood pressures in both sexes in the Libyan population were lower than those of Londoners. These lower figures in the Libyans, in comparison to those in developed countries, could be due to some genetic, environmental, geographic or dietetic factors and require investigation. (Author's abstract)

30. Kruizinga-Sabandar, A. "Young Moroccan and Turkish children in the hospital." Tijdschr. Ziekenverpl. 33(20), October 1980, pp 949-953. (Dutch)

Commonly encountered problems in young Morroccan and Turkish children during their hospitalization including such common ailments as childhood diarrhea, migraine headaches, and vitamin deficiencies. Use of vitamin supplements to counteract vitamin-deficient diets is urged. Psychosomatic illnesses in the children often caused by the stressful condition of being between two different cultures. Child abuse or "kinder-mishandeling" is a problem. Special methods of handling these cases and special training of workgroups of health personnel as "hospitalized child" teams are discussed.

31. Neumann, S. Z. "Childhood diarrhea and its treatment with indomethacin in Libya." Trop. Doct. 10(1), January 1980, pp 24-28.

The effect of indomethacin was studied in 355 children and infants suffering from childhood diarrhea admitted to a hospital in Libya from 1973 to 1977. The first 85 cases were rehydrated and fed soya milk. The next 270 cases were given this treatment and also given oral indomethacin. Those children not given indomethacin had diarrhea for an average of 4 days after treatment with an average of 8 stools per day. Those treated with indomethacin averaged only a few hours of diarrhea after treatment. The better results in the second group were considered to be due to the combination of rehydration, soya milk and indomethacin.

32. Simmonds, S. P. "Curative medicine or community health? Appropriate health services with refugees." J. Trop. Med. and Hyg. 83, 1980, pp 49-52.

A community health approach to serving the health needs of refugees in camps or settlements may be a superior alternative to traditional individual curative medical approaches. A strategy for meeting basic needs of food, water, sanitation, health services, clothing, housing, public transport, and education is presented as a strategy for health. Full participation by the refugee community in planning and managing the programme is urged, with pinpointing of priority health problems and specific disease problems. Initial and ongoing discussions between the refugee community, local community, local government, private and international agencies, and the health teams is urged to identify perceived health problems and needs, and to increase community commitment in resulting programmes. The need for proper evaluation, curative service, and training of unskilled health workers is stressed. In conclusion, the author urges a re-orientation of health workers working with refugees toward a greater emphasis on the community health approach.

33. Gunn, R. A., Kimball, A. M., Pollard, R. A., Feeley, J. C., Feldman, R. A., Dutta, S. R., Matthew, P. P., Mahmood, R. A., and Levine, M. M. "Bottle feeding as a risk factor for cholera in infants." Lancet 2(8145), October 6, 1979, pp 730-732.

To determine risk factors for cholera in infants, a retrospective matched-pair study of 42 cases and their controls was undertaken during an outbreak of El Tor cholera in Bahrain in the autumn of 1978. The highest attack-rate of cholera (125/10,000) occured in infants in the 6-11 month age-group, which corresponds to the weaning age in this community. Significantly more cases than controls were principally bottle fed (greater than 50% milk intake by bottle) than principally breast fed during the week before onset of illness (p-0.004). Analysis of various patterns of breast and bottle feeding did not determine whether the protection afforded by breast feeding was a negative effect (due to the lack of exposure to contaminated bottle feeding for breast fed infants) or a positive effect (due to protective functions of constitutents of human breast milk). Cholera infection (with or without symptoms) among mothers of either case or control infants was uncommon (case mothers 3, control mothers 5), and mean serum vibriocidal and antitoxic antibody levels were similar for the two groups of mothers. These observations suggest that maternal infection did not affect the relative risk of infants having symptomatic cholera. (Authors' abstract)

34. Kamel, K., Appesh, S., Worth, G., and Khalafallah, S. Emirates "Blood levels of selected nutritional status indicators in young men from a rapidly modernizing society in Abu Dhabi, United Arab Emirates." Am. J. Clin. Nutr. 32(10), October 1979, pp 2150-2153.

As the Bedouin society of Abu Dhabi is rapidly modernizing, the impact of urbanization and subsequent Westernization of the way of life of young male Bedouin recruits of the UAE Armed Forces was assessed nutritionally. Hematocrit, serum proteins, serum transferrin, serum calcium, serum iron, serum folate, and red blood cell folate were assessed in a control group of 10 male expatriate laboratory volunteers and in 30 Bedouin army recruits. Hematocrit, and serum proteins, transferrin, and calcium were found adequate in both groups. High milk and milk product consumption was thought responsible for the adequate calcium levels. Serium iron was adequate in all controls and in all but four of the recruits.

These four had serum iron less than 60 ug/dl. Average serum folate was similar in the two groups, with two recruits deficient at levels less than 3.0 ng/ml. 11 of 30 recruits and 5 of 10 controls had serum folate higher than 5.9 ng/ml. The remainder had borderline levels. Nine recruits had borderline red blood cell folate, (less than 200 ng/ml and more than 100 ng/ml). All others had values above 200 ng/ml. Lack of fresh vegetables historically contributed to low folate consumption. The current affluence has not affected dietary habits locally enough yet to raise the vegetable consumption rate and eliminate the borderline folate status.

35. Myntti, C. "Population processes in rural Yemen: temporary emigration, breastfeeding, and contraception." Stud. Fam. Plann. 10(10), October 1979, pp 282-289.

This report on North Yemen covers a two-stage study which consisted of a small demographic survey of all ever-married women (347) in three villages in different ecological and cultural zones, and an anthropological participant-observer research study of demographic trends and medical beliefs and practice in the village of Bani Ghazi in Hujariyya border district near South Yemen. The three most important intermediate fertility variables, temporary emigration with spousal separation, breastfeeding, and use of contraception were examined. Although as many as 1/3 to 1/2 of adult Yemeni men worked outside North Yemen, the spousal separation was not seen as important to smaller family size decision-making as attitudinal changes due to exposure to other societies and rural economic changes. Increasing ability of Yemeni families to pay for powdered milk was an underlying factor in increasing use of bottles to feed infants. Shortened birth intervals and higher fertility was thought to follow from this trend. Increased use of contraception by men and women was viewed as the result of multifactorial pressures. Conflicting effects of the above trends require further studies to elicit a fuller picture of the overall population trends in North Yemen.

36. Almedal, C. "Report from Redd Barnas hospital in North Yemen." Sykepleien 65(18), November 1978, pp 1138-1140. (Norwegian)

Calle Almedal gave this report on behalf of the Norwegian health care staff at "Redd Barnas Hospital" in Ibb, which was opened in 1977. The hospital was founded to help and educate the people of North Yemen, especially the women who were 99 percent illiterate.

As in most developing countries, the need for both curative and preventive medical care was immense in Yemen. Fundamental knowledge of disease prevention was considered especially crucial. Malnutrition and poor nutritional practices were often due to lack of information, not poverty. (Adapted from author's abstract, translated by Elizabeth Gustavsson.)

37. Burhani, H. A. "Epidemiological study in child dental health -- nutritional survey." Quintessence Int. 9(3), March 1978, pp 65-71.

18 girls and 20 boys 11 to 12 years of age in primary schools in Damascus and Daraya village were examined to determine the real DMF-T and dental plaque. A questionnaire with 35 questions on child knowledge, attitude, and behavior toward nutrition dental problems, and diseases of the mother and child when he was less than 5 years old was given. Fluoride content of Damascus water was

from .07 to .15 PPmF, and of Daraya was 1.14 PPmF. 60.72% of Damascus children had fluoride levels in urine between .27 and .25 PPm, whereas 70% of Daraya children had fluoride urine between 1 and 1.6 PPm. 65.79% of children visiting the dentist came to have the following: 47/37%-extraction, 2.63%-filling, and 7.89%-cleaning. Good knowledge of dental health was indicated by 60.52% knowing sweets and sugar to be cariogenic, and 36.84% relating dental caries to lack of oral hygiene. 60.52% of the children did not eat snacks, and 81.6% of the children did not eat sugar and sweets.

38. Eid, A. M. "Osteomalacia as a contributing factor in fracture of the femoral neck in the elderly in Quatar." Clin. Orthop. and Rel. Res. (132), May 1978, pp 129-135.

The presence of osteomalacia was investigated in 87 hospital patients suffering from femoral neck fractures. Results divided the patients into two types. In the first group, the patients had either sustained the fracture following a severe injury, or were less than 50 years old. There were eighteen patients in this group, and they showed no evidence of osteomalacia. In the second group, 69 patients, either a trivial injury or no injury at all was indicated in conjunction with the femoral neck fracture. In this group, 16 people, or 23.2%, displayed evidence of osteomalacia, and in another 7, or 10.1%, osteomalacia was suspected. Women showed more osteomalacia than men, and they also showed more trochanteric fractures than cervical fractures.

39. Parikh, S. D., and El-Ghamrawi, K. A. "Cancer of the naso-pharynx in Kuwait." J. Laryngol. Otol. 92(8), August 1978, pp 681-691.

A clinico-pathological study of 143 cases of malignancy of the naso-pharynx diagnosed and treated at the E.N.T. and Radiotherapy Departments of Al-Sabah Hospital, Kuwait, between the years 1963 to 1974 inclusive is presented. The entire population of Kuwait is served and also a variable but small number of Nomads. During the years of the survey the population has been steadily increasing from about 500,000 in 1963 to about a million in 1974. It is composed of 45% Kuwaitis of pure Arab stock and 55% of immigrant workers, largely of Arabic origin. Cancer of naso-pharynx is the commonest of all head and neck cancers (18.3%) and comprises 4.2% of all malignancies. This is comparable with the 5.1% in the Arab population of North Africa. The sex incidence is 2.2 Kuwaiti males and 0.8 females per 100,000; non-Kuwaitis 2.0 male and 1.2 female per 100,000, giving an approximate ratio of 2.9 to 1 in both groups. The age distribution shows two peaks in male patients, Kuwaitis and non-Kuwaitis in the 2nd decade (11.1%) and fifth decade (28.8%). In females, the graph shows a plateau pattern from the 3rd decade onwards. Cervical lymphadenopathy (83%) was the commonest presenting symptom. The commonest histological finding was undifferentiated carcinoma and squamous cell carcinoma (28% each). The hypotheses of the aetiology are reviewed. (Authors' abstract)

40. Anonymous "An Islamic twist." (Editorial) Lancet 2(8031), July 30, 1977, pp 232.

Duke and Yar in Afghanistan reported, during a period of 13 months, 26 Pushtoon men with primary small-bowel volvulus, of whom 19 started suffering from the condition during Ramadan. The Pushtoon's susceptibility to the condition to very high-fibre diets was attributed to the strict observance of the fasting rules of Ramadan. The comparative ease of corrective surgery for small-bowel volvulus compared to volvulus of the sigmoid was also discussed.

41. Morcos, S. R., Gabrial, G. N., and El-Hafez, M. A. "Nutritive studies on some raw and prepared leguminous seeds commonly used in the Arab Republic of Syria." Z. Ernsehrungswiss 15(4), December 1976, pp 378-386. Dr. Dietrich Steinkopff Verlag.

A nutritive analysis of raw Syrian lentils (Lens esculentus) and red chick pea (Cicer arietinum) variety balady was done. The protein contents of the two raw seeds were 23 and 22 g% for lentils and chick peas, respectively. Ethereal extract, fiber, ash, calcium, phosphorus and iron content of the two raw seeds were assayed. The levels of most of the amino acids were also estimated in the raw and cooked seeds. It was found that tryptophan- and sulphur-containing amino acids were the most limiting. Cooking the seeds by the same methods commonly used in Syria resulted in the loss of most of the amino acids, with the exception of lysine and tryptophan which were slightly increased. Trypsin inhibitors and saponins were detected in the raw seeds. Haemagglutinins were present in raw lentils only. Cooking the seeds destroyed the trypsin inhibitors and haemagglutinins but did not affect the saponins. The net protein utilization (NPU) of whole lentils and chick peas were 38 and 53, respectively. Decortication of lentils or cooking without decortication had no effect on the NPU values. Cooking the decorticated lentil seeds raised its NPU value from 38 to 56. Cooking chick peas resulted in a slight increase in NPU. Supplementation of the raw and treated seeds with methionine and tryptophan raised NPU values markedly. (Adapted from authors' abstract)

42. Abdel Kader, M. M., Adham, K., Maamoun, A., Mansour, M., and Rizk, A. M. "Biochemical studies on the Syrian broad beans 1. - Biochemical analysis." Egypt. J. Nutr. 1(1), January 1975, pp 17-34.

The Syrian broad bean (Vicia faba), the main component of several Syrian dishes, was sampled from four localities of the cultivated area in Syria. The samples were powdered and analyzed for moisture, ash, fiber, starch, sucrose, reducing sugars, fats and proteins. The amino acids of the bean-protein were fractionated by paper chromatography and the chemical score was calculated. Roasted and autoclaved samples were also analyzed for amino acid content to demonstrate the effect of heat on these amino acids.

Vitamins, thiamine, ascorbic acid, minerals, Na, K, Ca, Mg and P were also determined, and the effect of heat and germination on vitamin C content was demonstrated. (Authors' summary)

43. Abdel Kader, M. M., Adham, K., Rizk, A., and Maamoun, A. "Biochemical studies on the Syrian broad bean 3. - The biological value of roasted, autoclaved and supplemented Syrian broad bean." Egypt. J. Nutr. 1(1), January 1975, pp 35-42.

The biological value of the raw Syrian broad bean was found to be close to that of the roasted and autoclaved samples. This was explained by the fact that the destructive effect of heat on the bean protein amino acids was offset by certain beneficial effects of heat on the bean protein.

Supplementing the raw bean with skimmed cheese raised the PER to a very satisfactory level, and corrected the histopathological changes that result from the raw bean alone. Accordingly, it was concluded that a small amount of this cheese, which is cheap and quite available, is enough to make the Syrian bean an adequate diet. (Authors' summary)

44. Anonymous "Heights and weights of children in Southern Tunisia." Nutr. Rev. 33(8), August 1975, pp 235-236.

This is a review article on measurements done on children 6 to 11 years of age in Southern Tunisia and a comparison of their measurements with those of American children of corresponding ages. Lowenstein and O'Connell in 1974 measured 205 children, all boys, in six villages. The study's authors had argued that the differences seen between Tunisians classified as high socioeconomic groups and American children could be ascribed to true genetic attributes, but the reviewer questions the interpretation. Basically, he contends that no well-defined yardsticks of socioeconomic classes can be defined. The reviewer also takes exception to the discussion of protein deficiency without including the question of caloric adequacy in the Tunisian children.

45. Jahn, W., and Legel, S. "Studies on climate factors influencing the effectiveness of cattle production in the Syrian Arabic Republic. I. Effect of climate factors; climatic conditions in the SAR". Bietr. Trop. Landwirtsch. Veterinsermed 13(3), 1975, pp 279-288. Article in German, abstract English.

No previous investigations are available on climatic influences on the performance in cattle production in the Syrian Arab Republic. The reports found in the literature on the effect of the climate, especially of temperature and atmospheric moisture, are classified into physiological compatibility ranges for cattle. This makes it possible to compare different climatic regions. In the second part of the paper, the values found for temperature and moisture in an experimental cowshed in the SAR will be assessed. (Authors' abstract)

46. Young, H. B. "Factors and poverty in the families of young children." At Risk Factors and the Health and Nutrition of Young Children Publication of the International Conference held in Cairo, June 23-27, 1975, pp 247-261. Printed by Al-Shaab Printing House.

The social, maternal, family, and child-related at-risk factors in young childhood malnutrition were studied in the area of Greater Tunis, which holds 20% of Tunisia's population. Examination at birth and determination of gestational age and presence of handicaps took place. From 4 months of age, 4 groups were given varying nutritional supplementation regimens, and a fifth group received only medical care. Developmental examinations at 4, 8, 12, and 18 months were also done.

The control group 6 had a subgroup of 20 children who were also examined at the same times as experimental groups. Anthropometric measures showed differences between groups 1 through 5 and group 6 by 12 months which continued through 18 months. Group 5 at 18 months showed inferior total serum protein, and group 6 showed inferiority in all biochemical measures. Group 2, supplemented with supramine, was most superior in development overall. Girls were superior to boys in osseous development at 12 months.

Psychological data showed significant differences between experimental and control groups at 12 months, and less difference by 18 months.

47. Coulter, P. "Mother and child health care in the Yemen." Nurs. Times 70(46), November 14, 1974, pp 1764-1765.

The author described the problems in maternal and child health care existing in the Yemen, and the role that village health centres could have on local health care, particularly in child feeding practices. She noted that the most serious nutritional problems were found among infants and pre-school children, and deplored the rising use of bottles to feed infants in place of breastfeeding. She suggested nutrition education of the mothers as to the excellence of the traditional method of breastfeeding. The preferability of using a glass to feed an infant who cannot be breast-fed in place of a bottle was discussed in terms of ease of cleaning and ease of recording total consumption.

48. Hijazi, S. S. "Patterns of protein-energy malnutrition in early childhood in Jordan". Am. J. Clin. Nutr. 27(11), November 1974, pp 1254-1258.

Ninety-nine malnourished children in Ashrafieh Hospital, Amman, Jordan, were assessed for type of malnutrition, sex and age. Criterion for inclusion in the study was weight for age 80% or less of expected weight for age by Boston standards. A control group of 24 children with weight for age above 90% of Boston standard was selected from the outpatient clinic. The Wellcome Trust classification for protein-energy malnutrition was applied. Among the children classified as malnourished, 67% were non-edematous type (35% marasmus, 32% underweight) and 32% edematous type (21% kwashiorkor, 11% marasmic kwashiorkor). Marasmus affected 62% of the children by 3-6 months of age and resulted in up to 30% mortality. The Wellcome classification produced results very consistant with those from other countries. (Authors' abstract)

49. Hijazi, S. S. "Social and cultural aspects of hospitalized malnourished children in Jordan." J. Trop. Pediatr. 20(6), December 1974, pp 280-283. (Environ. Child Health)

The social and cultural factors and dietary features of protein-energy malnutrition in Jordan are discussed.

When comparing the malnourished group with the controls, the former has lower incomes, more sibling deaths, earlier weaning and earlier introduction of bottle-feeding. The weaning foods of the controls provided a fairly balanced diet with ample amounts of protein, while the weaning foods of the malnourished group were mainly starchy, with poor protein content.

The need for rehydration centres and proper vaccination programmes is discussed. (Author's abstract)

50. Legel, S. "Chemical composition and nutritional value of feed in the Syrian Arab Republic." Arch. Tierernaehr. 24(9-10), December 1974, pp 711-719. (German) Akademic Verlag

A study was made of 370 samples of 74 feed-stuffs obtained in different areas of the Syrian Arab Republic. The feed-stuffs included green forages grown on irrigated land, conservation products of these crops, cereal grains and seeds (leguminous and gramineous plants), the straw, chaff, hulls and husks of these crops and their industrial by-products (milling products and by-products of the oil and sugar industries). In this study the crude nutrient content of these foods was estimated and, additionally, their energetic feeding value was calculated. The characteristic data of the feeding value thus obtained were compared with the tabular values of the GDR system of food evaluation. Deviations from these values are discussed. The content of digestible crude protein, crude fibre, and nitrogen-free extractives in the different feed-stuffs was generally the same as that in the tabular values, although deviations above and below the tabular values were also noted. The crude fat content was equal or higher. The crude ash content was considerably higher than the tabulated value. The content of EFr in the green forages and their conservation products was generally in the range of the tabular values. In the case of cereals and seeds the data largely coincided, with certain exceptions. A general tendency towards a higher content in EFr was observed in industrially manufactured products. (Author's abstract in English)

51. Lowenstein, F. W., and O'Connell, D. E. "Selected body measurements in boys ages 6-11 years from six villages in Southern Tunisia: An international comparison." Human Biol. 46(3), September 1974, pp 471-482.

Mean heights and weights for 205 boys aged 6-11 years in South Tunisia are compared with mean heights and weights of boys in the same age groups from India, Egypt and the U.S.A. Generally, boys from India rank lowest, Tunisian boys second lowest, followed by the Egyptians and the U.S.A. boys with the highest means. Duncan Multiple Range Test was used to group each of the mean weights and heights of all ages from all countries into homogeneous subsets of similar magnitude. A similar height and weight is reached by the American boys about two years earlier than by the Tunisian boys. Skinfold comparisons for the triceps and subscapular skinfolds between the Tunisian and U.S.A. boys show that the Tunisian boys have between 16% and 49% lesser skinfold measurements, with differences increasing with age.

In comparing mean heights and weights of a Tunisian privileged group with the average U.S.A. group on the one hand and the Tunisian village group on the other hand, differences are much greater between the two Tunisian groups of the same racial background but different socio-economic status than between the privileged Tunisians and the U.S. Americans of similar socio-economic status but different racial backgrounds. (Authors' abstract)

52. Mokhtar, N. A., and Ghaly, I. M. "Lactose intolerance, a cause of recurrent diarrhea in Kuwait." Gaz. Egypt Paediatr. Assoc. 22(2), April 1974, pp 113-118.

A comparative study was carried out on 198 patients convalescing from gastroenteritis.

Cases were divided into 2 groups: group I was given 1/2 cream milk formula and group II received 1/2 cream lactase free formula. The incidence of diarrhea was higher (28%) in the first group compared to the second (12.3%). Diarrhea was accompanied by the appearance of reducing substances in the stools in 22% of cases and acid stools in 37% of cases of Group I compared to zero and 9% respectively in group II. Transient lactose intolerance must be considered a possible cause of recurrent diarrhea.

The administration of a lactose-free formula to patients convalescent from severe gastroenteritis is thus recommended to diminish the incidence of recurrent diarrhea and stop the vicious cycle. (Adapted from authors' abstract.)

53. Forslund, J. "Public health services in a starvation-stricken desert country." Laekartidningen 69(4), January 19, 1972, pp 309-311. (Swedish)

From "Radda Barnens" (Save the Children) help activity in Yemen. A report by Jorgen Forslund, medical doctor at the hospital in Saffle, who was sent to Yemen to map out the need for help when the country was struck by famine in 1970. The help project is being continued--a new famine is expected this spring. (Author's abstract translated by Elizabeth Gustavsson.)

54. Kimmance, K. J. "Failure to thrive and lactation failure in Jordanian villages in 1970." J. Trop. Pediatr. 18(4), December 1972, pp 313-316.

313 Jordanian infants were assessed at three months of age for relationships between lactation failure and certain medical and social factors. There was a disturbingly high incidence of lactation failure in the series (36%).

Heavy mothers had a greater likelihood of failure, but apart from this, the aim of identifying at-risk factors was not realised. One interesting finding was the slightly lower incidence among primiparae. Another was the marked preponderance of failure to thrive among girls when the children were reassessd at six months of age. (Author's abstract)

55. Samadi, A. R. "Protein-calorie malnutrition among children in Kaboul." Ann. Pediatr. (Paris) 19(8), September 1972, pp 631-635. (French)

In a study of 595 cases of protein-energy malnutrition, approximately half showed kwashiorkor and half marasmus. Those with kwashiorkor were more likely to show clinical signs of deficiences in vitamins A, D, and B, were more likely to be irritable, and were shorter for age. The main contributors to malnutrition were chronic diarrhea and prolonged breastfeeding with inadequate supplementation.

56. Reitz, L. P. "New wheats and social progress." Science 169(949), September 4, 1970, pp 952-955.

This paper reviews the history of the development of new, improved wheat strains, both conventional types and semi-dwarf types, and their use by various countries around the world. Topics included are: the manipulation of several hundred known genes into desired combinations, including shorter, stiffer straw, greater adaptability, and more resistance to diseases and insects; the use of the Gaines variety and the subsequent development of the Mexican semi-dwarf varieties by Borlaug of the Rockefeller Foundation; FAO and CIMMYT's research, testing, and training program; introduction of the new semi-dwarf varieties for higher national yields, such as in Turkey, Mexico, India and West Pakistan; how extensive planting of the new varieties in such developing countries as Afghanistan, Nepal, Iran, Lebanon, Morocco, and Tunisia, as well as in America and Europe, has resulted in a narrowing of the genetic base of much of the world's production; and the development of the seed bank of the U.S.D.A. to counteract this effect.

57. Ali-S. A., al-Yusuf, A. R., Salem, S. N., el-Ghamrawy, E., and Zagulaul, S. "Pernicious anaemia among Arabs in Kuwait." J. Clin. Pathol. 23(7), October 1970, pp 577-579.

During the period 1967 to 1969, three cases of pernicious anaemia were found among 55 cases of macrocytic anaemia seen in Arabs and Al-Sabah Hospital and the Emerie Hospital, Kuwait. A 65-year-old Jordanian woman, 1 35-year-old Jordanian male, and a 40-year-old Egyptian male each presented with peripheral macrocytosis, frankly megaloblastic bone marrow, and a Schilling test typical of pernicious anaemia. Vitamin B_{12} therapy resulted in improvement of all three patients. They have maintained a normal haemoglobin level since. No gastric cancer was indicated in any case. A careful dietary history excluded nutritional vitamin B_{12} deficiency. The physician concluded that the patients suffered from Addisonian pernicious anaemia, which is thought to be very rare in Arabs.

Non-Country Specific

1. Guy, C., Annino, M. C., Danis, C., Durr, F., and Frederich, A. 25-Hydroxyvitamin D in children 3 to 6 years old followed at the Service de Protection Maternelle et Infantile." Pediatrie 41(3), April-May 1986, pp 205-214.

25 OH-D calcium, phosphorus and alkaline phosphatase serum levels were measured in 53 children. Three forths of the children were immigrants 3 to 6 years of age. They were in good health, and usually followed the medical advice of the PMI. During the months of February, March and April half of the immigrant children had a serum 25 OH-D deficiency and high alkaline phosphatase levels, when European children had a normal 25 OH-D level and a low alkaline phosphatase. After a stay during September and October in their country of origin, the children had normal 25 OH-D levels. Differences between winter and autumn levels were very significant. The risk factors of a vitamin D deficiency are studied.

2. Gilat, T., Horwitz, C., Halpern, Z., Bar Itzhak, A., and Feldman, C. "Gallstones and diet in Tel Aviv and Gaza." Am. J. Clin. Nutr. 41(2), February 1985, pp 336-342.

In two populations in Tel Aviv and Gaza with presumed differences in both the possible association between diet and gallstones were investigated. Gallstones were more frequent in Jews in Tel Aviv than in Arabs in Gaza, 12.1% versus 3.8% (p less than 0.001). The 60+ age groups in both populations fully accounted the difference. There were no significant differences in the frequency of gallstones among the 20-39 and 40-59 age groups. Both populations had numerous and marked differences in diet composition. Energy, carbohydrate and fiber intake was higher in Gaza. The consumption of unsaturated fats was greater in Gazans and their P/S ratio was higher, 0.92 versus 0.70 in Tel Aviv. Poultry was more frequently consumed in Tel Aviv than Gaza which usually consumed more beef and fish. There were also differences in vitamin and mineral consumption. It cannot be determined which, if any, of these dietary differences is related to the lower frequency of gallstones in the older population of Gaza.

3. Naeye, R. L., and Tafari, N. "Biologic bases for international fetal growth curves." Acta. Paediatr. Scand. suppl, 319, 1985, pp 164-169.

To control for nutrition in the development of fetal growth curves for diverse populations, a simple, inexpensive method for assessing maternal nutritional status during pregnancy was sought. 60 Ethiopian women's triceps skinfold thickness was measured at intervals throughout pregnancy. In normally nourished pregnancies this measurement increases in the first two trimesters and decreases in the third, reflecting early pregnancy storage of fat and its release in late gestation to meet the increasing energy needs of the fetus. The Ethiopian women who had skinfold thickness similar to those in the United Kingdom (UK) had neonates as heavy as those in the UK. This may mean that Ethiopian fetuses have the same growth potential as those in the UK and that the same growth curves can be used for the two populations. Skinfold thickness measurements may be the means by which nutrition can be controlled as a growth factor in determining the intrinsic fetal growth potentials of diverse populations.

4. Hendrickse, R. G. "The influence of aflatoxins on child health in

the tropics with particular reference to kwashiorkor." Trans. R. Soc. Trop. Med. Hyg. 78(4), 1984, pp 427-435.

Aflatoxins which contaminate food are a common environmental hazard in all the underdeveloped countries of the tropics. Similarities in the geographical and climatic prevalence of kwashiorkor and aflatoxins and similarities in the metabolic derangements caused by aflatoxins and those observed in kwashiorkor, prompted investigation of the relationship between aflatoxin and kwashiorkor in the Sudan and elsewhere in Africa. Analysis of foods from markets and in homes revealed widespread aflatoxin contamination. Aflatoxins were found more frequently and at higher concentrations in the serum of children with kwashiorkor than in those with other types of malnutrition or in normal children. Autopsy liver samples from West and Southern Africa have shown aflatoxins in all cases of kwashiorkor but not in marasmus. These findings establish relationships between aflatoxin and kwashiorkor the nature of which remains obscure but includes the possibility of a causal association.

5. Fantino, M., Baigts, F., Cabanac, M., and Apfelbaum, M. "Effects of an overfeeding regimen--the affective component of the sweet sensation." Appetite 4(3), September 1983, pp 155-164.

In parts of North Africa, an ancient Berber custom of imposing an overfeeding regimen on young girls before marriage, to achieve an obesity which is regarded as aesthetically pleasing exists. The effect of such a regimen, lasting 12-16 weeks, on blood lipids and on the affective reactions to sweet tastes in nine subjects was studied. Only three subjects gained weight (by 3, 5 and 8 kg), in spite of the strong pressure to overeat. No change in plasma lipid concentrations were observed. Nevertheless, at the end of the regimen every subject showed a highly significant decrease in the rated pleasantness of sweet stimuli when they were tested fasting. However, the reduction in sweet pleasantness induced by ingestion of a 200 ml load of 1.4 M glucose solution was not changed by the overfeeding. Thus, pressure to overfeed can reduce hunger, as seen in the attractiveness of sweet foods in fasted subjects, without modifying glucose-induced satiety.

6. Jordan, P., and Rosenfield, P. L. "Schistosomiasis control: Past, Present, and Future". Ann. Rev. Public Health 4, 1983, pp 311-334.

The authors describe the schistosome's life cycle through ova, miracidium, cercariae, and adult worm stages, and its transmission and habitat in each life stage. Past reliance on snail control measures and, more recently, increasing use of chemotherapy are discussed, as are "nonspecific" control methods such as use of latrines, safe water provisioning, and health education efforts. Locally appropriate and effective, practical control methods are needed based on study of each of the world's infested areas. Techniques of investigation, including quantitative parasitology, biological studies, and water contact studies, permit evaluation of the control method's efficiency and cost effectiveness through use of mathematical models which have been developed. Various past national control programs and research-oriented programs are listed and described.

7. Prasad, A. S. "Zinc in Human Nutrition." CRC Press, Boca Raton, Florida 1983.

It appears that nutritional zinc deficiency may be prevalent in inhabitants of many developing countries subsisting on a high cereal protein intake. Recent reports indicate a marginal zinc deficiency may be widespread even in developed countries such as the U.S., probably related to self-imposed dietary restrictions, use of alcohol, and cereal proteins and increasing use of refined food materials. (Author's abstract)

8. Keusch, G. T., and Migagena, P. "Biological implications of polyparasitism." Rev. Infect. Dis. 4(4), July-August 1982, pp 880-882.

Polyparasitism appears to be the rule, rather than the exception, both in populations and in individuals in the developing countries of the world. Thus, polyparasitism represents coendemicity in the epidemiologic sense and simultaneous infections in individual patients in the clinical sense. The effects of polyparasitism are often clinically inapparent. In some situations, however, combined infections may exacerbate clinical manifestations. Coexistent infections may also, under some circumstances, suppress disease symptoms. The possibility of either synergistic or antagonistic effects must therefore be considered in planning public health intervention programs, and the priorities on strategies selected may need to be altered accordingly. There are few available data at present that are suitable for evaluation of the real consequences of polyparasitism, in part because of the many confounding variables involved and the lack of prospective studies. Therefore, future intervention programs should be accompanied by an epidemiologic research component designed to detect clinical or laboratory changes in parasitic and other infections or in host responses. (Authors' abstract)

9. Barreveld, W. H. "FAO's action programme for the prevention of food losses, its scope and objectives." Prog. Food Nutr. Sci. 4(3-4), 1980, pp 41-45.

The action programme for the Prevention of Food Losses (PFL) started operations in early 1978 under the auspices of the FAO's Agricultural Services Division. The objective is to assist developing countries to make more food available to the people by reducing losses from harvesting to consumption. This paper delineates the program, criteria, funding, and mode of operation. Examples are given of projects in Cyprus, the Philippines, Egypt, Liberia, and Peru. The programme for loss reduction in staple foods is to be expanded to cover perishable plant foods, and roots and tubers will be re-emphasized.

10. Riordan, J., and Countryman, B. A. "Basics of breastfeeding. Part I: Infant feeding patterns and present." Jogn Nurs. 9(4), July-August 1980, pp 207-210.

One of the great medical advances of the past decade has been the scientific validation of the importance of species-specific milk. This "discovery" has led to a growing general awareness of the value, during the first year of life, of the milk of the baby's own mother for optimal physical and emotional development. These benefits of breastfeeding may last a lifetime. The need to understand and assist the mother in maintaining this relationship presents a major challenge to the nurse. Beginning with this issue of JOGN and continuing in two subsequent issues a series of six articlesis being presented that gives an overview of breastfeeding, from historical perspectives to specific problems nursing mothers may encounter. The initial installment consists of "Infant Feeding Patterns Past and Present" and "The Anatomy and Psychophysiology of Lactation". Following in September/October and November/December will be "The Biologic Specificity of Breast Milk", "Preparation for Breastfeeding and Early Optimal Functioning", "Self-Care for Continued Breastfeeding", and "Some Breastfeeding Problems and Solutions". The cultural pattern of breastfeeding in ancient and contemporary cultures are compared, and changes during the Industrial Revolution that led to the decline in breastfeeding are outlined. Also described are the consequences of the trend away from breastfeeding in Third World countries and current breastfeeding patterns in the United States. (Authors' abstract)

11. Scrimshaw, N., and Garb, M. (Editors) "Practical Approaches to Combat Malnutrition with Special Reference to Mothers and Children". Summary Repot of IUNS Conference, Professor I. Badran, chairman. Published by Ministry of health, Cairo, Egypt. Conference held May 25-29, 1977 in Cairo.

One-hundred-forty conferees, representing 31 countries, met to share information on current research and methodology to combat malnutrition. Plenary session topics included current information on nutritional problems in Egypt, Africa, and the Middle East; the relationship of malnutrition to associated problems; interactions of malnutrition and infection, diarrheal diseases, fertility, and national development and planning. Working groups addressed the reliability of available data and additional data needed for planning the prevention of malnutrition; ongoing surveillance of nutritional status; nutritional requirements for mothers and children under prevailing environmental conditions, and an analysis of methods of approach to combat malnutrition in mothers and children. Practical discussions on policies and programs to improve nutrition included a range of direct intervention programs covering nutrition education, basic health care, family wellbeing, improved environmental conditions, new feeding programs for vulnerable groups, supplementary feeding programs, fortification of staple foods, and nutritional surveillance.

12. Lechat, M. F. "The epidemiology of disasters." Proc. R. Soc. Med. 69(6), June 1976, pp 421-426.

Emphasis is moving from post-disaster improvisation to predisaster preparadness. The League of Red Cross Societies encourages predisaster planning. A United Nations agency - United Nations Disaster Relief Office (UNDRO) - is headquartered in Geneva. Coordination and exchange of information between agencies engaged in disaster relief is becoming the rule rather than the exception; a number of groups have started with the specific objective of making professional expertise available for disaster management. Private initiatives are taken, meetings are organized, research centers set up, and research projects launched. The study of disasters needs to be approached on a multidisciplinary basis, the more so since the health component is only one part of the broad disaster problem and, perhaps not the major one. Social scientists, psychologists, administrators, economists, geographers, conduct studies on natural disasters which provide new insights and prove useful in preparing for disasters and increasing the effectiveness and acceptance of relief operations. This vital and challenging field is wide open for research: epidemiologists and community health scientists can provide information on which a rational, effective and flexible policy for the management of disasters can be based. (Adopted from author's abstract)

13. Bavandi, M. "Industrial growth and nutrition." Ciba Found Symp. (32), 1975, pp 73-88.

The historical sequence of industrialization in developing countries by which the industrial sectors have enlarged at the expense of agriculture, and cash crops have supplanted subsitence crops, is shown to have resulted in local shortages of foods for local consumption. Maldistribution of food stores in various developing countries is also discussed. The need for a different pattern of development, which aims for generation of income and even distribution among needy groups, involving them in the development process, is highlighted. A discussion follows the paper text. (Author's abstract)

14. Day, N. E. "Some aspects of the epidemiology of esophageal cancer." Cancer Res. 35(11 Pt. 2), November 1975, pp. 3304-3307.

The worldwide occurrence of esophageal cancer is reviewed, together with the epidemiological information on its causation. The data strongly suggest the factors associated with poverty and specific limitations of dietary intake increase susceptibility for this disease. (Author's abstract)

15. Gori, G. B., and Peters, J. A. "Etiology and prevention of Cancer." Prev. Med. 4(3), September 1975, pp 239-246. Academic Press.

A review of the epidemiological literature on cancer shows that most cancers are of environmental origin, although genetic factors may increase or decrease susceptibility or resistance in some cases. In addition, some rare forms of cancer may have direct genetic determinants. Environmental factors are often prime factors in cancer etiology. Nutritional imbalances, occupational hazards, cigarette smoking, and various toxic agents such as alcohol, nitrosamines, polycyclic hydrocarbons, heavy metals, and aflatoxins, are chief among these. Since the cancer incidence has increased alarmingly in the Western world in the past few decades, it behooves those concerned to continue to garner knowledge on the etiologica agents involved. In addition, education of the public to encourage healthier life styles, the adoption of legislation regulating the use and disposal of known etiologic agents, and emphasis on cancer prevention rather than just cure among health professionals is urged.

16. Jelliffe, D. B. "Unique properties of human milk (remarks on some recent developments)." J. Reprod. Med. 14(4), April 1975, pp 133-137.

The suitability of the biochemical composition of human milk for infants includes high lactose content and high levels of linoleic acid and cystine, thought to be related to the human infant's rapid brain growth needs. Human milk has important immunologic properties such as the bifidus factor, and the presence of secretory IgA and other antibodies, lymphocytes and the interferon they produced, and active corpuscles such as macrophages. Advantages include the low cost of human milk vs. cow's milk, the convenience aspect, and contraceptive property of breastfeeding, the lower incidence of obesity in infants who were breastfed vs formula-fed, and the emotional bonding of mother and child during breastfeeding. In conclusion, the author urged use of the unique human resource of breast milk for human infants as their logical optimal food.

17. Osman, A. A. "Etiology of venous disorders." Int. Surg. 60 (10), October 1975, pp. 540-543.

We have investigated the role played by the bulk and transit time of food in the bowel and the squatting position characteristically adopted by Africans and Asians for defecation in the causation of venous disorders. Refinement of carbohydrates leads to low residue diets and consequent prolonged transit time through the intestines. This, together with abandonment of squatting, as the use of water closets increased, has contributed to the increase in incidence of venous disorders among Westerners. (Author's abstract)

18. McLaren, D. S. "The great protein fiasco." Lancet 2(872), July 1974, pp 93-96.

The historical development and promulgation of the popular concept of a world protein problem was traced from its inception with the description of kwashiorkor in young children in the Gold Coast of Africa by Cicely Williams in 1932. This common assumption, which became widespread in scientific circles and was acted upon by the U.N., ignored the rising significance of marasmus, or total starvation, which occurs with the rapid social change experienced worldwide in recent decades. The emphasis on biochemical test batteries to detect protein and/or amino acid deficiencies rather than on anthropometric measures to detect overall stunting and emaciation of malnutrition and the resources and time spent on development of various commercial high protein foodstuffs rather than on emphasizing maternal use of indigenous food mixtures are cited as two examples of misguided efforts resulting from the protein fiasco. The scientific establishment has come to the recent realization that the focus on protein has not produced gains in world child nutritional status, and that the energy or total food gap is the crucial one which needs to be solved.

19. Vakil, V., and Morgan, R. W. "Etiology of breast cancer II. Epidemiologic aspects". C.M.A. Journal 109, August 4, 1973, pp 201-206.

A number of studies suggest that differences in breast cancer incidence are associated with differences in marital status, number of pregnancies, age of menarche, age at menopause, height and weight, socioeconomic status, geographic location, and residence. However, in no case is the evidence adequate to establish a "cause and effect" relationship. The genetic component of these associations may be of primary importance, while other conditions such as marital status are probably indirect reflections of the operation of more fundamental factors. There is a general consensus that endocrine factors play an important part in mammary cancer occurrence. At present, the association between breast cancer and the presence of the virus-like (type B) particles in human milk is not established. (Authors' abstract)

20. Pearson, L. S. "The role of livestock in developing economics." Adv. Sci. 26(129), March 1970, pp 289-297.

Livestock production can be a positive contributor to the ecomomy of developing countries and thereby be a valuable contributor to the nutrition of the populations. There are different advantages and disadvantages of tropical vs temperate-zone vs mixed-breed cattle. Increased irrigation and grass strains which increase the grazing seasons in tropical zones, night feeding and feeding cattle with high energy feeds, and replinishing lands with minerals all increase productivity. Frequent inspections for evidence of oestrous and use of artificial insemination are beneficial. Highly productive systems are in use in Puerto Rico and Israel, and improved genetic pastures in East Africa, Australia, and the Caribbean. Livestock use can be a potentially valuable tool for developing economies.

Subject Index

Entries list duplicate page numbers when a topic appears in more than one entry on that page.

TURKEY

ALL OTHER COUNTRIES

NON-COUNTRY SPECIFIC

Author Index

Entries list duplicate page numbers when the author has contributed to more than one entry on that page.

About the Compilers

GAIL G. HARRISON is a Professor in the Department of Family and Community Medicine of the University of Arizona's College of Medicine. She is the coauthor of *Nutrition, Behavior and Change* and of *Nutrition and the Cell.*

OSMAN M. GALAL is Chairman, Board of Directors of the Nutrition Institute in Cairo, Egypt and Visiting Professor in the Department of Family and Community Medicine, University of Arizona. He specializes in nutrition and pediatrics, and is the author of numerous articles and monographs.

MARY E. MOHS is a Graduate Research Associate at the Department of Family and Community Medicine at the University of Arizona. She has contributed chapters to *Nutrition and Heart Disease in the Aged* and *Handbook of Nutrition in the Aged* and has published articles in *Physiology and Behavior* and *Federation Proceedings.*

www.ingramcontent.com/pod-product-compliance
Ingram Content Group UK Ltd.
Pitfield, Milton Keynes, MK11 3LW, UK
UKHW041639031026
15587UKWH00001B/387

9 780313 261886